MILADY'S
ART & science
of
NAIL TECHNOLOGY

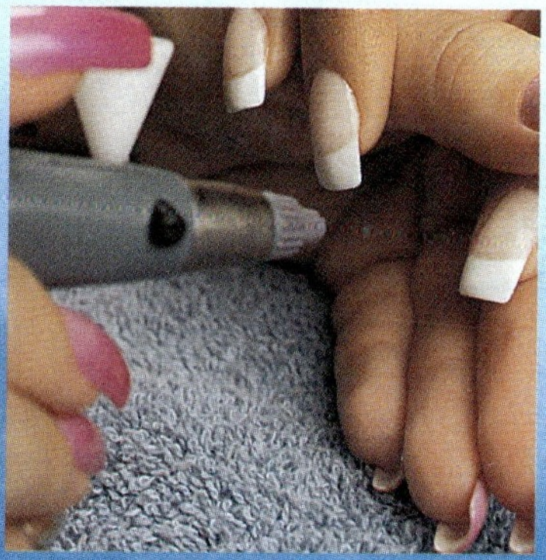

Second Edition

MILADY'S
Art & Science of
NAIL TECHNOLOGY

Second Edition

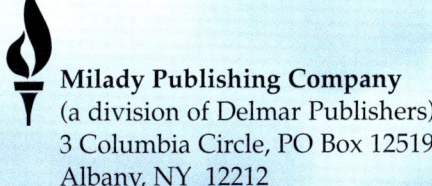

Milady Publishing Company
(a division of Delmar Publishers)
3 Columbia Circle, PO Box 12519
Albany, NY 12212

NOTICE TO THE READER

Publisher does not warrant or guarantee any of the products described herein or perform any independent analysis in connection with any of the product information contained herein. Publisher does not assume, and expressly disclaims, any obligation to obtain and include information other than that provided to it by the manufacturer.

The reader is expressly warned to consider and adopt all safety precautions that might be indicated by the activities herein and to avoid all potential hazards. By following the instructions contained herein, the reader willingly assumes all risks in connection with such instructions.

The Publisher makes no representation or warranties of any kind, including but not limited to, the warranties of fitness for particular purpose or merchantability, nor are any such representations implied with respect to the material set forth herein, and the publisher takes no responsibility with respect to such material. The publisher shall not be liable for any special, consequential, or exemplary damages resulting, in whole or part, from the readers' use of, or reliance upon, this material.

Milady Staff:
Publisher: Gordon Miller
Editor: Joseph Miranda
Freelance Developmental Editor: Martha S. Deschaines
Project Editor: Nancy Downey
Production Manager: Brian Yacur
Art Coordinator: Suzanne Nelson
Photo Director: Catherine Frangie
Photographers: Michael A. Gallitelli on location at the Austin Beauty School with Dino Petrocelli
             Steven Paul Knox
Technical Consultant: Tanya Severino
Medical Photographer: Elvin G. Zook, M.D., Division of Plastic Surgery,
             Southern Illinois University School of Medicine
Artists: Shizuko Horii
        Ron Young

COPYRIGHT © 1997
Milady is an imprint of Delmar, a division of Thomson Learning. The Thomson Learning logo is a registered trademark used herein under license.

Printed in the United States of America
    9 10 XXX 05 04 03 02

For more information, contact Milady, 3 Columbia Circle, PO Box 15015, Albany, NY 12212-0515; or find us on the World Wide Web at http://www.Milady.com

All rights reserved Thomson Learning 1997. The text of this publication, or any part thereof, may not be reproduced or transmitted in any form or by any means, electronics or mechanical, including photocopying, recording, storage in an information retrieval system, or otherwise, without prior permission of the publisher.

You can request permission to use material from this text through the following phone and fax numbers. Phone: 1-800-730-2214; Fax 1-800-730-2215; or visit our Web site at http://www.thomsonrights.com

Library of Congress Cataloging-in-Publication Data:
Milady's art and science of nail technology. — 2nd ed.
        p. cm.
    Rev. ed. of: The Art and science of nail technology. c1992.
    Includes index.
    ISBN 1-56253-326-6
    1. Manicuring. I. Milady Publishing Company. II. Title: Art and science of manicuring.
TT958.3.M55   1997
646.7'27—dc20   96-35281
                                                CIP

Contents

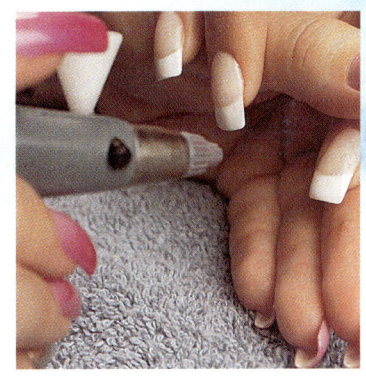

PREFACE xiii
ACKNOWLEDGMENTS xvii
INTRODUCTION 1

PART I GETTING STARTED

Chapter 1
YOUR PROFESSIONAL IMAGE
Introduction 7
Professional Salon Conduct 7
• Professional Salon Conduct Toward Clients 7
• Professional Salon Conduct Toward Employers and Coworkers ... 9
Professional Ethics 10
• Professional Ethics Toward Clients 10
• Professional Ethics Toward Employer and Coworkers 11
Your Professional Appearance 12

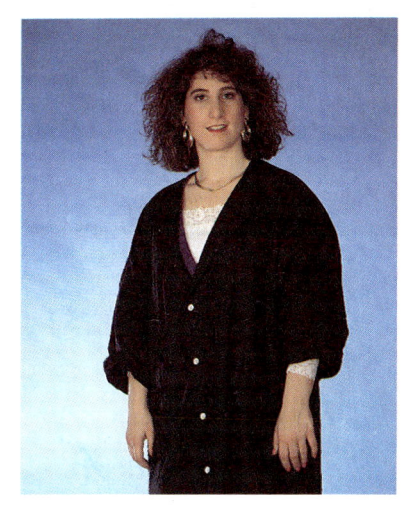

Chapter 2
BACTERIA AND OTHER INFECTIOUS AGENTS
Introduction 15
Bacteria 15
• Types of Bacteria 15
• Classifications of Pathogenic Bacteria 16
• Growth and Reproduction of Bacteria 17
• Movement of Bacteria 17
Viruses and Fungus 17
• Viruses 17
• Acquired Immune Deficiency Syndrome (AIDS) 17
• Fungus and Mold 18
• Nail Fungal Infections 18
• Mold and Mildew 19
• Exposing the Natural Nail 19
• Prevention 19
Parasites 20
• Rickettsia 20
Understanding Infection 20
• Immunity to Infection 20
• How Infections Breed in the Salon 21
• How Nail Technicians Can Fight Infections 22

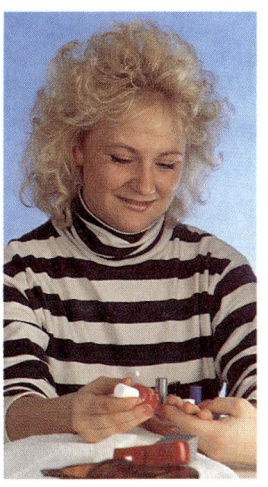

vi ◆ MILADY'S ART & SCIENCE OF NAIL TECHNOLOGY

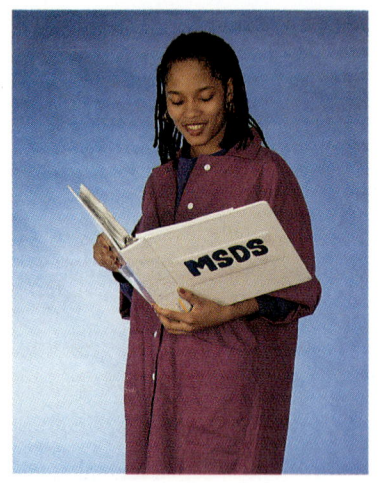

Chapter 3
SANITATION AND DISINFECTION
Introduction 26
Contamination Control 26
Sterilization 27
Sanitation 27
Disinfection 28
• Effective Use of Disinfectants 29
• Types of Disinfectants 30
Implements and Other Surfaces 31
Pre-Service Sanitation Procedure 32
Ultraviolet Ray Sanitizers 33
Bead "Sterilizers" 33
Beware of Formalin 34
Blood Spills 34
Disinfectant Safety 35
Universal Sanitation 35

Chapter 4
SAFETY IN THE SALON
Introduction 38
Common Chemicals Used by Nail Technicians 38
Learn About the Chemicals in Your Products 39
• What Is an MSDS? 39
• How You Can Get Material Safety Data Sheets 40
Avoiding Overexposure Is Easy! 41
• Ventilation Control 41
• Local Exhaust 42
• Preventing Overexposure to Dusts .43
A Dangerous Misconception 43
Protect Your Eyes 43
Other Tips for Working Safely 44
Cumulative Trauma Disorders 46
• What to Do? 46

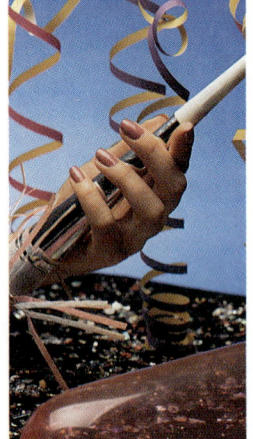

PART 2 THE SCIENCE OF NAIL TECHNOLOGY

Chapter 5
NAIL PRODUCT CHEMISTRY SIMPLIFIED
Introduction 51
Understanding Chemicals 51
• Matter and Energy 51
• Molecules and Elements 51
• Forms of Matter 51
• Chemical Reactions 52
• Catalyst 52
• Solvents and Solutes 52

CONTENTS ◆ **vii**

Adhesion and Adhesives 53
- Adhesives 53
- Primers 53
- A Clean Start 54

Fingernail Coatings 55
- Monomers and Polymers 55
- Understanding Polymerizations 56
- Simple vs. Cross-linking Polymer Chains 56
- Light and Heat Energy 57
- Evaporation Coatings 57
- "Better for the Nail" Claims 58

Avoiding Skin Problems 58
- Dermatitis 58
- Prolonged or Repeated Contact 59
- Irritant Contact Dermatitis 60
- Remember These Precautions 61
- Protect Yourself 62

The Overexposure Principle 62

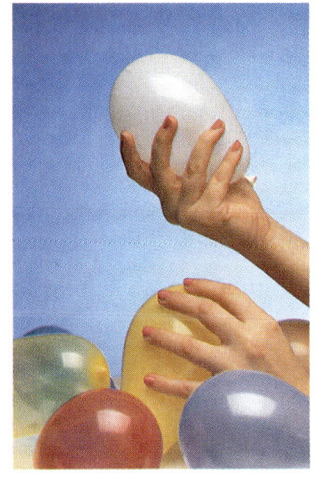

Chapter 6
ANATOMY AND PHYSIOLOGY

Introduction 65
Cells 65
- Cell Growth 66
- Cell Metabolism 66

Tissues 67
Organs 67
Systems 68
The Skeletal System 68
- Structure of Bone 69
- Joints 69
- Bones of the Arm and Hand 69
- Bones of the Leg and Foot 70

The Muscular System 71
- Muscle Parts 72
- Stimulation of Muscles 73
- Muscles Affected by Massage 73

The Nervous System 76
- The Brain and Spinal Cord 76
- Nerve Cells and Nerves 77

The Circulatory System 79
- The Heart 79
- The Blood 80

The Endocrine System 83
The Excretory System 83
The Respiratory System 84
The Digestive System 84

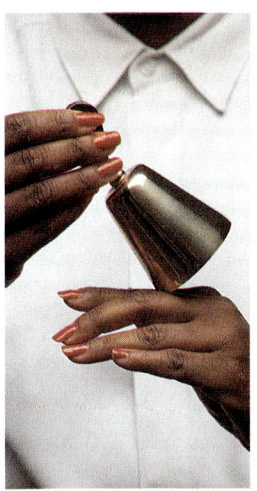

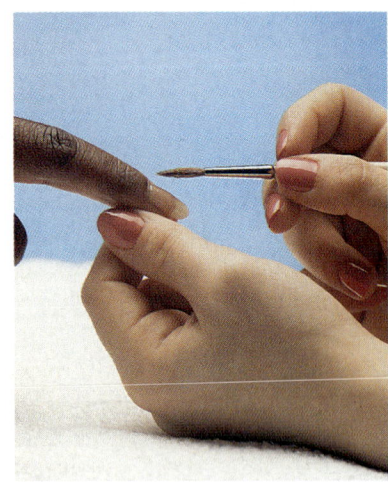

Chapter 7
THE NAIL AND ITS DISORDERS
Introduction 87
Parts of the Nail 87
  • Parts of the Nail 87
  • Structures Beneath the Nail 87
  • Skin Surrounding the Nail 88
Nail Disorders 88
  • Nail Disorders That Can Be Serviced by a Nail Technician 89
  • Nail Disorders That Cannot Be Serviced by a Nail Technician 93

Chapter 8
THE SKIN AND ITS DISORDERS
Introduction 97
Healthy Skin 97
  • Function of the Skin 97
  • Structure of the Skin 98
  • Nourishment of the Skin 100
  • Nerves of the Skin 100
  • Glands of the Skin 101
  • Elasticity of the Skin 102
Skin Disorders 102
  • Lesions of the Skin 103
  • Inflammations of the Skin 104
  • Infections of the Skin 105
Pigmentation of the Skin 105
Hypertrophies (New Growths) of the Skin 106

Chapter 9
CLIENT CONSULTATION
Introduction 108
Determining the Condition of Nails and Skin 108
Determining Your Client's Needs 109
Meeting Your Client's Needs 109
Completing the Client Health/Record Card .110
Maintaining the Client Service Record 113

PART 3 BASIC PROCEDURES

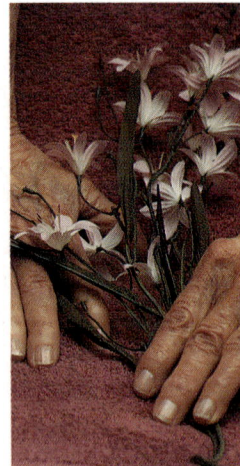

Chapter 10
MANICURING
Introduction 117
Nail Technology Supplies 117
  • Equipment 117
  • Implements 118
  • Materials 120
  • Nail Cosmetics 121

CONTENTS ◆ ix

Procedure for Basic Table Set-Up 124
Choosing a Nail Shape 125
Water Manicure 126
• Water Manicure Pre-Service 126
• Water Manicure Procedure 127
• Water Manicure Post-Service 132
French Manicure 133
Reconditioning Hot Oil Manicure 133
• Supplies 134
• Reconditioning Hot Oil Manicure Pre-Service 134
• Reconditioning Hot Oil Manicure Procedure 134
Man's Manicure 135
• Procedure 135
Electric Manicure 139
Paraffin Wax 140
Hand and Arm Massage 140
• Hand Massage Techniques 141
• Arm Massage Techniques 142

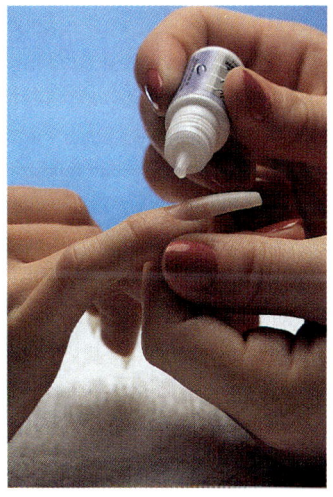

Chapter 11
PEDICURING
Introduction 145
• Supplies 145
Pedicure 146
• Pedicure Pre-Service 146
• Pedicure Procedure 147
• Pedicure Post-Service 150
Foot Massage 151
• Foot Massage Techniques 151

PART 4 THE ART OF NAIL TECHNOLOGY

Chapter 12
NAIL TIPS
Introduction 157
Supplies for Nail Tips 157
Nail Tip Application 158
• Nail Tip Application Pre-Service 158
• Nail Tip Application Procedure 158
• Nail Tip Post-Service 161
Maintenance and Removal of Tips 162
• Maintenance 162
• Tip Removal 162

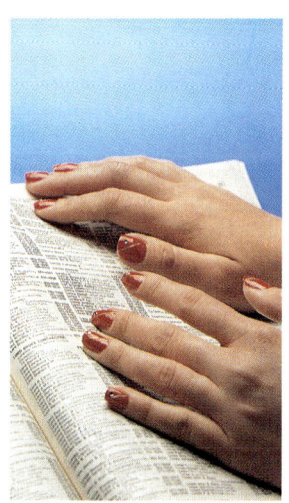

Chapter 13
NAIL WRAPS
Introduction 165

Fabric Wraps 165
- Supplies 165
- Nail Wrap Pre-Service 165
- Nail Wrap Procedure 166
- Nail Wrap Post-Service 168
Fabric Wrap Maintenance, Removal, and Repairs 169
- Fabric Wrap Maintenance 169
- Repairs with Fabric Wraps 171
- Fabric Wrap Removal 171
Paper Wraps 172
- Supplies 172
Paper Wrap Application Procedure 172
Liquid Nail Wrap 173

Chapter 14
ACRYLIC NAILS
Introduction 176
Acrylic Nails Over Forms 176
- Supplies for Acrylic Nails 176
- Acrylic Nail Pre-Service 177
- Acrylic Nail Procedure 177
- Acrylic Nail Post-Service 181
Acrylic Nails Over Tips or Natural Nails 182
- Procedure 182
Acrylic Nail Application Over Bitten Nails 184
- Procedure 184
Acrylic Nail Maintenance and Removal 186
- Acrylic Maintenance 186
- Acrylic Removal 189
Odorless Acrylics 190

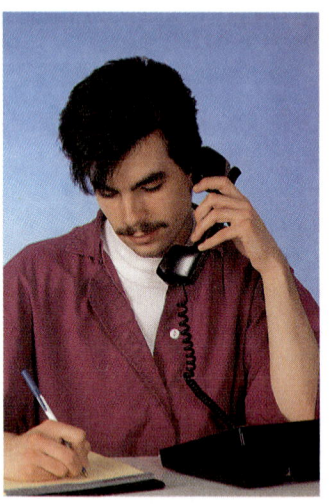

Chapter 15
GELS
Introduction 193
Light-Cured Gel on Tips or Natural Nails .193
- Supplies 193
- Gel Application Pre-Service 193
- Light-Cured Gel Procedure 194
- Gel Application Post-Service 196
Light-Cured Gel Over Forms 196
No-Light Gel Application 198
Gel Maintenance and Removal 199
- Gel Maintenance 199
- Gel Removal 199

Chapter 16
THE CREATIVE TOUCH
Introduction 202

CONTENTS ◆ **xi**

Creating Nail Art 202
- Gems 202
- Striping Tape 203
- Foil 203
- Nail Tape Application 203
- Gold Leaf Application 205
- Freehand Painting 206
Using an Airbrush for Nail Color and Nail Art 206
- Airbrush Equipment and Operation 207
Getting Started and Finished 209
- Set-up and Practice 209
- Real People 211
Two-Color Fade 213
Traditional French Manicure (with Optional Lunula) 216

PART 5 THE BUSINESS OF NAIL TECHNOLOGY

Chapter 17
SALON BUSINESS

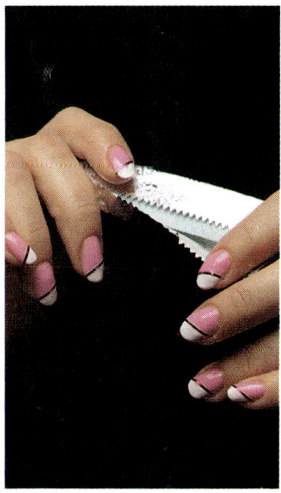

Introduction 221
Your Working Environment 221
- The Full-Service Salon 221
- The Nails-Only Salon 221
- Make Your Decision 222
Keeping Good Personal Records 223
- Income 223
- Expenses 223
- Appointments 223
Understanding Salon Business Records 224
- Using Business Records 224
- Keeping Client Records 225
- Keeping Inventory Records 225
Booking Appointments 225
Advertising Yourself 226
Collecting Payment for Services 226

Chapter 18
SELLING NAIL PRODUCTS AND SERVICES
Introduction 229
Know Your Products and Services 229
- Features 229
- Benefits 230
Know What Your Client Needs and Wants 230
Present Your Products and Services 231
- Sell While You Work 231
- Display a List of Your Services 231
- Display Your Products 231

Answer Questions and Objections 232
- Questions 232
- Objections 232

Close the Sale 232
- Suggestion Selling 232
- Wrap-Up 233
- Scheduling Another Appointment 233

ANSWERS TO REVIEW QUESTIONS 234

GLOSSARY/INDEX 259

Preface

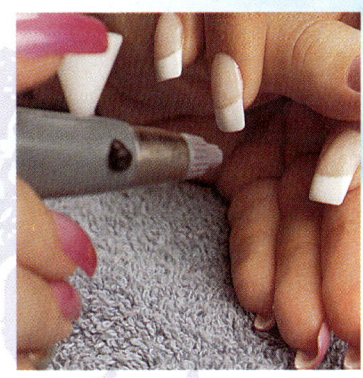

Nail technology is an exciting and rewarding profession. Each year professional nail technicians perform more than $3 billion worth of manicuring, pedicuring, and artificial nail services for millions of fashion-conscious clients.

Milady's Art and Science of Nail Technology, is the complete guide to basic nail technology that every professional nail technician has been waiting for. When the staff at Milady began the revision process, we surveyed **you**, the users of the book. Through hundreds of surveys, formal focus groups, and detailed written critiques, you told us what you wanted in a new nail technology book, **and we listened**.

FEATURES OF THIS EDITION

In response to **your needs**, this exciting new edition of *The Art and Science of Nail Technology* includes the following features:

- *Chapters and Parts*. The book is divided into eighteen chapters and five parts so it is much easier to use.
- *Full-Color Art*. All art is in **full color**, with actual photographs to show you step-by-step procedures for manicuring, pedicuring, tips, wraps, acrylic nails, and basic nail art procedures.
- *Learning Objectives and Review Questions*. Learning objectives provide goals for the students in each chapter. These objectives are reinforced by review questions that assess how well the student has mastered the goals established in the learning objectives. The answers to these review questions are conveniently located at the back of the book. They can be used by students to study for exams.
- *Actual Photos of Nail Disorders*. For the first time in any nail technology or cosmetology book, full-color photos are included to help students identify nail disorders more accurately.
- *Client Consultation Guidelines*. A complete chapter focuses on client consultation and gives suggestions for identifying and meeting the needs of each individual client.

- *Chemical Safety Coverage.* A complete chapter is devoted to the important topic of chemical safety in the nail salon. Students will learn to identify the chemicals commonly used in the nail salon, how they can cause harm, how to protect themselves and their clients, and how to read an MSDS (Material Safety Data Sheet).
- *State Licensing Exam Topics.* The topics required for state licensing examinations are presented in a complete, easy-to-read fashion.
- *Safety Cautions.* Highlighted safety cautions alert students to services that include potentially dangerous procedures. These cautions explain how to avoid dangerous situations and how to provide services in a safe, clean environment.
- *Sanitation Cautions.* Highlighted sanitation cautions give specific suggestions for maintaining proper sanitation at all times.
- *Procedural Tips.* Procedural tips provide hints on the most efficient and effective way to complete step-by-step procedures. These tips help students improve their nail technology skills
- *State Regulation Alerts.* Because state regulations vary, state regulation alerts remind students to check with their instructors for specific regulations in their state.

SUPPLEMENTS FOR THE STUDENT AND INSTRUCTOR

The *Art and Science of Nail Technology*, revised edition, features four entirely new supplements:

Milady's Nail Technology Workbook

This workbook is a valuable student supplement that coordinates chapter-by-chapter with the textbook. It strengthens the students' understanding of nail technology by reinforcing the material covered in the textbook. The workbook includes short answer, short essay, sentence completion, matching, definition, labeling, and word review activities. The workbook also includes a final exam review made up of multiple choice questions and a series of situational tests that ask students what they would do in a difficult situation if they were the nail technician

Answers to Milady's Nail Technology Workbook

This is an easy-to-use teacher's edition of the workbook that provides answers for all workbook questions and activities.

Milady's Nail Technology Course Management Guide
This step-by-step, simple-to-use course guide has been designed specifically to help the nail technology instructor set up and operate a successful nail technology training program. It includes:
- Guidelines for starting and implementing a nail technology program
- Detailed lesson plans for each chapter in the book
- Handouts ready for use in the classroom
- Transparency masters for easy-to-create visual aids
- A Chemical Safety Program that can be implemented in the nail technology classroom

State Exam Review for Nail Technology
This book of exam reviews contains questions similar to those that may be found on state licensing exams for nail technology. It employs the multiple-choice type question, which has been widely adopted and approved by the majority of state licensing boards. Groups of questions are arranged under major subject areas.

Nail Technology Video Series
Each of the six videos listed below emphasizes key actions by professional nail technicians involved in specific procedures, to help students master their own hand movements. Graphics illustrate vital points, while safety precautions are highlighted for student technicians.
- The Basic Manicure and Hand and Arm Massage
- The Pedicure and Foot and Leg Massage
- Nail Tips and Wraps
- Acrylic Nails
- Gel Nails: Light and No-Light Cured
- Nail Art and Design

Advanced, Reference and Continuing Education Material
- *Airbrushing for Nails*, Elizabeth Anthony — A comprehensive resource that provides components and directions for assembling and maintaining an airbrush system. Application techniques, from color fades and French manicures all the way to detailed nail art picture work, are given in step-by-step instructions through photographs, illustrations and written procedures.
- *Guide to Owning and Operating a Nail Salon*, Joanne Wiggins — Includes well-organized, step-by-step tips for starting a salon, business features specific to nail salons, and

tips on developing a long-term plan. (Book also available on audio cassette.)

◆ *Nail Art & Design*, Tammy Bigan — Provides a thorough, detailed resource for creating achievable, wearable, and commercial nail art. Full-color photography and illustrations show techniques in explicit detail and focus. Features the latest trends og glitter art, gold leafy application, pierced nail charms, among others.

◆ *Nail Q & A Book*, Vicki Peters — This book has over 500 questions and answers for nail technicians ranging from nail preparation to business practice tips.

◆ *Nail Structure and Product Chemistry*, Douglas D. Schoon — Topics cross the spectrum of nails from anatomy to salon safety, with particular attention to basic product chemistry and how it affects the nails.

◆ *The Professional's Reflexology Handbook*, Shelley Hess — Offers a full spectrum of treatments using pressure points of the foot, hand and ear. This guide provides clear, concise instructions and background on how reflexology treatments can be used in selected areas of service.

◆ *Technails: Extensions, Wraps and Nail Art*, Tammy Bigan — Chapters include preparing for services, nail tips, wraps, gels, repairs, and fill-ins. Also explores the business side of nail services.

◆ *30 Nail Designs*, Susan Tumblety — Step-by-step techniques to execute 30 of the latest nail art designs. Special attention is given to more imaginative and creative designs, helping students develop their own personal style. Plus, unique coverage on developing and photographing a portfolio, offers numerous tips for guaranteed success.

Acknowledgments

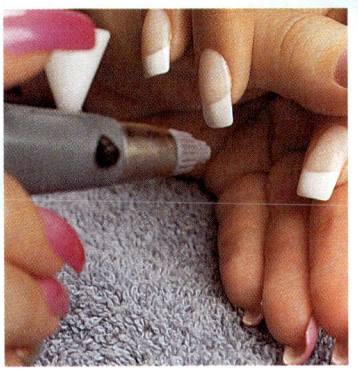

The staff of Milady Publishing Company wishes to acknowledge the many individuals and organizations who helped shape this edition of *Milady's Art and Science of Nail Technology*. Their input enabled us to produce a book that will be a valuable resource for both students and professionals in the field of nail technology. To all those who contributed to this edition we extend our sincere thanks and appreciation.

- Barbara Abramovitch
New England Hair Academy
Malden, MA

- Evelyn Adams
Jan-Mar Beauty Academy
Newport News, VA

- Elizabeth Anthony
Progressive Nail Concepts, Inc.
Palatine, IL

- Suzanne Arduini
Albany, NY

- Jan Austin
Austin Beauty School
Albany, NY

- Giselle Bohamde
Austin Beauty School
Albany, NY

- Dale Bona
C.H. McCann Vocational
Technical High School
North Adams, MA

- Jason Boulla
Albany, NY

- Bich Ly
Albany, NY

- Teresa K. Bryant
Carousel Beauty College
Middletown, OH

- Gayle Bryner
Oklahoma State Board
of Cosmetology
Oklahoma City, Oklahoma

- Burmax Co.
Hauppauge, NY

- Patricia Castro
College of San Mateo
San Mateo, CA

- Alice Ciurlino
P & B Beauty School
Gloucester, NJ

- Deborah Clark
Albany, NY

- Elizabeth Coleman
Albany, NY

- Howard Conlon
Bellaire Beauty College
Bellaire, TX

- Suzanne Council
Van Michael Salon
Atlanta, GA

- Van Council
Van Michael Salon
Atlanta, GA

- Matthew Creo
Austin Beauty School
Albany, NY

- Nancy Court
Arnold Beauty College, Inc.
Fremont, CA

- Wilma Curry
Bellaire Beauty College
Bellaire, TX

- Brenda De Angelo
Daytona Beauty School
Daytona Beach, FL

- Arnold DeMille
Milady Publishing Consultant
Continuing Education Specialist
New York, NY

- Christine DeRusso
Albany, NY

- Peggy Dietrich
Laredo Beauty College
Laredo, TX

- Luciano Di Paolo
Euclidian Beauty College Inc.
Euclid, OH

- Barbara Dorsey
Baltimore Stud. of Hair Design
Baltimore, MD

- Cindy Drummy
Nails Magazine
Redondo Beach, CA

- Carol Duffy
Alameda Beauty College
Alameda, CA

- Roslyn Duncan
Debbie's School of Beauty Culture
Houston, TX

- Dana Ennello
Mechanicville, NY

- Barbara Feiner
NailPro Magazine
Van Nuys, CA

- Flo Finch
Northland Pioneer College
Holbrook, AZ

- Marion Ford
Albany, NY

- Laverne Foster
Pat Goins Beauty Schools
Monroe, LA

- Nehme Frangie
Albany, NY

- Jamal Frangie
Albany, NY

- Wadad Frangie
Austin Beauty School
Albany, NY

- Anne Fretto
Stanton, CA

  Nancy Gallitelli
Albany, NY

- Ray Gambrell
South Carolina State Board of Cosmetology
Greenwood, SC

- Anthony Gardy
Albany, NY

- Sharon Gil
Garden State Academy
South Bound Brook, NJ

- Cynthia Gimenez
Arnold Beauty Colleges, Inc.
Remont, CA

- Anne Golloway
Ossining, NY

- Aurie Gosnell
National Interstate Council
of Cosmetology
Aiken, SC

- Constance Gregg
Boca Raton Institute
Boca Raton, FL

- Ann Harrell
St. Petersburg, FL

- Linda Harris
Maxims Beauty Academy
Blaine, MN

- Danielle Hasberry
Albany, NY

- Helen Heine
South Eastern College of Beauty Culture
Charlotte, NC

- Michael Hill
Arkansas State Board of Cosmetology
Fayetteville, AR

- Frances Hoffman
Manatee Area Vocational Technical Center
Bradenton, FL

- Barbara Hogue
Arizona Academy of Beauty
Tucson, AZ

- Linda Howe
Pittsburgh, PA

- Sally Hudson
Tampa Bay Career Academy
Tampa, FL

- Karen Iolli
Ailano School of Cosmetology
Brockton, MA

- Frank Jacobi
Citrus Community College
Glendara, CA

- Janice Jaynes
Institute of Cosmetology
Houston, TX

- Julia Jefferson
Vogue College of Hair Design
Highland Heights, KY

- Dorothy Johnson
Yuma School of Beauty
Yuma, AZ

- Spring Kelsey
Earlton, NY

- Glenn Kewley
Drome Sound Music Store
Schenectady, NY

- Paulette Know
Antioch Beauty
Antioch, CA

- L. Jean Lake
Elaine Steven Beauty College
St. Louis, MO

- Carol Laubach
San Jacinto College
Pasadena, TX

- Denise Leach
Oakland Technical Center
South East Campus
Royal Oak, MI

- Yvonne Lowenstein
Margate International School of Beauty
Margate, FL

- Inna Lozhkin
Albany, NY

- June A. Lyle
Lyle's School of Hair Design
Nashville, TN

- Charles Lynch
International Beauty School
Lancaster, PA

- Deborah A. Mack
Pivot Point International, Inc.
Chicago, IL

- Tina Macki
Albany, NY

- Laura Manicho
Nationwide Beauty Academy
Cols, OH

- Sharon Matern
Albany, NY

ACKNOWLEDGMENTS

- Patricia Mc Daniel
Bellaire Beauty College
Bellaire, TX

- Robert McLaughlin
Maine State Board of Cosmetology
Cape Elizabeth, ME

- John Mickelbank
Albany, NY

- Louise Miller
Lamson Academy of Hair Design
Phoenix, AZ

- Ruth Miller
Quincy Beauty Academy
Quincy, MA

- Marcia Miller
Federico Beauty College
Fresno, CA

- Peggy Moon
Georgia State Board of Cosmetology
Lavonia, GA

- Pauline Moram
Innerstate Beauty School
Bedford Heights, OH

- Mary Ann Morris
House of Heavilin
Blue Springs, MO

- Eileen Morrissey
Maison de Paris Beauty College
Haddon Field, NJ

- Florence Nebblett
Washington, DC

- Neka Beauty Supplies
Albany, NY

- Pat Nix
Past President,
National Interstate Council of Cosmetology
Booneville, IN

- Theda O'Brien
Albany, NY

- John Olsen
Phagan's Beauty School, NW
Tigard, OR

- Stephanie Pedersen
New York, NY

- Susan Peters
Lansdale School of Cosmetology
Lansdale, PA

- Dino Petrocelli
Albany, NY

- Nilsene Privette
College of Beauty and Art and Science
Sedona, AZ

- Lois Purewal
Spring Branch Beauty College
Houston, TX

- Irma Quezada
Pipo Academy of Hair Design
El Paso, TX

- Sarah Rainey
St. Augustine Technical Center
St. Augustine, FL

- Jennifer Rhatigan
Albany, NY

- Cleolis Richardson
Philadelphia, PA

- Jim Rogers
Milpitas Beauty College
Milpitas, CA

- Betty Romesberg
The Head Hunters
Cuyahoga Falls, OH

- Sue Sansom
Executive Director,
Arizona State Board of Cosmetology
Phoenix, AZ

- Richard Scher, MD
College of Physicians and Surgeons
Columbia University
New York, NY

- Douglas Schoon
Chemical Awareness Training Service
Irvine, CA

- Regina Schrenko
Northhampton, PA

- Joan Sesock
Austin Beauty School
Albany, NY

- Tanya Severino
Albany, NY

- Sandra Skoney
Toledo Academy of Beauty Culture
Toledo, OH

- Jenny Smith
Vogue Beauty College
Idaho Falls, ID'

- Kenneth J. Smith
Nail Tech Academy
Brown Deer, WI

- Alicia Solazzo
Bronxville, NY

- Bertha Stanko
Menands, NY

- Linda Stark
Michigan College of Beauty
Troy, MI

- Judith Stewart
PJ's College of Cosmetology
Carmel, IN

- Alma Tilghman
North Carolina Board of Cosmetology
Beaufort, NC

- Sandy Tirpak
Albany, NY

- Mona Townsend
Backscratchers Nail Care Products
Sacramento, CA

- Wendy Trainor
Schuylerville, NY

- Veda Traylor
Arkansas State Board of Cosmetology
Mayflower, AR

- Peggy Turbyfill
Mike's Barber and Beauty Salon
Hot Springs, AR

- Barbara Turman
School of Nail Technology Inc.
Coral Gables, FL

- Beverly Venable
Loudonville, NY

- Judy Ventura
Greensboro, NC

- Dave Welsh
J & D Supply
Albany, NY

- Barbara Wetzel
Nail Splash, Inc.
LaGrange Park, IL

- Renee Wilson
Argyle, NY

- Lois Wiskur
South Dakota Cosmetology Commission
Pierre, SD

- Victoria Wurdinger
New York, NY

- Jack Yahm
Milady Publishing Consultant Emeritis
"Father of Cosmetology Accreditation"
Lauderdale Lakes, FL

- Linda Zizzo
Milwaukee Area Technical College
Milwaukee, WI

- Elvin Zook, M.D.
Southern Illinois University
School of Medicine
Springfield, IL

The Milady staff would like to thank the following individuals and organizations for their assistance:

For the use of photographs:

Salon on pages 2 and 221 courtesy of
Takara Belmont U.S.A., Inc.
Harvey Allen Salon
Merrick, NY
(Award of Special Distinction,
Modern Salon of the Year Award, 1991)
Thomas Stanwood, Photographer

Manufacturer's representative of page 2 courtesy of
Backscratchers Nail Care Products Inc.

Model on page 2 courtesy of
OPI Products, Inc.
Nail Fashion by OPI International Design Team

Salon manicuring area on page 221 courtesy of
Takara Belmont U.S.A., Inc.
Urban Retreat
Houston, Texas
(Grand Prize, Modern Salon of the Year Award, 1991)
James F. Wilson, Photographer

Photographs of onycholysis caused by trauma and onycholysis on page 94 courtesy of
Orville J. Stone, M.D.
Dermatology Medical Group
Huntington Beach, California
and NAILS Magazine

For help with supplies:

Carl J. Mione
Vice President/School Sales
Burmax
Hauppauge, NY 11788

Neka Beauty Supplies
Albany, New York

OPI Products, Inc.

Dave Welsh
J & D Supply
Albany, New York
(Safety glasses)

Introduction

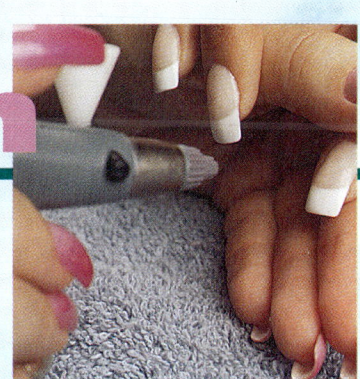

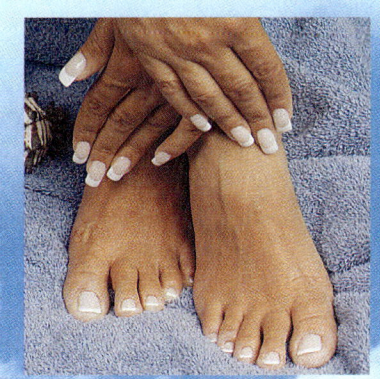

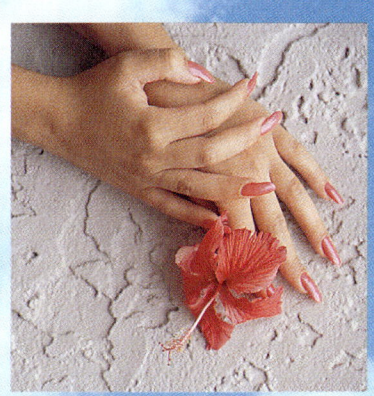

NAIL TECHNOLOGY OVERVIEW

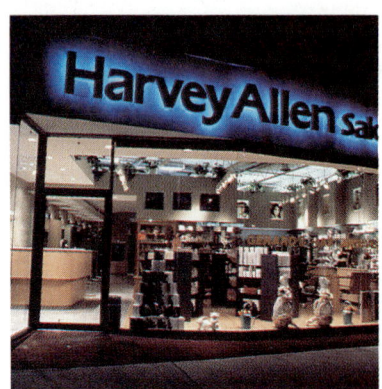

Welcome to the exciting world of nail technology.

You have chosen to become a nail technician, one of the fastest-growing and most creative, rewarding, and high-paying professions in cosmetology today. As a nail technician you will use the latest technology to apply artificial nails. You will use your artistic abilities to create original designs on nails. Your work will be relaxed and comfortable, with many successful and fashionable clients, some of whom may pay as much as $125 an hour for a service. You will be part of the booming manicuring, pedicuring, and artificial nail industry, with combined sales of more than $3 billion a year. This figure represents more than a 25 percent increase over previous years in some areas, and continues to climb.

Because nail technology is a complex, changing profession you will want to continue learning even after you receive a license. You may start your career as a nail technician in a salon. As you develop your knowledge and skills, you may want to move into other career areas in nail technology. These careers include teaching nail technology in cosmetology schools or demonstrating manufacturer's nail products at shows, conventions, or stores. You can become a salon owner or even the personal nail technician for fashion models or actors on the stage, in movies, or on TV. You can write, edit, or be a consultant for nail technology books and magazines.

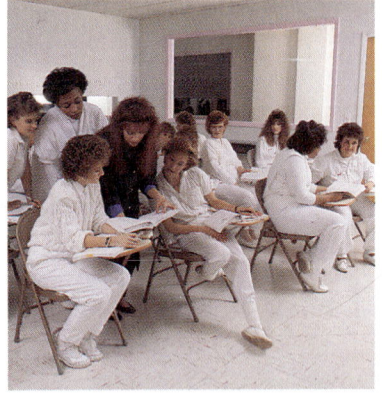

You could teach nail technology.

Nail technology has changed in the 5000 years since the first manicure was recorded. Manicures used to be a luxury enjoyed only by rulers and the wealthy, and were performed by servants. Today, nail technology is enjoyed by millions of fashion-conscious people from many social and economic groups. In most states today nail technology services are performed by licensed professionals who have completed up to 500 hours of classroom instruction. During instruction they learn to improve the health of their

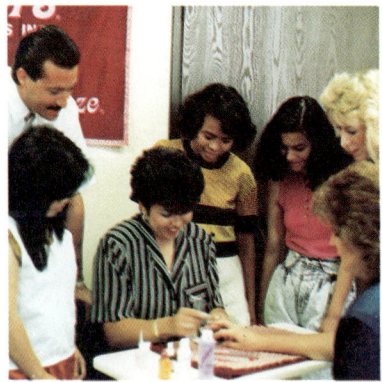

You could be a manufacturer's representative.

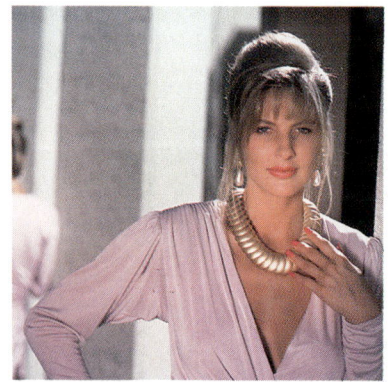

You could be a personal nail technician for a fashion model.

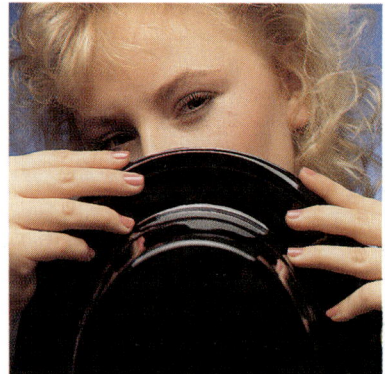

You could be a nail technician for actors in the theater.

INTRODUCTION ◆ 3

clients' nails and recognize healthy nails and skin, as well as possible nail and skin disorders. They become skilled in using the latest nail technology while following proper sanitation and safety procedures to protect both themselves and their clients. Today's professional nail technicians learn how to give pedicures to enhance the look of their clients' feet, improve health, and relieve stress. They also learn how to handle the business aspects of their profession.

The first manicures did not require formal instruction. The word "manicure" comes from the Latin "manus" (hand) and "cura" (care). The first evidence of nail care recorded in history was before 3000 BC in Egypt and China. Ancient Egyptian men and women of high social rank stained their nails with red-orange dye called henna, which comes from a shrub. The color of a person's nails in ancient Egypt was a sign of importance. Kings and queens wore deep red, while people of lower rank were allowed to wear only pale colors. Around 3000 BC the Chinese developed a nail paint made from beeswax, egg whites, gelatin, and gum arabic. In 600 BC, Chinese royalty wore gold and silver paint on their nails. In the 15th century, leaders of the Chinese Ming Dynasty painted their nails black and red. Military commanders in Egypt, Babylon, and early Rome spent hours before a battle having their hair lacquered and curled and their nails painted the same shade as their lips.

As a 20th Century nail technician, you can give your clients many more choices for nail care than the privileged people of ancient civilizations had. You can offer your clients a basic manicure or pedicure and information about nail care. They can also choose from a variety of artificial nail services shaped, colored, and designed specifically to their needs. You will become a successful nail technician by studying hard and learning the skills and professional manner to make all your clients feel like 20th Century kings and queens. Let's get started studying this exciting field.

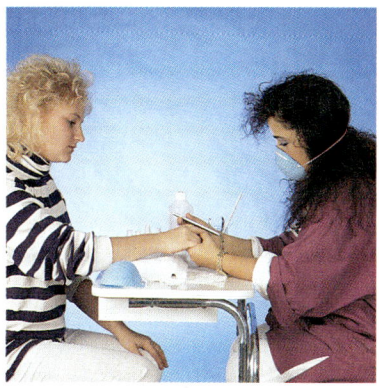

You will learn proper sanitation and safety procedures.

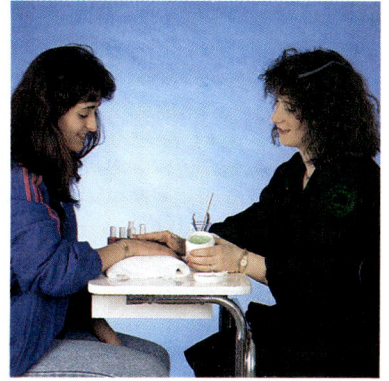

You can help your clients select the products and services that meet their needs.

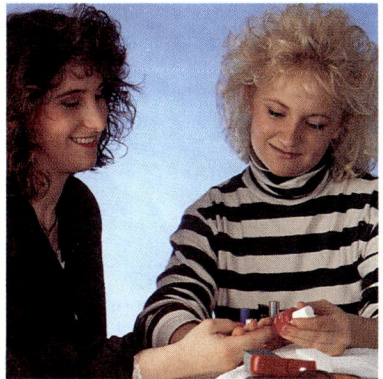

You can offer your clients a variety of nail technology services.

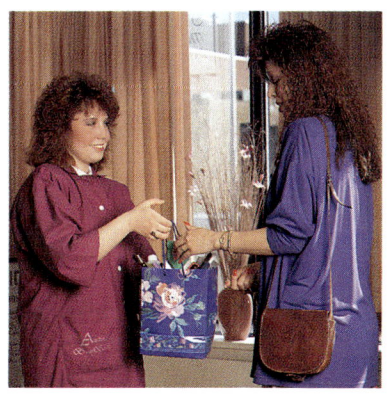

You can use your skills to build a steady, happy clientele.

Part 1

GETTING STARTED

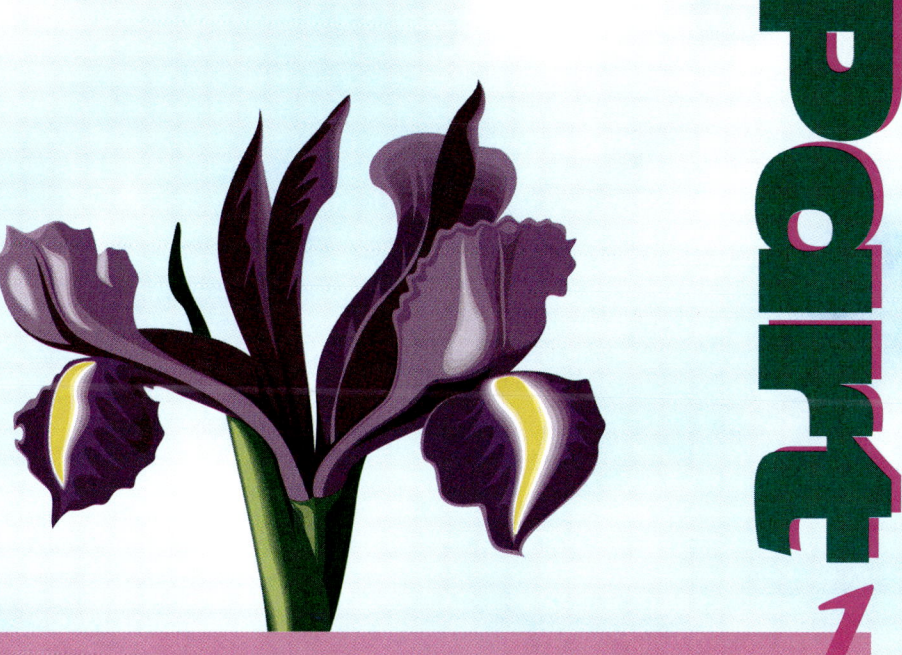

- ◆ CHAPTER 1 - Your Professional Image
- ◆ CHAPTER 2 - Bacteria and Other Infectious Agents
- ◆ CHAPTER 3 - Sanitation and Disinfection
- ◆ CHAPTER 4 - Safety in the Salon

Chapter 1

YOUR PROFESSIONAL IMAGE

LEARNING OBJECTIVES

After you have studied this chapter, you should be able to:

1. Define salon conduct.
2. Give examples of professional salon conduct toward clients.
3. Give examples of professional salon conduct toward employers and coworkers.
4. Define professional ethics.
5. Give examples of professional ethics toward clients.
6. Give examples of professional ethics toward employers and coworkers.
7. Describe the type of appearance you should have as a professional nail technician.

INTRODUCTION

When you are a successful nail technician you will be able to do more than give an expert manicure, create natural-looking artificial nails, or paint original designs on a client's nail. You will know how to behave in a professional manner. You will follow the rules for professional behavior with clients, employers, and coworkers. You will also develop good personal health and grooming habits. In this chapter, you will learn the rules of professionalism for nail technicians. They include proper salon conduct, professional ethics, and how to present yourself to clients as an attractive and well-groomed representative of the nail technology industry. If you practice these rules, you will quickly build a satisfied clientele that will lead to your success.

PROFESSIONAL SALON CONDUCT

Salon conduct is the way you behave when you are working with clients, your employer, and coworkers in a salon.

PROFESSIONAL SALON CONDUCT TOWARD CLIENTS

Set high standards for proper salon conduct. You can create an environment in your salon that is relaxed and pleasant for clients and makes them want to come back and bring their friends.

1. **Be on time.** You will appear relaxed, competent, and concerned about your clients' needs if you are on time, waiting to serve them when they arrive. Being late can make you seem disorganized or uncaring. It is discourteous and can annoy and inconvenience your clients.

2. **Be prepared.** Before your clients arrive, make sure your station is completely set up with an adequate supply of materials and equipment. Make sure your implements are sanitary and ready to use.

3. **Plan your day.** Keep an appointment schedule near you for each day so that you know what you are supposed to do every hour. The schedule should include your client's name, service to be performed, time of appointment, and client's phone number. Call your clients by name when they arrive. When you know what service you are to perform, you can begin without hesitation and give your clients a feeling of security. (Fig. 1.1)

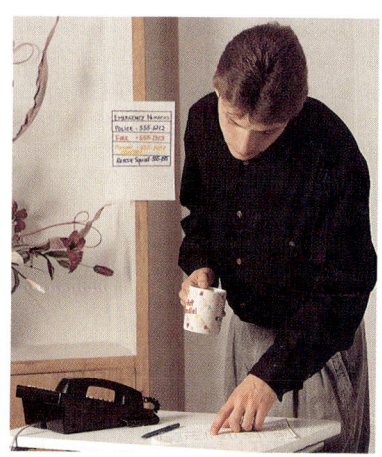

1.1 — Plan your day carefully.

4. **Plan in advance.** Except in emergency situations, nail technicians should not reschedule appointments to accommodate their personal life. You should know about important events three or more weeks in advance. Be sure to put them on your calendar and set your schedule accordingly. This career offers flexibility in scheduling, if you can be organized and plan weeks in advance.

5. **Arrange appointments carefully.** Schedule your appointments so that each client has enough time. If you schedule too many clients during your day, you won't have time to serve them and some will have to wait or be rescheduled for another day. If the receptionist makes appointments for you, be sure to give him or her a neat list of the services you offer and the time you need to complete each one.

6. **Keep clients informed of schedule changes.** Contact clients if your appointments are running very late or if you have to reschedule their appointments. They will appreciate your honesty and they will be grateful that you haven't wasted their time.

7. **Be courteous.** Have a cheerful, friendly, and helpful attitude. This attitude will tell your clients that you care for them. Before you perform any service, you can make your clients feel comfortable and relaxed. Help them take off their coats and show them where to sit for the service. All new clients can be given a tour of the salon and shown where the rest rooms and phones are. You may also tell them how to book future appointments, how to reschedule an appointment, and what forms of payment your salon accepts.

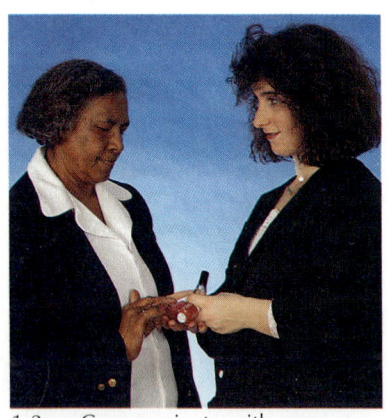

1.2 — Communicate with your client.

8. **Perform all tasks willingly and efficiently.** Never make your clients feel their appointments inconvenience you.

9. **Communicate with your clients.** Explain the services you will perform for your clients and the retail products needed to maintain these services. Listen to their concerns with undivided attention and answer their questions. No matter how successful you become, always keep your attitude humble when dealing with your clients. (Fig. 1.2)

10. **Never complain to, or argue with, a client.** Try to keep any conversation on a professional level at all times. While you are performing nail services, you can use the time to explain what you are doing and why. You can also suggest and discuss other salon services or products that could help your client.

11. **Use good judgment.** Do not share information about your personal life or personal stories about other clients, your coworkers, or your employer with your client. Discussion of politics or religion should be avoided. While the nail technician and client or coworker may share the same views, others in earshot may not and may be offended. Concentrate on your client's needs.

12. **Never chew gum, smoke, eat, or take personal telephone calls where you can be seen by clients.** These habits can be extremely annoying to clients and smoking can be dangerous around nail chemicals. (Fig. 1.3)

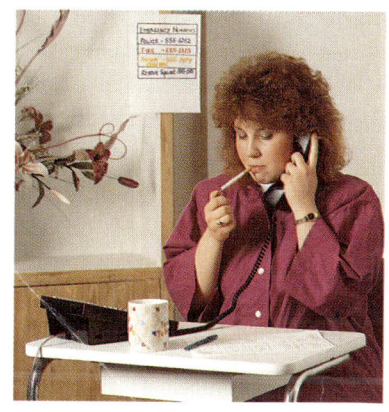

1.3 — Never chew gum, smoke, eat, or take personal telephone calls where you can be seen by clients.

PROFESSIONAL SALON CONDUCT TOWARD EMPLOYERS AND COWORKERS

It is important to work closely with your employer and coworkers because it will help create a strong, successful salon that will eventually secure your future in this industry. To be competitive, the entire staff must work together. You want to create an atmosphere that will make your clients enjoy their visits to your salon so much they will not want to go to another.

Below are guidelines to follow for dealing with employers and coworkers.

1. **Communicate.** Establish an open, honest line of communication between yourself and your employer. Be perfectly honest about your strengths and weaknesses. Make sure your work meets the standards the salon expects.

2. **Be willing to learn.** Keep an open mind and be willing to accept suggestions. Don't automatically assume that your way of doing something is the only correct way. Nail products and services are improved often; be prepared to update your skills.

3. **Give credit to others.** Never take credit for another person's ideas. Try to acknowledge contributions made by others.

4. **Respect the opinions of coworkers.** Your ideas and opinions are important, but yours are not the only ones. Frequently, the ideas of many people create the best solution.

5. **Take the initiative.** Never be afraid to offer help or suggestions to make things better or easier for your employer or coworkers.

6. **Use good judgment.** If you have a problem or question about your job, discuss it directly with your employer, not with your clients or coworkers.

7. **Leave personal problems at home.** Do not tell your personal problems to your employer, fellow employees, or clients.

Personal problems are distractions that interrupt the concentration needed to do a good job. You should not take telephone calls from family or friends while you are working unless it is an emergency.

8. **Never borrow money from employers or coworkers.** This is a practice that can result in a very awkward work situation. Eventually your coworkers may lose respect for you.

9. **Promote the salon**. Learn about the other services offered at your salon, such as hair care, skin care, and cosmetic consultations so you can promote the entire salon to clients.

10. **Develop your ability to sell.** Explain the benefits of products and services to clients without pressuring them.

PROFESSIONAL ETHICS

Professional *ethics* (**ETH**-iks) is your sense of right and wrong when You interact with your clients, employer, and coworkers. The essential values in professional ethics are honesty, fairness, courtesy, and respect for the feelings and right of others.

PROFESSIONAL ETHICS TOWARD CLIENTS

High ethical standards for treating clients will earn you a good reputation. your clients will trust you, keep coming back, and bring their friends. Your best source of advertising is through the recommendations of clients who respect and trust you.

1. **Suggest services that meet your clients' needs.** Never suggest or give clients services they don't need or want, or ones that could harm them. Explain what you recommend for your clients and why, so they will feel comfortable with your services.

2. **Keep your word and fulfill all obligations.** Always do what you have promised the client and what the client wants you to do. Don't take short cuts because you are rushed or substitute other services because they are more convenient for you.

3. **Treat all your clients fairly.** Never offer special discounts or services to one client and not to another.

4. **Follow your state regulations for sanitation and safety.** Always follow provisions of the state laws covering nail technology. Regulations may seem inconvenient at times, but they are created to protect you and your clients. To be an ethical nail technician, you must always be knowledgeable about current laws concerning your profession.

5. **Be loyal.** Never complain, gossip, or talk to your client about other clients, your employer, or coworkers. Your clients will not trust you if you talk about other people to them because they will think you will talk about them the same way.

6. **Don't criticize others.** Never criticize the services offered by other nail technicians or other salons. Even if the client insists on discussing another colleague's or salon's service, you may listen, but remain neutral in your responses.

7. **Don't abandon your clients.** If you leave the manicuring field or move to another community, give your clients enough notice to find another nail technician or recommend a coworker or colleague you trust. If you have a large clientele, consider training someone to take your place. You want your clients to experience the least amount of discomfort.

PROFESSIONAL ETHICS TOWARD EMPLOYER AND COWORKERS

By using professional ethics to support the efforts and morale of your coworkers and employers, you will help contribute to the success of your salon. As the salon becomes more successful, so will you.

1. **Be honest.** Never blame a coworker for your mistakes. Take responsibility for your own actions.

2. **Fulfill your obligations.** Keep any promises you make to an employer and coworker, such as coming in on your day off to help with a special client. If you cannot possibly keep a promise, contact your employer or coworker ahead of time and ask if you can help to make other arrangements.

3. **Respect the talents of your employer and coworkers.** Praise them and encourage them when they do a good job. Try not to criticize.

4. **Don't invite criticism of coworkers.** When you hear a client complain about another technician, do not take sides. You don't know all the facts and it is not your business. Suggest that the client speak directly to the coworker involved. Never criticize someone else's work. Let your standards and work speak for themselves. If another's work is exceptionally poor, offer to repair your client's nails without placing blame on another nail technician.

5. **Never gossip or start rumors among coworkers.** Some people think these tactics can get them ahead in business, but they only serve to make you look bad and alienate your associates.

Know the Competition

Your clients want what's best for their nails, and they rely on you to tell them which products will keep their hands looking beautiful in between manicure appointments. In order to reinforce the belief that professional products are best for maintaining nails' health and beauty, you must thoroughly educate yourself about the points of difference between salon and drugstore formulas. You must also be able to explain the differences to your clients. For instance, if you know that mass market emery boards are very abrasive and can cause problems by tearing up layers of nail plate, you'll know to prescribe professional boards, which have a softer abrasive and don't rip the layers.

YOUR PROFESSIONAL APPEARANCE

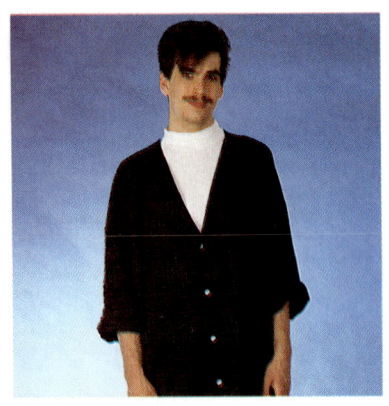

1.4 — A professional male nail technician

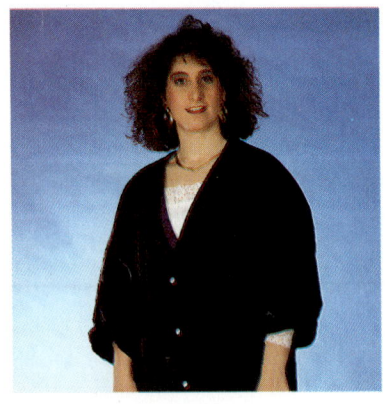

1.5 — A professional female nail technician

You should be a model of good grooming for your clients because you are a member of the beauty industry. Your clients expect you to look your best. You should be pleasant to be around. You must be clean and pleasant-smelling so clients will not object to having you touch them while you perform nail services. They should find it pleasant to sit across from you while you perform nail services. (Fig. 1.4)

1. **Be clean and fresh.** Bathe or shower daily and use an effective deodorant.

2. **Have fresh breath and healthy teeth.** Make sure your breath is fresh at all times. Do not eat garlic or spicy foods that can give you bad breath during the working day. Keep a toothbrush, toothpaste, and mints with you so you can freshen your breath when needed. Keep your teeth and gums healthy by regular brushing and dental check-ups.

3. **Wear clean clothes that are appropriate for the salon.** You should look your best in stylish, professional clothes that reflect your dedication to the industry without inhibiting your ability to work. (Fig. 1.5)

4. **Pay attention to your hair, skin, and nails.** Make sure your hair is neat, you have on just enough make-up to enhance your natural beauty, and your nails are well-manicured.

REVIEW QUESTIONS

1. What is salon conduct?
2. Give ten examples of professional salon conduct toward clients.
3. Explain why a salon might lose clients if nail technicians do not exhibit professional salon conduct.
4. Give ten examples of professional salon conduct toward employers and coworkers.
5. Define professional ethics.
6. Give seven examples of professional ethics toward clients.
7. Give five examples of professional ethics toward employers and coworkers.
8. Describe the type of appearance you should have as a professional nail technician.
9. Explain why a salon might lose clients if it employs nail technicians who have an unprofessional appearance.

Chapter 2

BACTERIA AND OTHER INFECTIOUS AGENTS

LEARNING OBJECTIVES

After you have studied this chapter, you should be able to:

1. Define and understand bacteria.
2. Explain the difference between pathogenic and non-pathogenic bacteria.
3. Identify and describe the main groups of pathogenic bacteria.
4. Give examples of common infections caused by viruses and bacteria.
5. Understand which types of infections are likely to occur on the fingernail.
6. Name the various types of immunities.
7. Name some common sources of infection in the salon.

CHAPTER 2 BACTERIA AND OTHER INFECTIOUS AGENTS ◆ 15

INTRODUCTION

Just about any kind of job can be performed safely. This is certainly true for the work done by professional nail technicians. However, even the most skilled professionals know they must follow guidelines and rules if they expect to protect themselves and others from harm. This is especially important when it comes to proper sanitation. If you are not cautious, both you and your clients may needlessly suffer from infection by bacteria, viruses, fungi or parasites. Not surprisingly, certain kinds of infections may be transmitted during nail services. In this chapter, you will learn what causes infection and how to prevent its spread. Then you will learn how easy it is to avoid these problems with proper disinfection and sanitation procedures.

BACTERIA

Bacteria (bak-**TEER**-ee-ah) are one-celled *microorganisms* (meye-kroh-**OR**-gah-niz-ems) that are so small they can only be seen through a microscope. A microorganism is any living thing that is too small to be seen by the eye. Many bacteria are so tiny that fifteen hundred of them barely cover the head of a pin. A thimble of soil can contain as many as five billion bacteria. Bacteria are the most plentiful organisms on earth. There are 15,000 known species of bacteria, and they can exist nearly everywhere. They multiply at an incredible speed. A single bacterial cell can produce 16,000,000 copies of itself in only half a day.

Bacteria are found in water, air, dust, lint, and decaying matter. They are on the skin of the body, in the secretions of body openings, on clothing, on your manicuring table, on your implements, and under nails. Most bacteria are harmless, but some can cause problems.

TYPES OF BACTERIA

Bacteria are classified into two types, depending on whether they are beneficial or harmful.

1. *Nonpathogenic* (non-path-o-**JEN**-ik) (non-disease-causing) bacteria can't harm us and are often beneficial. About 70 percent of all bacteria are nonpathogenic. Some forms of nonpathogenic bacteria help produce food and oxygen. Others are used in compost piles to improve the fertility of the soil. In humans, nonpathogenic bacteria are most numerous in the mouth and intestines where they help the digestive process by breaking down food.

2. ***Pathogenic*** (path-o-**JEN**-ik) (disease-causing) bacteria are harmful. Though less than 30 percent of all bacteria are pathogenic, they are the most common cause of infection and disease in humans. Pathogenic bacteria are also called ***germs.*** They invade living plant or animal tissues and feed on living matter. They breed rapidly and spread disease by producing ***toxins***, or poisons, in the tissue they invade. ***Sepsis*** is the presence in the blood or other tissues of pathogenic microorganisms or their toxins, and ***asepsis*** is freedom from disease-producing bacteria.

CLASSIFICATIONS OF PATHOGENIC BACTERIA

There are three main groups of pathogenic bacteria. They include:

1. ***Cocci*** (**KOK**-si). These are round, pus-producing bacteria. Cocci appear singly or in groups as follows: (Fig. 2.1)

    a) ***Staphylococci*** (staf-lo-**KOK**-si) grow in clusters and are present in local infections, such as abscesses, pustules, and boils. (Fig. 2.2)

    b) ***Streptococci*** (strep-to-**KOK**-si) grow in chains. They cause strep throat and infections or diseases that spread throughout the body such as blood poisoning and rheumatic fever. (Fig. 2.3)

    c) ***Diplococci*** (deye-ploh-**KOK**-si) grow in pairs and cause pneumonia. (Fig. 2.4)

2. ***Bacilli*** (bah-**SIL**-i). These are the most common bacteria. They are rod-shaped and produce such diseases as tetanus, influenza, typhoid, tuberculosis, and diphtheria. (Fig. 2.5)

3. ***Spirilla*** (spi-**RIL**-a). These are spiral or corkscrew-shaped bacteria. One example of these bacteria is treponema pallida (trep-o-**NE**-mah **PAL**-i-dah), which causes syphilis. (Fig. 2.6)

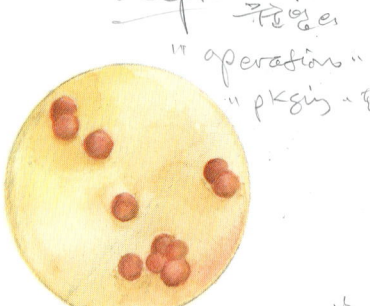
2.1 — Cocci

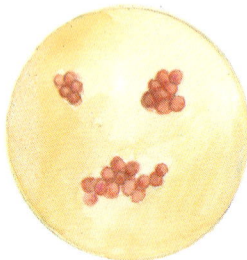
2.2 — Staphylococci

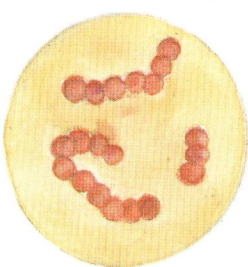
2.3 — Streptococci

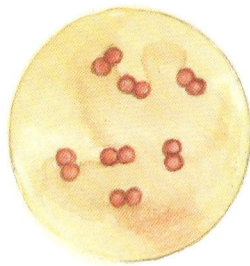
2.4 — Diplococci

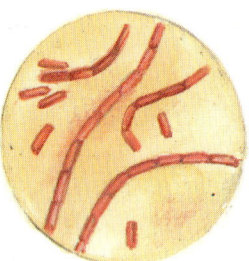
2.5 — Bacilli

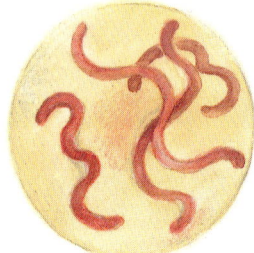
2.6 — Spirilla

GROWTH AND REPRODUCTION OF BACTERIA

Bacteria live, grow, and multiply best in warm, dark, damp, unsanitary conditions. The drawer of your manicuring table is a perfect place to breed bacteria on dirty implements.

Each bacterium, or bacteria cell, has the ability to grow and reproduce. As bacteria are nourished, each bacterium grows in size. When it reaches maturity, it splits in half and forms two identical cells. This type of reproduction is called *mitosis* (meye-**TOH**-sus). These two cells will grow and divide again, forming four cells. It is easy to see how one bacterium can reproduce into as many as 16 million bacteria in 12 hours.

When conditions become unfavorable for growth and reproduction, some types of bacteria form a tough outer covering called a spore. Then they remain dormant, or in a state of rest. Some bacteria remain in very harsh conditions for long periods. Spores can be blown about in the dust and they are not harmed by even the most powerful disinfectants. When conditions become favorable, they again begin to grow and reproduce.

MOVEMENT OF BACTERIA

Bacteria travel very easily. They are spread through air or water, or through contact with contaminated objects. Bacilli and spirilla are the only bacteria that can propel themselves. They have hairlike projections known as *flagella* (flah-**JEL**-ah) or *cilia* (**SIL**-ee-a), which they move in a whiplike motion to propel themselves in liquid.

VIRUSES AND FUNGUS

VIRUSES

Viruses are pathogenic (disease-causing) agents that are many times smaller than bacteria. Viruses enter a healthy cell, grow to maturity, and reproduce, often destroying the cell. Hepatitis, chicken pox, influenza, measles, mumps, and the common cold are examples of viral infections that can be transferred through casual contact with an infected person. Infection spreads when the person sneezes or coughs.

ACQUIRED IMMUNE DEFICIENCY SYNDROME (AIDS)

Acquired Immune Deficiency Syndrome (AIDS) is a disease caused by the HIV virus. HIV attacks and usually destroys the body's immune system. The disease usually lies dormant for many years. Some people have been infected for more than 15 years without showing symptoms. Luckily, it is very difficult to transmit HIV.

Unlike other viruses, HIV cannot be transferred through casual contact with an infected person, sneezing, or coughing, etc. HIV is passed from one person to another through the transfer of bodily fluids such as semen or blood.

The most common methods of transmitting HIV are:

1. sexual contact with an infected person
2. the use of dirty hypodermic needles for injectable drugs

HIV can also be transferred from mother to child during pregnancy and birth. In the early 1980s HIV was transmitted during transfusions of infected blood. However, this rarely happens anymore.

Fortunately, it is virtually impossible to transfer HIV in the salon. HIV isn't spread through salon services. You should make sure your clients are aware of this. Many are needlessly frightened and will look to you for reassurance. This doesn't mean that preventing disease transmission in the salon is not important. It simply means that HIV prevention is *NOT* the reason for proper sanitation and disinfection.

FUNGUS AND MOLD

Fungi (**FUN**-gi) is the general term for plantlike *parasites*, including all types of fungus and mold. Both are contagious, but only fungi are a risk to clients receiving nail services. Fungi can spread from nail to nail on the client and from the client to the nail technician.

NAIL FUNGAL INFECTIONS

Certain common types of fungus may appear as white or discolored areas under the nail plate. They may appear to spread toward the cuticle. As the condition matures, the discoloration becomes darker. Fungus may affect the hands, feet, and nails. Clients with nail fungus must be referred to a physician. (Fig. 2.7)

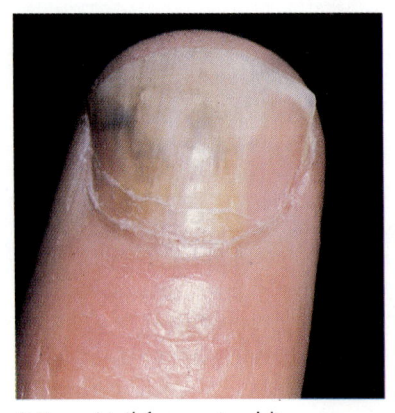

2.7 — Nail fungus (mold)

MOLD AND MILDEW

One of the biggest misconceptions in the nail industry is that molds or mildews can infect fingernails. These organisms rarely, if ever, appear on the fingernails. They are generally confused with the more common greenish bacterial infections. Improperly prepared nail plates harbor bacteria which survive on the moisture and oils found between an unsanitized natural nail and enhancements.

A bacterial infection can be identified in the early stages as a yellow-green spot that becomes darker in advanced stages. The green is caused by the bacteria's waste products. These wastes stain the nail plate causing a green discoloration long after the bacteria is gone. If the infection is destroyed, the green stain will remain.

If the nail has been infected for a period of time, the discoloration becomes black and the nail may soften or smell bad. Neglect is the major reason that this condition advances to this stage. Clients should be warned that the infection could become serious. A qualified medical doctor can quickly treat the problem.

EXPOSING THE NATURAL NAIL

You should not provide nail services for a client who has nail fungus or other infections, but the client may want you to remove any artificial nail covering to expose the natural nail. After the natural nail is exposed, the client should be referred to a physician.

You should wear gloves during removal of artificial nails and follow the manufacturer's directions for removal. When the artificial nail has been removed, discard orangewood sticks, abrasives, and any other porous product used. Disinfect all other implements and the table surface before and after the procedure.

PREVENTION

Bacterial and fungal infections are easily avoided by following sanitary precautions. In most cases, these problems are caused by the nail technician. Do not perform nail services for a client who has discoloration on his or her nails. Do not take short cuts or omit any of the sanitation steps when performing an artificial nail service. If you find that your clients are suffering from such infections you should reexamine your procedures and application techniques for the cause. No one should suffer from nail infections. These problems are bad for the client, a poor reflection on your services and a black eye for the entire nail industry.

PARASITES

Parasites (**PAR**-ah-syts) are tiny, multi-celled animal or plant organisms. They live off living matter without providing any benefits to their hosts. An example of plant parasite infection is ringworm. Animal parasites are responsible for such contagious diseases as scabies, itch-mite, and pediculosis (lice).

RICKETTSIA

Rickettsia (rik-**ET**-see-ah) are much smaller organisms than bacteria, but larger than viruses. They cause typhus and Rocky Mountain spotted fever. Fleas, ticks, and lice carry rickettsia.

UNDERSTANDING INFECTION

An *infection* occurs when body tissue is invaded by disease-causing microorganisms such as bacteria, viruses, and fungi. Microorganisms establish themselves and multiply in body tissue to produce tissue damage. At first, the infection is usually localized. Infection that spreads to the bloodstream is called a general infection. Blood poisoning is a type of general infection.

IMMUNITY TO INFECTION

All living organisms have defenses or immunity against infection. *Immunity* (i-**MYOO**-ni-tee) is the ability of the body to resist disease and destroy microorganisms when they have entered the body. Immunity against disease is a sign of good health. Immunity can be natural, naturally acquired, or artificially acquired.

1. *Natural immunity.* By keeping our bodies healthy, we are able to fight off microorganisms before they can grow and cause disease. Our bodies fight infection in three ways.

    a) We have a protective layer of unbroken skin.

    b) We naturally secrete perspiration and digestive juices that discourage the growth of pathogens.

    c) Our blood contains white blood cells that kill pathogens.

2. *Naturally acquired immunity.* After fighting off a disease, antibodies (a type of protein molecule) remain in the bloodstream ready to fight another attack of the microorganisms should they return.

3. *Artificially acquired immunity.* This immunity is one produced by the injection of a serum or vaccine. The injection introduces a small dose of dead or disabled pathogens into the body. This small dose fools the immune system into making antibodies that can fight that particular disease.

HOW INFECTIONS BREED IN THE SALON

Most bacteria, viruses, fungi, and other pathogens enter the body through the nose, the mouth, and small breaks in the skin. They can also enter your body through your eyes or ears. You are at risk of becoming infected or transmitting infection to your clients because you come in constant contact with pathogens in the salon. Some of the common sources of infections include:

1. **Contaminated manicuring tools and equipment**. Bacteria and other pathogens multiply at a very rapid rate in places such as dirty nail files, cuticle nippers, manicuring tables, trash cans, and towels. (Fig. 2.8)

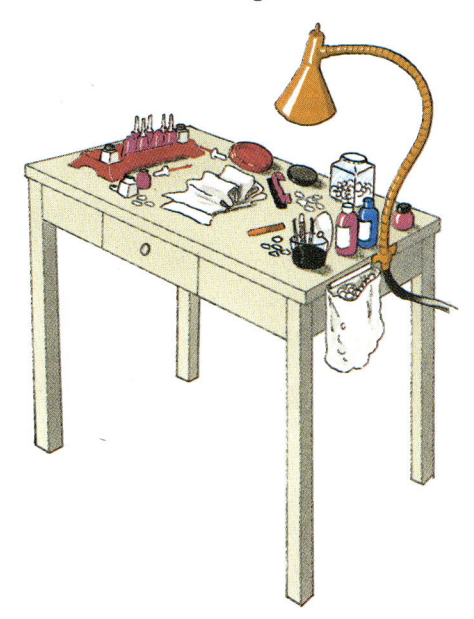

2.8 — Bacteria multiply rapidly on a messy manicuring table.

2. **Your clients' nails, hands, and feet.** Each client who walks into the salon brings in a whole new set of microorganisms and possibly parasites. When you perform a service on this client, you risk being infected. When you perform artificial

nail services, you risk trapping pathogens between the natural nail plate and the enhancement or overlay.

3. **Your clients', coworkers', and your own mouth, nose, and eyes.** Anyone in the salon who has a cough, is sneezing, or has a runny nose is like a fountain of bacteria or viruses.

4. **Open wounds or sores on you or your client.** Infected fluids can be transferred from one person to another through open wounds.

5. **Objects throughout the entire salon.** Pathogens collect on chairs, telephones, cash registers, tables, towels, bottles, brushes, and everything else that is exposed to the air in the salon. They also collect on the fixtures in the restroom—especially the door handle.

HOW NAIL TECHNICIANS CAN FIGHT INFECTIONS

As a professional, you are responsible for keeping yourself and your clients safe from infection. Here are the steps to take:

1. **Learn proper sanitation and disinfection procedures and follow them.** Chapter 3 in this book describes the procedures to follow for proper sanitation. It is your professional responsibility to learn these procedures and follow them faithfully. If you decide to short-cut sanitation and disinfection, you could easily become infected or transmit infection to your clients.

2. **Do not work in contagious conditions.** You should not work with clients while they are *contagious* (kon-**TAY**-jus), or have an infection that can easily be transmitted from one person to another. Someone with a severe cold, influenza, or chicken pox, for example, should not receive nail services. The same holds true for nail technicians. You should also stay home and rest if you are contagious. Working with the public, you could easily start your own local flu or cold epidemic.

3. **Do not work near an open wound.** Refer clients who have an open wound to a physician and make sure they return with a written release before you perform any services for them.

4. **Do not cause wounds.** Be very careful when you are performing nail services. It is easy to cut a client while manicuring cuticles or to break the skin if you file too deeply. Overfiling with heavy abrasive and drills can also cause wounds and bruises to the sensitive nail bed.

It is your job to provide a safe haven for your clients. You can only do this if you understand how. In the next chapter you will learn how to ensure that you are protecting the health of every client, as well as yourself.

Reassuring Your Clients About Safety

Your clients belong to today's "protection generation": at the doctor's office they are examined with a gloved hand and when they go to the dentist office they see individually-wrapped tarter scrapers. As a result, clients are interested in knowing what precautions you are taking to prevent the spread of harmful bacteria, viruses and fungi that grow in the salon and can affect their health. Reassure them by showing them the sanitation measures that you take. When speaking with your clients, remember, you're trying to create a feeling of security. Say something like, "this is how I disinfect my tools and wipe down by table for your safety."

REVIEW QUESTIONS

1. What are bacteria? What do bacteria look like?
2. Are all bacteria harmful? Give examples to explain your answer.
3. What are the three main groups of pathogenic bacteria? Describe them.
4. Why can bacteria reproduce so quickly?
5. Give examples of common infections caused by viruses.
6. Is it likely that salon services can cause AIDS?
7. Describe the appearance of bacterial infection on the nail plate.
8. Do molds and mildew grow on or under the nail plate?
9. What is immunity? Name three types of immunity.
10. Name five common sources of infection in the salon.

Chapter 3
SANITATION AND DISINFECTION

LEARNING OBJECTIVES
After you have studied this chapter, you should be able to:

1. Understand contamination control and identify common salon contaminants.
2. Explain why sterilization is not important in the professional salon.
3. Define sanitation and disinfection and know when each is appropriate.
4. Know how to effectively use disinfectants on implements and hard surfaces.
5. Perform Universal Sanitation procedures in your salon.

INTRODUCTION

When you become a nail technician, you will be licensed to apply professional products to the hands, feet, and nails of the general public. Whenever you work with the public there is the possibility of infection or injury to you and to your clients. The risks are much greater if your implements and work area are not properly cleaned or you do not use disinfection products correctly. States have strict rules for sanitation and disinfection procedures at manicuring work stations. These regulations are to protect both you and your clients.

In this chapter, you will learn the proper procedures to enable you to pass state licensing exams and become a licensed nail technician. However, you will learn much more. You will learn why and when you should disinfect and what the consequences are if you do not.

> **STATE REGULATION ALERT**
>
> *You must obey the rules issued by your local Health Department and your state cosmetology regulatory agency. Be alert for changes in the rules and regulations in your area. For your own safety and that of your clients, it is extremely important that you obtain and obey sanitation rules and regulations.*

CONTAMINATION CONTROL

What do floors, door knobs, table tops and implements have in common? Each of these has a surface. The problem with a surface is that eventually it will become *contaminated*. Any surface that is not completely free of all foreign substances is contaminated. A substance that causes contamination is called a *contaminant.*

Filings and dust are contaminants. Even liquid monomer in a towel is a contaminant. Implements may appear to be clean when they are covered with bacteria.

In the last chapter you learned that disease-causing microorganisms are called *pathogens.* Your duty as a professional is to control pathogens. **Decontamination** is the elimination of contaminants, including pathogens, from implements or other surfaces. There are three types of decontamination.

CHAPTER 3   SANITATION AND DISINFECTION   ◆   **27**

STERILIZATION

Sterilization destroys all living organisms on an object or surface. Sterilization is a difficult, multi-step process. Some sterilization techniques are far too dangerous to be used in the salon. It is impractical and virtually impossible to sterilize tools and surfaces in the salon. Sterilization is only required for surgical procedures.

The word "sterilize" is often used incorrectly. For instance, it is impossible to sterilize the nail plate or cuticle. Sterilizing would destroy the nail plate and kill the skin. There is no need to sterilize anything in the salon. It is not possible to kill all microorganisms in the salon, nor should you try. You only have to control pathogens so they can't cause infection or illness.

SANITATION

The lowest level of decontamination is called **sanitation** or **sanitizing**. Sanitation will significantly reduce the number of pathogens on a surface. Normally, low levels of pathogens are considered safe, so sanitation can be a very effective form of decontamination.

Cleaning with detergent and water is an example of sanitizing. Putting antiseptics on skin or nail plates is sanitizing. **Antiseptics** reduce the number of pathogens in a cut and the immune system kills those that remain. So, antiseptics are sanitizers that help prevent skin infections.

Hand washing is also a form of sanitation. (Fig. 3.1) Frequent hand washing is an important way to control the spread of dangerous organisms. Hand washing removes many types of contaminants. Dirt, oils, monomer, other product residues and pathogens are all removed by frequent hand washing.

Sanitation is a vital routine that must not be ignored. Sanitation is a critical part of maintaining a professional establishment. Below are some simple guidelines that will help keep the salon clean and sanitary.

- Floors should be swept clean whenever needed.
- Deposit all waste materials in a metal waste can with a self-closing lid.
- Waste cans must be emptied regularly throughout the day.
- Mop floors and vacuum carpets every day.
- Dust and nail filings can carry pathogens so they must be controlled.
- Windows, screens, and curtains should be clean.

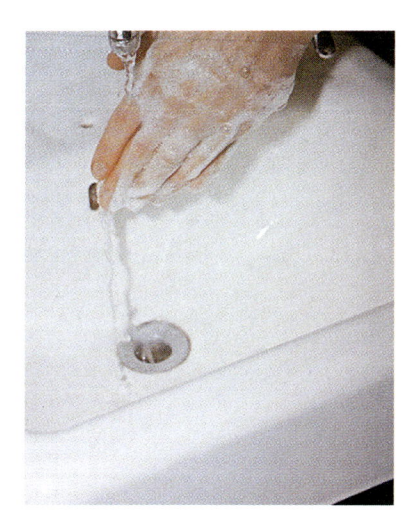

3.1 — Hand washing is a form of sanitation.

- Salons need both hot and cold running water.
- Rest rooms must be clean and tidy.
- Toilet tissue, paper towels, and liquid soap must be provided.
- Wash hands after using the rest room and between clients.
- Clean doorknobs often, especially in the bathroom.
- Clean sinks and drinking fountains regularly.
- Separate or disposable drinking cups must be provided.
- The salon must be free from insects and rodents.
- Salons should never be used for cooking or living quarters.
- Food must never be placed in refrigerators used to store salon products.
- Eating, drinking and smoking in the salon is prohibited by federal regulations.
- Employees must wear clean, freshly washed clothing.
- Always use a freshly laundered or disposable table towel for each client.
- All containers must be clearly marked, tightly closed, and properly stored.
- The outside of all containers, pumps, and dappen dishes should be kept clean.
- Soiled linen is to be removed from the workplace and properly stored for cleaning.
- Do not place any implements or tools in your mouth or pockets.
- Implements must be properly cleaned, disinfected, and stored *after each use*.
- Professionals should avoid touching their face or eye area during services.
- Wash hands before touching the face, eyes, eating or using the bathroom.
- No pets or animals should ever be allowed in salons, except for trained, seeing eye dogs.

These are only a few of the things you must do in order to safeguard yourself and clients. Contact your local State Board of Cosmetology or Health Department for a complete list of regulations.

DISINFECTION

Sterilization is not practical in salons and sanitation may not kill all pathogens. How can nail technicians prevent the spread of dangerous organisms? Disinfection is the answer! **Disinfection** controls microorganisms on nonliving surfaces, such as implements. Disinfection is the second level of decontamination. It is a much higher level than sanitation. Disinfection is almost **identical to sterilization, except disinfection does not kill bacterial spores**. Fortunately, bacterial spores cause no harm in salons. Therefore, disinfection is just as effective in the salon as sterilization, but without the expense, danger and hassle.

Disinfectants are substances that destroy pathogens on implements and other nonliving surfaces. Disinfectants are not safe for use on skin or nails. Disinfectants are designed to kill pathogens. Substances powerful enough to destroy pathogens will certainly damage skin. Disinfectants are serious, professional-strength tools which may cause irritation and skin damage with prolonged or repeated contact.

Of course, manufacturers of these products are careful to make disinfectants as safe as possible. However, disinfectants are potentially dangerous if used incorrectly. Like all of your tools, disinfectants must be used properly. Disinfectants are only safe if used *exactly* as the manufacturer instructs and if kept out of the reach of children. Federal law requires that you be given directions for proper use, safety precautions, a list of active ingredients and a list of the virus that the product is effective against. You must also receive a **Material Safety Data Sheet** or **MSDS** for short. More will be said about the MSDS in Chapter 4.

EFFECTIVE USE OF DISINFECTANTS

Each disinfectant is different. The best way to learn about them is to read the manufacturers' instructions. You should also periodically review these directions in case new information is added.

High quality disinfectants must perform a variety of special jobs in the salon. They must be:

bactericides (kill harmful bacteria)

viricides (kill pathogenic viruses)

fungicides (destroy fungus)

A *hospital-level disinfectant* must perform all of these functions and pass special EPA registration tests. EPA registered, hospital-level disinfectants are perfect for salons. In fact, they exceed requirements for salon disinfection. Unless you are cleaning up blood spills, no other disinfectant is required.

Always clean implements before placing them into the disinfectant. Dirty implements will contaminate the disinfecting solution. Nail filings, oils, and lotions will lessen the effectiveness of the solution. The glass, metal, or plastic jars or containers used to disinfect implements are often incorrectly called *wet sanitizers.* They should really be called *disinfection containers.* (Fig. 3.2) The purpose of these containers is not to sanitize, but instead, to disinfect.

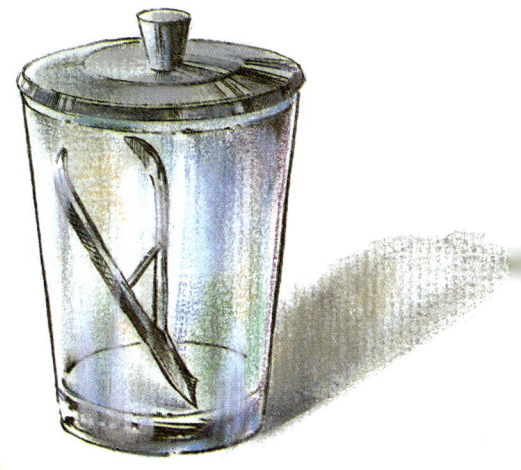

3.2 — Disinfection container

Cloudy disinfectant solution must be changed immediately. Change the solution according to manufacturer's instructions regardless of its appearance. If you think that using cloudy, contaminated disinfectant is, "...better than nothing," think again! Microorganisms can live in contaminated disinfectant solutions. Besides, if clients see implements in a jar of cloudy liquid, they will not think highly of you. Also, be sure that the implement is properly placed in the disinfecting solution. The EPA recommends that implements be *fully immersed for a minimum of ten minutes*.

TYPES OF DISINFECTANTS

Quats

There are several types of salon disinfectants. **Quaternary ammonium compounds (quats)** are the most commonly used. Quats have the advantage of being safe and fast-acting. Most disinfectants of this type are blends of many different kinds of quats. This dramatically increases effectiveness. Quats are the most cost effective of all professional disinfectants. Most quat solutions disinfect implements in ten minutes with total immersion. A 1:1000 solution of quats requires a one to five minute immersion time. Leaving them in for too long may damage metal implements. However, most formulas contain corrosion and rust inhibitors. Quats are also very effective for cleaning table and counter tops.

Phenolics

Like quats, phenolics have been used for many years to disinfect implements. They too can be safe and extremely effective if used according to instructions. Some materials such as rubber and certain plastics are not compatible with these disinfectants. Phenolics can soften and destroy these materials over time. Care should be taken to avoid skin contact with phenols. The concentrated liquid can cause serious skin irritation and is corrosive to the eyes. Avoid uncontrolled spraying of phenolic-type disinfectants. Inhalation of the mists can be extremely irritating to the sensitive lining of the nose, throat and lungs. Phenolics are highly effective, but they are the most expensive of all common, professional salon disinfectants. Some states have expressed concern over disposal of phenolic disinfectants because of their high alkaline pH (usually greater than pH 11). You should check your state regulations to see if special disposal restrictions exist for phenolic disinfectants. As with all disinfectants, you must exactly follow manufacturer's instructions.

Alcohol and Bleach

Common alcohol and bleach are sometimes used for disinfecting implements. To be effective disinfectants, implements must be completely immersed for ten minutes. A simple wipe with alcohol is completely ineffective as a disinfectant. There are many disadvantages to using alcohol and bleach. Alcohol is extremely flammable, evaporates quickly, is slow acting and less effective than professionally designed disinfectant systems. They cannot be diluted below 70% or they lose effectiveness. Alcohol will corrode tools and cause sharp edges to become dull. Household bleach is effective as a disinfectant, but shares some of the same drawbacks of alcohol. Neither bleach nor alcohol are professionally designed and tested for disinfection of salon implements. Bleach can discolor some materials and has almost no cleaning power. Bleach was used extensively in the past, but has since been replaced by more advanced and effective technologies.

IMPLEMENTS AND OTHER SURFACES

There are many things that require disinfection, for example, table and counter tops, mirrors, telephone receivers, door handles, etc. Implements such as clippers, nippers, cuticle pushers, scissors, reusable forms, manicure and pedicure bowls must be disinfected between each client.

> **PROCEDURAL TIP:**
>
> Make sure you have at least two complete sets of implements. On busy days, one set can be disinfecting while you continue your work.

Some files and buffers can be disinfected. Check with the manufacturer for disinfection recommendations. Buffers, files, porous drill bits and wooden sticks which absorb water cannot be disinfected. Instead of throwing these items away, you may wish to keep them in an envelope with the client's name on the outside. Brushes used in applying acrylics and gels do not require disinfection.

To decontaminate other surfaces such as counter tops, wash them thoroughly with a detergent, then spray or wipe on a disinfectant recommended for this purpose. Wipe up the disinfectant and spray again. Then allow the surface to air dry. Be sure to wear gloves while disinfecting surfaces. Also, if using a spray bottle, wear a mask and take care to avoid inhalation of the mists.

PRE-SERVICE SANITATION PROCEDURE

Before your service begins you should perform the following steps:

1. **Wash implements.** Thoroughly wash all implements with soap and warm water.

2. **Rinse implements in plain water.** Rinse away all traces of soap with plain water. Dry thoroughly with a clean towel.

3. **Completely immerse implements in disinfectant solution.** Immerse implements in a container holding an EPA registered, hospital level disinfectant for the required time (usually ten minutes). If it is cloudy, the solution is contaminated and must be replaced. Make sure to avoid skin contact with all disinfectants. Use tongs or rubber gloves.

4. **Wash hands with antibacterial liquid soap.** Thoroughly wash your hands with antibacterial liquid soap, rinse, and dry with clean towel. Liquid soaps are more sanitary than bar soaps and should be used whenever possible. A soap dish can breed bacteria.

5. **Rinse implements and dry with clean towel**. Remove implements from disinfectant solution with tongs or while wearing rubber gloves, rinse well in water, and wipe dry with clean towel to prevent rusting.

6. **Follow approved storage procedure.** Follow your state regulations for storage of sanitized manicuring implements. The regulations will tell you to store sanitized implements in sealed containers, or to keep them in a cabinet sanitizer until ready to be used.

7. **Sanitize table.** To sanitize, wipe manicuring table with disinfectant or sanitizing solution.

8. **Disinfect surface.** To disinfect, spray surface with any EPA registered disinfectant that is allowed by your state regulations. Allow surface to remain wet for ten minutes and wipe dry, then spray again and let air dry.

9. **Wrap client's cushion in clean towel.** Put a clean towel over your manicuring cushion. Be sure to use a clean towel for each client.

10. **Refill disposable materials.** Put new emery board, orangewood stick, cotton balls, and other disposable materials on manicuring table. These materials are discarded after use on *one* client.

11. **Use a sanitizing hand wash.** Clients like to see that you practice sanitation. Make a ceremony of this and they will trust you. When the client sits at your table use a waterless hand sanitizer gel or wipe on your hands. Ask your client to do so, too. Several alcohol gels are available. They feel cool, don't dry the skin and make excellent sanitizers.

Now you are ready to begin your service.

ULTRAVIOLET RAY SANITIZERS

Once implements are properly disinfected, they must be stored where they will remain free from contamination. Ultraviolet (UV) sanitizers are useful storage containers, but the types sold to salons *will not disinfect salon implements*. They are not very effective against viruses and can't reach into crevices. Never use these devices to disinfect! However, they make useful storage cabinets for properly disinfected implements. (Fig. 3.3) Another alternative is to store your implements in an airtight container, i.e. Rubber Maid™ or Tupper Ware™, etc.

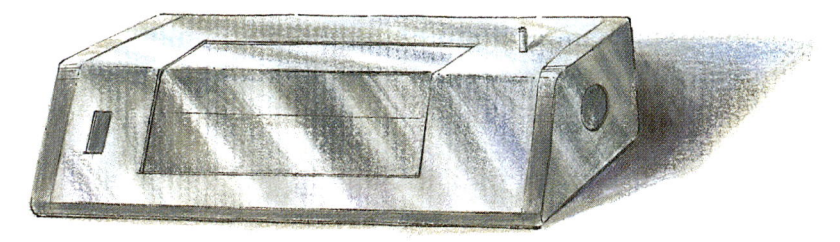

3.3 — Ultraviolet sanitizer

BEAD "STERILIZERS"

These devices do not sterilize or disinfect implements. They only give users a false sense of security. Sterilizing an implement with dry heat would require heating to 325°F for at least 30 minutes. These units can't even come close to doing this. Also, to be effective, the entire implement, including handle, would have to be buried in the beads. These devices are a waste of money and a gamble with your client's health. Don't be fooled by claims suggesting that these are FDA registered devices. This means absolutely nothing. The FDA does not require any testing or proof, therefore, FDA registration is meaningless to salon professionals.

BEWARE OF FORMALIN

For many years, formalin was used as a disinfectant and fumigant in dry cabinet sanitizers. Formalin *is not safe for salon use* and cannot be used in some states. Formalin contains large amounts of **formaldehyde,** a suspected human cancer-causing agent. It is poisonous to inhale or touch and is very irritating to the eyes, nose, throat and lungs. It can also cause skin irritation, dryness and rash. Formaldehyde is a strong **allergic sensitizer.** Prolonged or repeated exposure can cause allergic reactions similar to chronic bronchitis or asthma. These symptoms may take months to appear and then worsen over time with continued exposure.

> **PROCEDURAL TIP**
>
> *After each procedure that involves artificial nails, discard your plastic trash bag. This will prevent the release of vapors from products you've used.*

BLOOD SPILLS

There are several pathogens (i.e., hepatitis B) that can be found in blood. Since health care professionals regularly deal with seriously ill people, they must be very careful cleaning up blood spills. Many health care regulations have been written about cleaning up blood. Recently, some State Cosmetology boards have borrowed from these hospital regulations and are making special recommendations concerning accidental cuts.

If a blood spill occurs, many state boards require the use of a tuberculocidal disinfectant to clean up the *visible* blood. These disinfectants are considered to provide a little extra protection where blood spills are involved. This doesn't mean that other disinfectants are weak. Any EPA registered, hospital-level disinfectant will easily exceed all normal salon requirements. Tuberculocidal disinfectants are not required for general use, only to clean up blood.

Tuberculocidal disinfectants will not prevent the spread of TB in salons. It is impossible to transmit TB on a salon implement. Tuberculocidal disinfectants are safe, but must be used with extra caution. Most are based on phenolic compounds. The potential hazards of such materials were described earlier in this chapter.

Most cuts occur from new files or emery boards. One way to prevent this is to rub the edges of new files against the abrasive side of another file. This will "break in" the file and soften sharp edges. If you are careful, you will rarely cut a client. But, accidents will happen. If you do cut a client with a file… never try to disinfect it!

CHAPTER 3   SANITATION AND DISINFECTION ◆ 35

Tell your client that you are sorry and give them the file to take home. They will see it as a nice gift, but you have just gotten rid of a difficult disinfection problem.

> **STATE REGULATION ALERT**
>
> *Consult your state cosmetology regulatory agency or the Health Department for a list of approved disinfectants in your state.*

DISINFECTANT SAFETY

Be sure to read and follow exactly the instructions provided with any professional salon product. Wear **gloves** and **safety glasses** when mixing and using any product, especially disinfectants. *Never* stick your fingers into a disinfectant. Your skin is a barrier between you and microorganisms. Keep that barrier healthy by wearing gloves and avoiding skin contact. Never pour alcohol, bleach or other disinfectants over your hands. This foolish practice can cause skin disease and increase the chance of infection. Wash your hands with an antiseptic liquid soap and dry them thoroughly.

Carefully measure everything when mixing disinfectants. Otherwise, you cannot expect peak performance. Never place any product or other chemical in an unmarked bottle. This is an invitation to accidents and could have disastrous consequences. Always use tongs to remove implements from disinfection solutions. Store all professional products away from food and in a cool, dark, dry location. Be sure they are tightly closed and out of the reach of children.

UNIVERSAL SANITATION

To make your salon a safe haven you must use gloves and safety glasses, disinfectants and detergents, personal hygiene and salon cleanliness, sanitizers and antiseptics. When all of these things are performed together, it is called Universal Sanitation. You're doing it all! Universal sanitation is one of many responsibilities you have as a salon professional. You have the responsibility to protect your clients from harm. They depend on your training and expertise. Today, clients are more concerned than ever about safety and health. You also have a responsibility to yourself. You must protect your safety, as well. Don't take short cuts when it comes to sanitation and disinfection. These important measures are also designed to protect you!

Finally, you have a responsibility to your profession. When any one acts unprofessionally in the salon, everyone's image is tarnished. Clients expect to see you act in a professional manner. This is how trust and respect are earned!

Promote Nail Health

Clients come to you not only for beautiful-looking hands, but to solve nail problems, such as strengthening too-soft tips or doing something about brittleness and cracking. This is why, in addition to learning about nail anatomy and growth, it's important to know how various circumstances affect nails—from pregnancy to diet to prescription drug use. Medical texts offer a good source of information about conditions affecting nails, as do dermatology and nutrition publications. Being knowledgeable about nail health lets you custom-tailor a manicure to solve an individual's problems and allows you to prescribe personalized homecare regimens. Your clients will appreciate your professional knowledge and your work will appear that much nicer on strong, healthy nails.'

REVIEW QUESTIONS

1. What is the difference between disinfection and sanitation?
2. Disinfection is almost identical to _____ except, disinfection does not kill bacterial spores.
3. What is an antiseptic?
4. What is the best type of disinfectant to use in a salon?
5. What are the two most commonly used types of disinfectants?
6. Once implements are properly _____, they must be stored where they will remain free from _____.
7. Can tuberculosis (TB) be transmitted by salon implements?
8. Formaldehyde is a strong _____.
9. What must you use to remove implements from disinfectant containers?
10. Describe Universal Sanitation in your own words.

Chapter 4

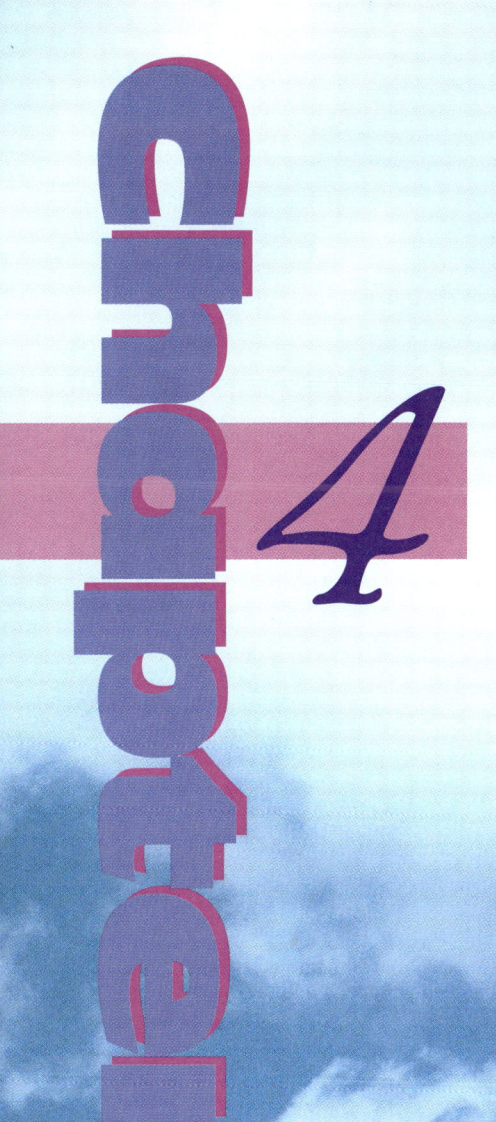

SAFETY IN THE SALON

LEARNING OBJECTIVES

After you have studied this chapter, you should be able to:

1. Understand and identify the early warning signs of overexposure.
2. Read and use Material Safety Data Sheets (MSDS).
3. List all three chemical "Routes of Entry."
4. Know how to achieve proper ventilation in the salon.
5. Avoid the risks of overexposure to vapors and dusts.
6. Recognize and avoid cumulative trauma disorders (CTDs).

INTRODUCTION

Today anyone can have long, beautiful nails thanks to the advances of chemistry and artistic talents of nail technicians. We can make short nails long, long nails strong, and we can turn anyone's nails into a work of art.

Most nail technicians are skilled in services such as nail tips, nail wraps, acrylic nails, and gel nails. For each of these services you will use "hi-tech" chemicals that could cause harm to both you and your clients. No product *need* harm your health, but all of them *can*. The key to working safely is in understanding your chemical tools.

In other chapters, you will learn step-by-step procedures for giving your clients advanced nail services. But first, you must learn to work safely with professional products. In this chapter, you will learn some basic rules for using nail chemicals wisely.

COMMON CHEMICALS USED BY NAIL TECHNICIANS

If you perform advanced nail services, your manicuring table is full of chemical products including:

- Nail polish and nail polish remover
- Liquid and powder for acrylic nails
- Primer for acrylic nails
- Temporary dehydrators
- Light cured gel nail supplies
- No-light gels and activators
- Cuticle oils and creams
- Adhesives for fabric wraps and much more.

All of these products can be safe, but all can be dangerous if used incorrectly. Luckily, you need not be afraid of these chemicals. Simply coming in contact with a chemical will not harm you. **Overexposure** is a danger you need to avoid. Overexposure for prolonged periods causes most of the problems. How can you tell if you have been overexposed? Your body will usually give you some *early warning signs of overexposure*. Some of these are listed below:

- Rash and other skin irritation
- Lightheadedness
- Insomnia
- Runny nose

- Sore, dry throat
- Watery eyes
- Tingling toes
- Fatigue
- Irritability
- Sluggishness
- Breathing problems

If you do suffer from any of these problems, there is good news. You don't have to take it! All of these are easily avoided and will completely reverse themselves in a short time, if you do your part. Working correctly and safely will eliminate these side effects and allow you to work comfortably. That is what working safely is all about.

LEARN ABOUT THE CHEMICALS IN YOUR PRODUCTS

Manufacturers try to make products as safe as possible. But they can only do so much. Their best efforts can be undone by a single careless act. It's up to you to learn about the chemicals in your professional products and how to handle them safely.

One excellent way to learn about working safely with a chemical is to read the *Material Safety Data Sheet (MSDS)* for that product.

WHAT IS AN MSDS?

The United States government requires that product manufacturers make Material Safety Data Sheets available to people who use their products. (Fig. 4.1) Each MSDS must contain basic items of information. MSDSs are written for everyone, not just nail technicians. Doctors, fire fighters, postal employees, truckers and many others use MSDSs. Some of the information on the MSDS is more important for them. While looking at MSDSs you will discover that there is no standard format. However, each MSDS must contain the following information:

1. **Identity of chemicals presenting physical or chemical hazards.** You can get information concerning potentially hazardous ingredients found in each product.

2. **Physical hazards.** You learn about how the product reacts with other chemicals, potential for explosion, fire hazards and how easily it will evaporate into the air.

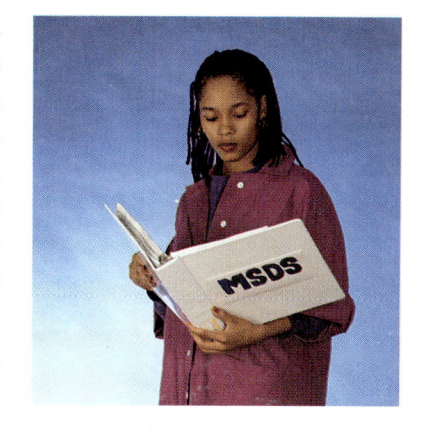

4.1 — Read your MSDS sheets.

3. **Health hazards.** You can learn the signs and symptoms of overexposure, and illnesses that might be caused by the product or existing medical conditions that might be made worse. There is also information concerning overexposure on the skin, eyes and respiratory system, as well as, problems caused if the product is accidentally swallowed. Both the short and long term health effects of overexposure (if any) are listed.

4. **Primary routes of entry into the body.** This explains how the products ingredients may enter your body. Usually chemicals gain entry through the skin, mouth or lungs. The MSDS will warn you of any such risks so that you can prevent overexposure.

5. **Permissible exposure limits.** Recommended safe limits in the air to prevent overexposure by inhalation.

6. **Carcinogen hazard of the chemical.** Information about whether any ingredient over 1/10th percent is suspected of causing cancer.

7. **Precautions and handling procedures.** Tips on safe handling of the product to prevent overexposure and how to properly clean up leaks or spills.

8. **Control and protection measures.** How to protect yourself and clients against the potential hazards of the product. Suggested ventilation needed, type of glove and eye wear protection required, and so on.

9. **Emergency and first aid procedures.** What to do in case of accidents and how to respond in emergencies related to product use. This section is one of the most important since it will give information for treating problems. Emergency first aid advice and emergency phone numbers are given.

10. **Storage and disposal information.** The best and safest way to get rid of old or unused products without causing injury to yourself, others or the environment. Also, you can get information on proper and safe storage.

HOW YOU CAN GET MATERIAL SAFETY DATA SHEETS

Your local distributor of beauty supplies is required by federal law to supply you with an MSDS for each product you buy from them. It is your legal responsibility to collect these sheets and keep them available for reference. If you have difficulty collecting the MSDSs you need, send a formal written request to the distributor.

CHAPTER 4   SAFETY IN THE SALON   ◆   41

AVOIDING OVEREXPOSURE IS EASY!

It is easy to work safely. Remember, health hazards are created by overexposure. You only have to learn how to avoid overexposure and you will be able to work safely.

Luckily, products can only enter your body in three ways:

You **breathe** them *(inhalation)*.

You **absorb** them through your skin *(skin contact)*.

You **eat** them *(ingestion)*.

If you control these routes of entry, you will greatly lessen the chance of overexposure.

VENTILATION CONTROL

Always work in a well ventilated area! This is one of the most important safety rules of nail technology. Your ventilation system must remove vapors and dusts from the building. Most systems just circulate them around the salon, for example, fans, open doors, windows, ceiling vents, air cleaners, and so on. The only effective way to ventilate in the salon is to vent vapors and dust to the outside. Vented manicuring tables are almost completely ineffective. Their flimsy charcoal filters absorb as much vapors as they can hold after about twenty hours of use. You cannot wash or shake these vapors out, the filter must be discarded. Devices that are designed to "clean the air" are ineffective and not practical in salons. The only sure method of removing vapors and dusts is to vent to the outside.

There is one place on earth that is more important to you than any other. That place is called your **breathing zone.** Your breathing zone is an invisible sphere about the size of a beach ball that sits directly in front of your mouth. Every single breath you take comes from your breathing zone. Your health and safety depend on what occurs in this small area. This is the real reason for ventilation.

PROCEDURAL TIP

Proper ventilation protects your breathing zone. Proper ventilation is a requirement for using professional products. Before you decide to work in a salon, you should make sure they have a good ventilation system.

Excessive inhalation of vapors is a problem for nail technicians. These vapors come from the evaporation of liquids. All liquid nail products evaporate and contribute to the total vapors in the air, even odorless acrylics, wraps, and light cured gels. Odors aren't the reason to ventilate. Ventilate to control vapors and dusts. What can you do to lower your exposure to vapors? Luckily, some of the most effective ways to eliminate vapors are the easiest and least expensive.

- Tightly seal all product containers immediately after use.
- Use a covered dappen dish or pump to limit the vapors in the air.
- Avoid using pressurized sprays. They create finer mists and are difficult to control.
- Empty your waste container often. It is one of the best sources of vapors.

PROCEDURAL TIP

Don't buy systems that ventilate odors. Devices that claim to eliminate odors are useless. Eliminating odors doesn't mean the air is clean. Vapors and dusts are what need to be removed and controlled. Do this properly and there will be no odor problem.

LOCAL EXHAUST

The only complete answer to salon vapor and dust control is *local exhaust.* These devices are based on a simple concept. They capture vapors and dusts at the source and expel them from your breathing zone. Local exhaust uses an exhaust vent, hose or tube to capture vapors, dusts and mists. A moveable exhaust tube can be placed where needed, for example, over your open containers or beside the hand while you file. Specially designed blowers pull contaminants from the breathing zone down the exhaust tube and expel them from the building.

Although venting to the outside is preferred, it is not always possible. If your salon has no outside access, the vapors and dusts can be filtered through a HEPA filter and at least a five gallon canister packed with activated charcoal. If you can vent to the roof, make sure your exhaust pipe is at least fifteen feet from any intake vents, especially your neighbors. The higher it is above the roof, the better. This will prevent odors from being drawn into nearby homes or businesses.

Custom systems based on these principles can be built fairly inexpensively. An expert capable of building such a system is as close as your phone book. Look under heating or air conditioning for a specialist that understands proper ventilation. You'll be surprised at how affordable a well designed local ventilation system can be.

PREVENTING OVEREXPOSURE TO DUSTS

Prolonged inhalation of excessive amounts of nail filings may be harmful. Not that nail filings are especially dangerous. Breathing large amounts of *any* dusts for long periods may be harmful, even house dust! Our bodies can remove a lot of the dusts that are inhaled. Problems occur only if you continually inhale more than the lungs can handle. Wearing a dust mask can prevent this. (Fig. 4.2) Nothing you can buy will do a better job of protecting your lungs against dusts. The large, visible particles are less harmful since they fall on the table top and are easily removed. The smaller, invisible dusts are far more hazardous. Smaller particles lodge deeper in the lungs increasing the risks. Dust masks filter air from your breathing zone before it enters the mouth. Never use these masks to prevent inhalation of vapors. They cannot block any of the vapors in the salon.

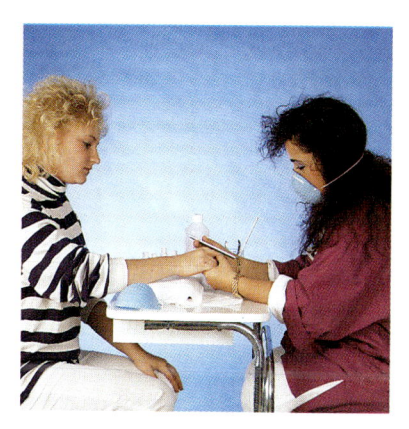

4.2 — Wear a dust mask when filing and offer one to your client.

PROCEDURAL TIP

Always wear a dust mask when filing, especially if you use a drill. Drills make much smaller, more hazardous dust particles than files or abrasive boards. Also, throw away dust masks every few days. They're disposable and become ineffective if used too long.

A DANGEROUS MISCONCEPTION

Many believe that they can tell how safe or dangerous a chemical is by its odor! A chemical's smell has absolutely nothing to do with its safety. Some very dangerous substances have sweet, pleasant fragrances. Products or ventilation systems that "cover-up" or "remove" odors will not protect your health. Odors are really the nail technician's friend. Odors can warn against overexposure danger. Odors are caused when vapors touch sensitive detectors in the nose. After the vapors leave the nose and enter the lungs, their odor is not important. You are asking for trouble if you use odor to judge product safety. The same is true for nice smells. Overexposure to nice smelling vapors can cause harm, too!

PROTECT YOUR EYES

Accidents involving the eyes are a serious danger in salons. Solvents in the eye can be very painful and may cause severe damage. Primer, wrap monomers and adhesives or phenolic

44 ◆ PART I GETTING STARTED

disinfectant solutions in the eyes are worse! Each of these can cause permanent eye injury or blindness. Imagine what it is like to be blind! It could happen if you are not careful to protect your vision.

Always use eye protection whenever there is the slightest chance that a liquid product could get into your eyes. (Fig. 4.3) Eye injuries account for approximately forty-five percent of the cosmetic related injuries seen in hospital emergency rooms. Many of these are students and salon professionals.

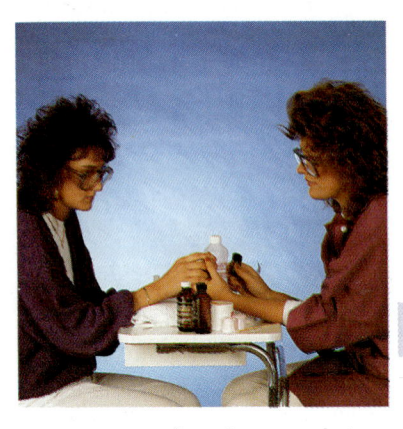

4.3 — Wear safety glasses and give your client a pair.

> **PROCEDURAL TIP**
>
> *Always wear approved safety glasses whenever you work with anything that can get into the eyes.*

Wearing contacts in the salon is risky. Vapors will collect in soft contacts and make them unwearable. Even if you wear safety glasses, vapors are still absorbed. The contaminated lens can etch the surface of the eye and cause permanent damage. Should an accidental splash occur, the liquid will "wick" under the lens. This will make proper cleaning of the eye more difficult.

OTHER TIPS FOR WORKING SAFELY

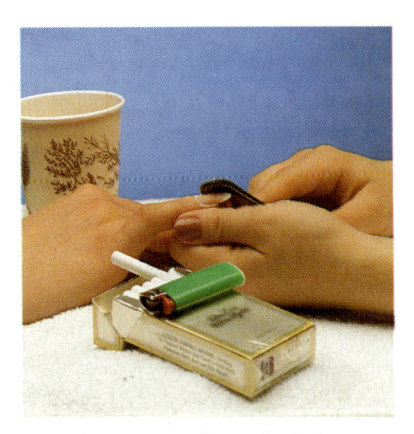

4.4 — Don't smoke in the salon; many nail products are highly flammable.

1. **Don't smoke in the salon.** Since nail technicians work with many flammable solvents and products, it is wise to take precautions to prevent fires in the salon. One way is by not allowing smoking in the salon. Smoking near flammable solvents is very risky. If smoking is permitted, it should be in an entirely different area. (Fig. 4.4)

2. **Always avoid skin contact.** Never touch any acrylic liquids, wraps or adhesives, light cure gels, etc., to the skin. This is one of the leading causes of service breakdown, lifting and allergic reactions. More will be said about adverse skin reactions in Chapter 5. The best rule to follow is, "if it isn't designed for skin application, keep it off the skin!"

3. **Never eat or drink in the salon area.** A cup of coffee is an excellent place for nail dust and vapors to collect. Hot liquids, like coffee and tea, can absorb vapors from the air. Dusts settle in any open container. The cup of coffee you or your client is drinking may be filled with contaminants.

CHAPTER 4   SAFETY IN THE SALON ◆ **45**

4. **Store and eat your lunch in a separate area of the salon.** If you put your food in the same refrigerator as chemical products, it will probably absorb a dose of chemical vapors before you can eat it. When you eat, you should leave the building or eat in a lunchroom that is separated from the rest of the salon by walls and a door. Federal law forbids eating in any area where professional chemicals are being stored or used.

5. **Always wash your hands before eating.** When someone offers you a piece of chocolate or when you dodge into the kitchen for a cookie, do you wash your hands first? If you forget to wash your hands before you grab a snack or eat lunch, you will probably end up eating the chemicals that are on your hands. (Fig. 4.5)

6. **Label all containers.** Every container, spray bottle, squeeze bottle, or tube in the salon must be properly labeled. This includes all cleaning products and any bulk purchased products in storage. Be sure the label is waterproof. If the container isn't labeled, *don't use it.* (Fig. 4.6)

7. **Store your products in a cool area.** Never store your professional products in a car trunk, by a window or near a pilot light, such as those for gas heaters or furnaces. Excessive heat will ruin them and some are more flammable than gasoline.

8. **Empty your trash can regularly.** Use a metal can with a self closing lid as a trash container. Vapors will escape from open trash and fill your air with vapors. Empty the trash several times a day and dispose of it properly. A metal can will also lessen the risk of fire.

9. **Keep caps on all products.** It may seem easier to leave caps off your products, but it isn't wise. Uncapped bottles on your table are very easy to spill. Keep your product containers closed to reduce the amount of vapor that escapes into the air. Capping will also make your products last longer. Uncapped nail polish thickens, solvents evaporate, and wrap glue starts to harden. (You will find that marbles are just the right size to cover the small dishes you use for acrylic powder and liquid.)

10. **Be prepared to handle accidents.** Don't wait until after an accident has happened to figure out how to handle it. Have the poison control center number and other emergency numbers near the phone. (Fig. 4.7) Keep the MSDS for each product in a convenient place. At salon meetings, discuss what you would do in case of an accident.

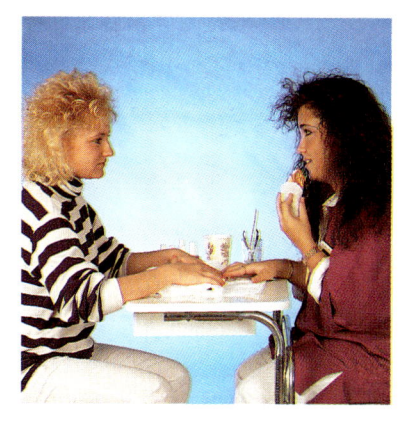

4.5 — Never eat or drink in the salon area. You may find that you're eating or drinking nail chemicals.

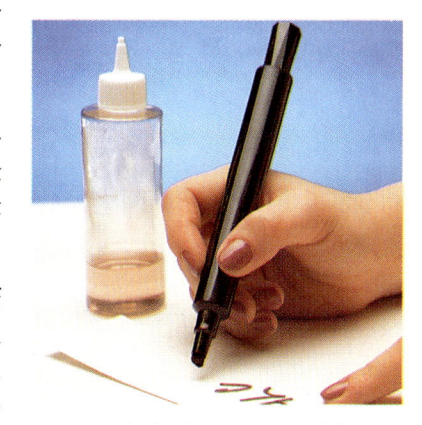

4.6 — Label all containers. If the container isn't labeled, don't use it.

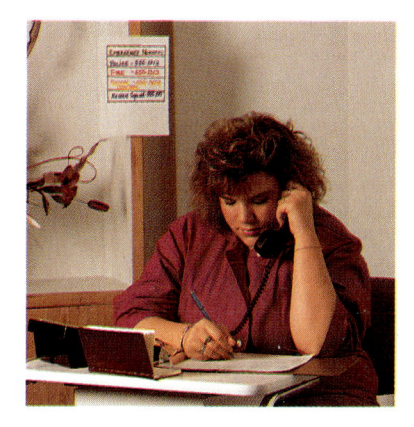

4.7 — Post important numbers close to the telephone.

CUMULATIVE TRAUMA DISORDERS

Cumulative trauma disorder (CTD) is also known as repetitive motion disorder. CTDs are the fastest growing type of injury for all occupations. CTDs cause painful and crippling illness that may become permanent if not treated. ***Carpal tunnel syndrome*** is the most common CTD. This illness affects the hands and wrists of many nail technicians. The carpal tunnel is a small passage in a wrist bone that carries a nerve from the fingers to the arm. Repetitive motions can create damaging pressure on the nerve.

Injury is usually caused by repetitive motions such as filing nails. Constant vibration from drills may also cause or aggravate the condition. Pain and numbness often spread into the arm and fingers. If ignored, the situation usually becomes worse. Continued injury can permanently damage the nerve. Other things can cause CTDs. Sitting or working in the same position, awkward reaching, stretching or twisting may damage the carpal tunnel nerve or similar nerves in the neck and back.

Symptoms of CTDs are:

- Pain
- Numbness
- Aching
- Stiffness
- Tingling
- Weakness
- Swelling

If you experience any of these symptoms, pay close attention to how you work. You can usually tell which repetitive motion is causing the pain. It is best to seek medical attention immediately before it is too late to correct the problem.

WHAT TO DO?

There are many things nail technicians can do to avoid CTDs.

- Always sit in a natural, unstrained position.
- Don't hunch over the client's nails. Change positions often.
- Stretch frequently, even if only for a few seconds.
- Avoid using tools that vibrate excessively.
- Hold wrists straight and avoid bending them while filing or using a brush.
- Stop work and stretch or shake out your hands.

Most importantly, take your time. Rushing through a service is hard on you and the client's nails. Quality is more important than speed! Dont sacrifice your health and your clients nails by speeding through a nail service. It is better to raise your prices and do great work on fewer clients.

PROCEDURAL TIP

An easy and effective exercise is to press your hand on a flat surface while stretching your finger and wrist for five seconds.

Ice and ibuprofen or aspirin will ease the pain, but if you think you have a CTD see a doctor! Your doctor will be able to make prevention recommendations that you might not think about.

Express Yourself Safely

Have a little fun with your safety goggles by turning them into a professional tool for nail art. They're a great vehicle for individual expression and they're sure to attract attention. Add hand-painted designs to goggle frames or edges and change them frequently to reflect seasonal themes, color trends, and personal preference. For mini test-marketing, determine which designs generate the most interest, then offer to create those designs on your client's nails. The bottom line is that you boost your profits and create interest in nail art while promoting safety.

REVIEW QUESTIONS

1. List five early warning signs of chemical overexposure.
2. What does MSDS stand for?
3. Name four simple and inexpensive things you can do to reduce vapors in the salon.
4. Define breathing zone.
5. Describe how a local exhaust system works. Why is it best?
6. What is the best and least expensive way to prevent excessive inhalation of dusts?
7. Why should products be stored away from heat and pilot lights?
8. Why should smoke not be allowed in the salon?
9. What is CTD? Explain how this happens.
10. List seven symptoms of CTD.

Part 2

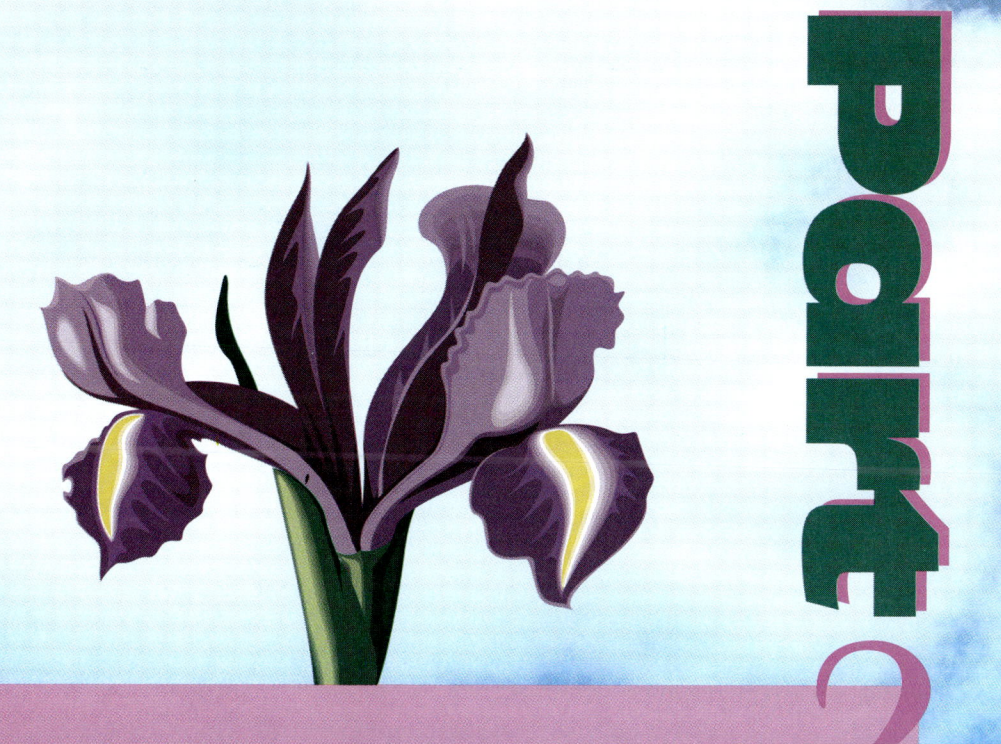

THE SCIENCE OF NAIL TECHNOLOGY

- ◆ *CHAPTER 5* - Nail Product Chemistry Simplified
- ◆ *CHAPTER 6* - Anatomy and Physiology
- ◆ *CHAPTER 7* - The Nail and Its Disorders
- ◆ *CHAPTER 8* - The Skin and Its Disorders
- ◆ *CHAPTER 9* - Client Consultation

Chapter 5
NAIL PRODUCT CHEMISTRY SIMPLIFIED

LEARNING OBJECTIVES
After you have studied this chapter, you should be able to:

1. Understand the basic chemistry of salon products.
2. Explain adhesion and how adhesives work.
3. Identify the two main categories of nail coatings.
4. Describe the basic chemistry of all enhancements
5. Determine the cause and prevention of skin disorders.

INTRODUCTION

Why do nail technicians need chemistry? Almost everything you do depends on chemistry. Even if you just want to "do nails," your success depends on having an understanding of chemicals and chemistry.

UNDERSTANDING CHEMICALS

It is incorrect to think all chemicals are dangerous or toxic substances. Most chemicals are completely safe. Everything around you is made of chemicals. The walls, this book, food, vitamins, even oxygen is a chemical. In fact, everything you can see or touch, except light and electricity, is a **chemical**.

Nail plates are 100% chemical. They are mostly protein made from chemicals called amino acids. Amino acids are composed of the chemicals carbon, nitrogen, oxygen, hydrogen and sulfur. The chemical sulfur is responsible for the sulfur cross-links that create strong natural nails. Nail plates also contain traces of iron, aluminum, copper, silver, gold and other chemicals.

MATTER AND ENERGY

Everything in the world is either matter or energy. **Matter** takes up space or occupies an area. For instance, books occupy space, therefore a book is made of matter. Very few things don't take up space. Even microscopic bacteria use a small amount of space.

Light, radio waves, and microwaves are examples of things that don't occupy space. These are not made of matter—they are **energy**. Energy has no substance. However, energy can affect matter in many ways.

MOLECULES AND ELEMENTS

A **molecule** is a chemical in its simplest form. A water molecule can be broken down in to hydrogen and oxygen, but it wouldn't be water any longer. Some molecules cannot be broken down at all. These are called **elements**. Oxygen and hydrogen are two of the 106 known elements.

FORMS OF MATTER

Matter can exist as a solid, liquid or gas. Water can be frozen into a solid, melted to a liquid and evaporated into a gas or vapor. When water freezes, thaws or evaporates it is **physically changed**. The water is simply changing form or appearance. It is not chemically altered.

Matter can be chemically changed, too. Burning sugar or paper makes a black substance. This is an example of a *chemical change* or one chemical changing into a completely different chemical substance.

Chemical molecules are like tiny tinker toys. They can be arranged and rearranged into an unlimited number of combinations. Petroleum oil can be chemically converted into vitamin C. Acetone can be changed into water or oxygen. Paper can be made into sugar. The possibilities are endless. In medieval times, alchemists searched in vain for ways to turn lead into gold. Today, even this is possible.

CHEMICAL REACTIONS

Under the right conditions a molecule can chemically change. This is called a *chemical reaction*. In general, a chemical reaction requires energy to occur. Most chemical reactions get this energy from heat or light. Artificial nail enhancements can use either heat or light energy to create the finished product.

CATALYST

A *catalyst* is a chemical that can make a chemical reaction go faster. Different chemical reactions require different catalysts. Catalysts are very important chemical tools. Many chemical reactions happen very slowly. For instance, graphite (pencil lead) will slowly change into diamond, but would take many thousands of years. Obviously, a graphite to diamond catalyst would be an important invention, if it were ever discovered.

Trillions of chemical reactions occur in our bodies every day. Most of these happen very quickly because of catalysts. Nail technicians use catalysts to make wraps, overlays and sculptured nails. Usually, these are found in the gel or liquid. In the case of wraps, they are sprayed on the surface.

SOLVENTS AND SOLUTES

A *solvent* is anything which dissolves another substance. Solvents are usually liquid. The substance that is dissolved is called a *solute*. Generally, solutes are solids. Water is a very good solvent. In fact, water is called the "universal solvent" because it will dissolve more substances than any other solvent. Acetone is frequently used as a polish remover and to dissolve nail enhancements. It is an extremely safe solvent to use for this purpose. When used as a polish remover, acetone dissolves old polish (the solute).

Acetone works quickly because it is a *good solvent*. A *poor solvent* dissolves solutes very slowly. Water is a poor solvent for nail polish. Otherwise, hand washing would remove the polish. Solvents only dissolve a certain amount of solute before they become *saturated.* Solvents become saturated with solute much like a mop becomes saturated with water. In other words, a saturated solvent cannot dissolve any more solute. Saturated solvents are very ineffective. Using a saturated solvent is a waste of time since fresh, clean solvents work much faster.

Gently warming solvents will also make them faster acting. This is especially true for removing artificial nail enhancements. Warming the solvent to 105°F (jacuzzi temperature) will speed removal time by thirty percent. Of course, warming solvents should be done with great care under hot, running water. Many are highly flammable! Never warm any flammable substances on a stove or in a microwave oven. Loosen the cap so that pressure doesn't build up in the bottle. Also, cover the dish and hand with a damp cloth while soaking to reduce vapors in the air. The products manufacturer will provide you with more safe handling information.

ADHESION AND ADHESIVES

Adhesion is a force of nature that makes two surfaces stick together. Adhesion is caused when the molecules on one surface are attracted to the molecules on another surface. Paste sticks to paper because its molecules are attracted to paper molecules. Oils, waxes and soil will contaminate a surface and block adhesion. This is why a clean, dry surface will give better adhesion.

ADHESIVES

An *adhesive* is a chemical that causes two surfaces to stick together. Adhesives allow incompatible surfaces to be joined. Scotch® tape is a plastic that is coated with a sticky adhesive. Without the adhesive the plastic would not stick to paper. The sticky adhesive layer acts as a "go between." It holds the tape to the paper. Adhesives are like a ship's anchor. One end of the anchor holds the ship, the other end attaches to the ground.

There are many types of adhesives. Different adhesives are compatible with different surfaces. *Glues* are a type of adhesive made by boiling animal hides, hooves and bones. Many white paper glues are this type of adhesive. True glues are low in strength and do not adhere well to the nail plate. What we often call "glue" is actually a high tech adhesive called *cyanoacrylate.* It is formulated specially for professional salon use on the nail plate.

PRIMERS

Primers are substances that improve adhesion. Nail polish base coats are primers. Why? Base coats make nail polish adhere better. Base coats act as the "go-between" or "anchor." They improve adhesion.

Other types of primers are sometimes required with artificial nail enhancements. They are especially useful if the client has oily skin. Primers act like double sided sticky tape. (Fig. 5.1) One side sticks well to the enhancement and the other side holds tightly to the nail plate. A common misconception is that nail primers "eat" the nail. This is completely false. Nail clippings can soak for many years in primer without dissolving. Still, nail primers must be used with caution. Some are very corrosive to soft tissue. A *corrosive* is a substance that can cause visible and possibly permanent skin damage. Nail primers, like most professional nail products, should never touch the skin! Primers are acids and can cause painful burns and scars to soft tissue.

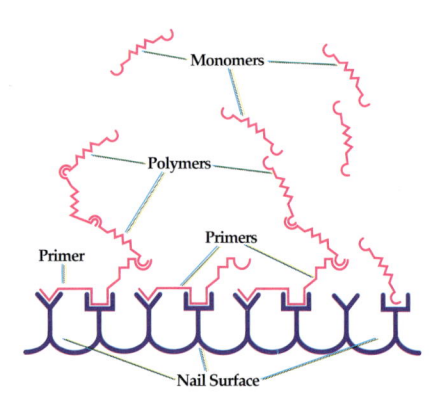

Even though primers will not damage the nail plate, they can burn the nail bed tissue. Overfiling the natural nail will excessively thin the nail making it more porous. If too much primer is used, the nail plate can become saturated. Small amounts may reach the nail bed causing sensitivity and painful burns. It may also lead to separation of the nail plate from the bed. Use primer sparingly! One very thin coat is enough for most clients. If you find that you rely on two or more coats to prevent lifting, something is wrong! Check your nail preparation and application procedure for problems. Primer can become a crutch, covering up improper application. In the long run, it is better to get to the root of the problem and improve your technique.

Some primers are not corrosive to skin. These are incorrectly called non-acid primers. They do contain acids. Like methacrylic acid primers, they will not damage the nail plate. These primers are designed to prevent burning of the soft tissue. They still must be used with caution and skin contact must be avoided. Prolonged or repeated exposure and incorrect application can cause skin problems over time. (Fig. 5.2)

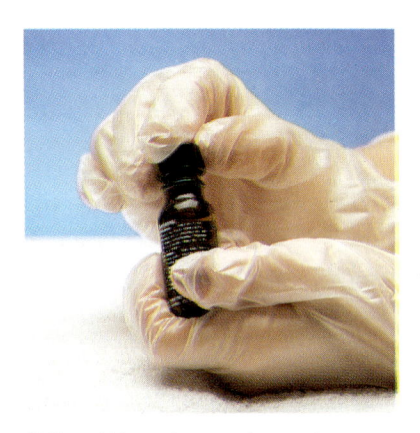

A CLEAN START

Good adhesion depends on proper technique and high quality products. The best way to ensure success is to start with a clean, dry surface. Washing the hands and scrubbing the nail plate removes surface oils and contaminants that interfere with proper adhesion. Scrubbing also gets rid of bacteria and fungal spores which lead to infections. Skipping this important step is the major cause of nail infections. It also causes enhancement to lifting at the cuticle.

A nail dehydrator temporarily removes moisture, which interferes with adhesion. To ensure proper adhesion always scrub the nail plate, dry thoroughly and dehydrate. It is a myth that enhancements and tips don't stick unless you "rough up the nail." This is absolutely false and very harmful for clients. Adhesion is best when the nail plate is clean and dry. Heavy abrasives and

5.1 — Primers act as "double-sided sticky tape" to anchor monomers firmly to the surface of the natural nail plate.

5.2 — Wear gloves when using primers, adhesives, wraps monomers, acrylics monomers and gels.

drills will strip away the natural nail plate, leaving it thin and weak. The result is a weak base for the enhancements which leads to breakage.

When artificial nails are removed, clients can see the damage caused by heavy filing. They mistakenly blame primers and nail enhancements for what they see. Rough filing damages both the nail plate and bed. Also, heavy abrasives and overfiling may cause the nail plate to lift and separate from the nail bed. Once this occurs, clients often develop infections under the nail plate.

Overfiling is a leading cause of nail technician and client problems. It promotes allergic reactions and causes painful burning sensations, infections, loss of the nail plate, product lifting and breakage. Roughing the plate causes dangerous and excessive thinning of the natural nail. This must be avoided at all cost!

If you need to rough up the nail plate to get good adhesion then something is wrong! Many nail technicians have great success without roughing up the nail plate. Why? The answer is simple, they properly prepare the nail plates, use correct application techniques and high quality products. Lifting problems can always be traced back to one of these areas.

FINGERNAIL COATINGS

As a nail technician, you must perform many tasks. The most important of these is to apply coatings to the nail plate. **Coatings** are products which cover the nail plate with a hard film. Examples of typical coatings are nail polish, top coats, artificial enhancements and adhesives. There are two main types of coatings:

1. Coatings that cure or polymerize (chemical reaction)

2. Coatings that harden upon evaporation (physical reaction)

Nail polish and top coats are examples of coatings created by evaporation. Artificial enhancements are created by chemical reactions.

MONOMERS AND POLYMERS

Creating a nail enhancement is a good example of a chemical reaction. Billions of molecules must react to make just one sculptured nail. Durable and long-lasting coatings or enhancements are all created by chemical reactions. All liquid and powder, UV gels, no-light gels and wrap products work in this fashion.

The molecules in the product join together into extremely long chains. Each chain containing millions of molecules. These gigantic chains of molecules are called *polymers* (**POL**-uh-murs).

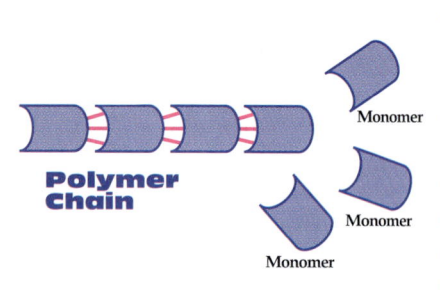

5.3 — A simple polymer chain grows in one direction by adding monomers in a head-to-tail fashion.

Polymers can be liquids, but they are usually solid. Chemical reactions that make polymers are called *polymerizations* (puh-lim-uh-ruh-**ZAY**-shuns). Sometimes the terms *cure, curing* or *hardening* are used, but they all have the same meaning.

There are many different types of polymers. Teflon®, nylon, hair and wood are polymers. Proteins are also polymers. Nail plates are made of a protein called keratin. So, nail plates are also polymers.

The individual molecules that join to make the polymer are called *monomers* (**MON**-uh-murs). In other words, monomers are the molecules that make polymers. For example, amino acids are monomers that join together to make the polymer we call keratin. (Fig. 5.3)

UNDERSTANDING POLYMERIZATIONS

If you understand the simple basics of polymerizations, you will be able to prevent many common salon problems. Liquid and powder systems, gels or no-light gels, wraps—they each seem very different, but they are actually quite similar. They each have a different type of monomer molecule. Monomers are like track runners mingling around the starting line, patiently waiting for the race to begin. The race starts when the proper signal is given. Once given, the runners don't stop until they reach the finish line.

The same is true for monomer molecules. They are like the runners, waiting for something to trigger the polymerization. This is done by a special ingredient called an *initiator.* Initiator molecule energize! They carry extra energy. Each time an initiator touches a monomer, the initiator excites it with a boost of energy. But, the monomer molecules don't like the extra energy and try to get rid of it. They do this by attaching themselves to the tail-end of another monomer and passing the energy along. The second monomer uses the same trick to get rid of the energy. As this game of tag continues, the chain of monomers gets longer and longer. A billion monomers can join in less than a second!

Soon, the many growing monomer chains begin to get in each other's way. They become tangled and knotted, which explains why the product starts to thicken. Eventually, the chains are much too long and crowded to freely move around. The product has become a teeming mass of microscopic-sized strings. When this occurs, the surface is hard enough to file, but it will be several days before the chains reach their ultimate lengths. This explains why enhancements become stronger during the first forty-eight hours.

SIMPLE VS. CROSS-LINKING POLYMER CHAINS

Normally, the head of one monomer reacts with the tail of another, and so on. The result is a long chain of monomers attached head to tail. These are called *simple polymer chains.* Wraps and tip adhesives form this type of polymer. In these polymers, the tangled chains are easily unraveled by solvents, which explains why they are easily removed. Polymer chains can also be unraveled by force. Products with simple polymer chains are easily damaged by sharp impacts or heavy stresses. Dyes and stains can also get lodged between the tangled chains. Nail polishes, marker ink, foods and many other things may cause unsightly stains on the surface.

To overcome these problems, UV gels and liquid and powder systems use small amounts of special monomers called cross-linkers. A *cross-linker* is a monomer that joins different polymer chains together. These cross-links are like rungs on a ladder. Cross-links create strong net-like polymers. The result is a three-dimensional structure of great strength and flexibility, which we call nail enhancements.

The nail plate and hair also contains cross-links which create a tough, resilient structure. Besides increased strength, the cross-linked nets prevent inks, dyes and nail polish from staining the surface. They are impervious to nail polish removers, as well. However, they are more resistant to all solvents, so removal is more difficult.

LIGHT AND HEAT ENERGY

Energy is the final key to understanding nail enhancement chemistry. Previously, you learned that monomers are energized by initiator molecules. Where does the initiator get the energy? You will recall that catalysts are used to make reactions happen more quickly. Catalysts give the initiator molecule its energy. Some catalysts use heat as an energy source while others use light. Whatever the source, catalysts absorb energy like a battery. At the appropriate time, they pass this energy to the initiator and the reaction begins. Light-cured enhancements generally use *ultraviolet* or *UV light.* All other products use heat energy. The heat from the room and client's hand is enough.

You can see why it is important to protect UV curing products from light. Sunlight and even artificial room lights can start polymerization in the container. The same can happen when heat-curing monomers are put in a hot car trunk, a store window or some other warm area. The high heat may also cause polymerization in the container. Products that require normal "incandescent" light bulbs are *not* light-curing monomers. They are using the extra heat released from the light bulb to speed evaporation of solvents.

EVAPORATION COATINGS

Nail polishes, top coats and base coats also form coatings. However, these products are entirely different. They do not polymerize. No chemical reactions occur and they contain no monomers. These products work strictly by evaporation. The majority of the ingredients are volatile or quickly evaporating solvents. Special polymers are dissolved in these solvents. These polymers are not cross-linked polymers, so they dissolve easily.

As the solvents evaporate, they leave behind a smooth polymer film. This film can hold pigments which give color. Artist paints and hair sprays work in the same fashion. Of course, the strength of uncross-linked polymers is much lower than cross-linked enhancement polymers. This explains why polishes are prone to chipping and are so easily dissolved by removers. Now you can see for yourself the great difference between coatings that cure or polymerize and those that harden upon evaporation.

"BETTER FOR THE NAIL" CLAIMS

Some believe that certain types of enhancement products are "better" for the natural nail. This is absolutely false! No one type of nail enhancement product is better for the nail plate than another. What is better for the nail? That is easy to answer. The best thing for the natural nail is highly skilled, educated and conscientious nail professionals. They are the natural nail's best friend. Good nail technicians protect and nurture the nail plate. Don't be fooled. Professional nail enhancement products don't damage the natural nail. Technicians are generally responsible for almost all their client's nail damage and disease. Any product can be applied and removed safely. It is up to *you* to use your knowledge and skill to see that it happens.

AVOIDING SKIN PROBLEMS

Skin problems are common in every facet of the professional salon industry. Nail, skin and hair services all can cause problems for the sensitive client. Fortunately, the vast majority of fingernail related problems can be easily avoided—if you understand how!

DERMATITIS

Dermatitis means skin inflammation. There are many kinds of dermatitis, but only one is important in the salon. **Contact dermatitis** is the most common skin disease for nail technicians. Contact dermatitis is caused by touching certain substances to the skin. This type of dermatitis can be short-term or long-term. Contact dermatitis can have several causes. The skin may be irritated by a substance. This is called **irritant contact dermatitis.** It is also possible to become allergic to an ingredient in a product. This is called **allergic contact dermatitis.**

PROLONGED OR REPEATED CONTACT

Allergic reactions are caused by prolonged or repeated contact. This type of skin problem does not occur overnight. Acrylic liquids, wraps and UV light gels are all capable of causing allergic reactions. In general, it takes from four to six months of repeated exposure before sensitive clients show symptoms.

Nail technicians are also at risk. Prolonged, repeated or long term exposures can cause anyone to become sensitive. This is called *overexposure.* Simply touching monomers doesn't cause sensitivities. It requires months of improper handling and overexposure. The most likely places for allergies to occur are:

1. Between a technician's thumb and pointer finger
2. On the nail technician's wrist or palm
3. On the nail technician's face, especially the cheeks
4. On the client's cuticles, finger tips or nail beds

If you examine the area where the problem occurs, you can usually determine the cause. For example, nail technicians often smooth wet brushes with their fingers. This is both prolonged and repeated contact! Eventually the area becomes sore and inflamed. The same occurs when technicians lay their arms on the towels contaminated with gel or monomer. The palms are overexposed by picking up containers that have traces of monomer on the outside. Small amounts of product on your hands are often transferred to the cheeks or face.

Touching a client's skin with any monomer or gel has the same effect. This is the most common reason for client sensitivities. With each service the risk of sensitization increases. *Sensitization* is a greatly increased or exaggerated sensitivity to products. It is extremely important that you always leave a 1/8" margin between the product and the skin. The most important rule of being a good nail technician is: **Never touch any nail enhancement product to the skin**.

Improper product consistency is the second most common reason for allergy. If too much liquid monomer is used, the result is an overly wet bead. Many technicians dont realize that the initiator in the polymer powder can only harden a certain amount of the liquid monomer. Wet beads are incorrectly balanced. Beads with too wet of a consistency will harden with monomer trapped inside. This extra monomer eventually works its way down to the nail bed and may cause an allergic reaction. The same thing occurs with gel enhancements. Many things can cause gels to harden incorrectly:

- Applying product too thickly
- Too short of a time under the light

- Dirty bulbs in the lamp unit
- Old bulbs that should be changed

Several thin coatings and long exposures lead to the best and most complete cure. If the UV bulb is dirty or old, it doesn't give enough energy to fully cure the enhancement. UV bulbs remain blue for years, but they lose effectiveness after four to six months of use. They should be cleaned daily and changed at least twice per year. The product will set faster, last longer and be less likely to cause allergy if you follow this advice.

Filings can also be too rich in gel or monomer. They can settle on the nail technicians arms or hands and cause skin problems. This is why it is critical to use medium wet beads and never use too wet of a consistency. The gooey layer on top of gel enhancements is mostly uncured gel. It must never come in contact with soft tissue. Also, never dip back into the dappen dish to get more liquid or clean up around the cuticle with monomer. If you do, chances are your clients will begin to develop skin problems in those areas. Avoid using extra large or oversize brushes. They usually make overly wet beads that are difficult to control. The belly of these large brushes can carry enough liquid for **four** normal size beads. Brushes that are too large don't save time—they cause allergic reactions.

Mixing product lines or custom blending your own "special" mixture can also create chemical imbalances which lead to allergic reactions. Don't take unnecessary risks. Always use products exactly as instructed and never mix your own products. If you do, don't be surprised when you or your clients develop skin problems.

Skin disorders of the hands affects forty percent of all nail technicians sometime during their careers. Skin problems and allergies force many good nail technicians to give up successful careers. Unfortunately, once you or a client become allergic to an ingredient, you are sensitive for the rest of your life. This is especially sad, because it is completely avoidable. No one should suffer from any work related allergy or irritation.

IRRITANT CONTACT DERMATITIS

Irritating substances will temporarily damage the epidermis. Corrosive substances are good examples of irritants. When the skin is damaged by irritating substances the immune system springs into action. It floods the tissue with water, trying to dilute the irritant. This is why swelling occurs. The body is trying to stop things from getting any worse. The immune system also tells the blood to release chemicals called **histamines** which enlarge the vessels around the injury. Blood can then rush to the scene more quickly and help remove the irritating substance.

You can see and feel all the extra blood under the skin. The entire area becomes red, warm and may throb. It is the histamines that cause the itchy feeling that often accompanies contact dermatitis. After everything calms down, the swelling will go away. The surrounding skin is often left damaged, scaly, cracked and dry. Fortunately, irritations are not permanent. If you avoid contact, the skin will usually quickly repair itself. However, continued or repeated exposure may lead to permanent allergic reactions.

Surprisingly, tap water is a very common salon irritant. Hands that remain damp for long periods often become sore, cracked and chapped. Avoiding the problem is simple. Always completely dry the hands. Regularly use moisturizing hand creams to compensate for loss of skin oils. Frequent hand washing, especially in hard water, can further damage the skin. Cleansers and detergents worsen the problem. They increase damage by stripping away sebum and other natural skin chemicals. Prolonged or repeated contact with many solvents will strip away skin oils, leaving the skin dry or damaged. Sometimes it is difficult to determine the cause of the irritation. One way to identify the irritant is by observing the location of the reaction. Symptoms are
always isolated to the contact area. The cause will be something that you are doing to this part of the skin.

REMEMBER THESE PRECAUTIONS

- *Never* smooth the enhancement surface with more liquid monomer.
- *Never* use monomer to "clean up" the edges, under the nail or sidewalls.
- *Never* touch any monomer liquids, gels or adhesives to the skin.
- *Never* touch the hairs of the brush with your fingers.
- *Never* mix your own special product blends.
- *Always* follow instructions—exactly!

Once a client becomes allergic, things will only get worse if you continue using the same products and techniques. It is best to discontinue use until you figure out what you are doing wrong. Otherwise, more clients will eventually be affected. Medications and illness don't make clients sensitive to nail products. These are just excuses. Only prolonged and repeated contact causes these allergies.

PROTECT YOURSELF

Take extreme care to keep brush handles, containers and table tops clean and free from product dusts and residues. Repeatedly handling these items will cause overexposure if the items are not kept clean. Enhancement products are not designed for skin contact! If you avoid contact, neither you nor your client will ever develop an allergic reaction.

Many serious problems can be related to contact dermatitis. Don't fall into the trap of developing bad habits. Many of these are ghosts from the early years of the nail industry when there was no proper education.

THE OVEREXPOSURE PRINCIPLE

We usually think of toxic substances as dangerous poisons. We hear the term "toxic" often, but should nail technicians try to avoid products that are toxic? The answer to this question may surprise you.

Paracelus, a famous 14th century physician, was the first to use the word "toxic." He said, *"All substances are poisons; there is none which is not a poison. Only the dose differentiates a poison and a remedy."*

The **Overexposure Principle** is the modern day interpretation of what Paracleus learned. This important principle says that *overexposure* determines toxicity. Scientists have found that Paracelus is correct. Everything is a poison! Do we have to avoid everything, including cuticle oils and skin creams? Isn't anything nontoxic? Scientists define toxic and nontoxic differently than the terms are commonly understood. They consider a chemical relatively nontoxic only if drinking a quart or more won't cause death.

Next time someone tells you a product is "nontoxic" think about this definition. Salt water is very toxic to drink. Still, we can safely swim in the ocean without fear of poisoning. Rubbing alcohol is also quite toxic, but we manage to use it quite easily.

Retail As You Work

A manicure provides the perfect opportunity to sell nailcare products. If, during a hand massage, the client comments that the lotion you're using feels good, selling it to her should be easy—just explain the lotion's benefits and ask her if she'd like some for home use. Even if the client seems uninterested in the products you are using, you can still sell her items. Show her something you are about to apply to her nails and try saying something like: "This is our latest high-shine top coat" (or whatever else you'd like to sell). Use it as part of the service, then at the end of the manicure place the item in her hand and ask if you can add it to her ticket. This last step is crucial to close the sale. If you make a recommendation early in the appointment but don't pursue it at the end, the client often forgets about it.

REVIEW QUESTIONS

1. Nail plates are mostly protein made from chemicals called _____ _____.
2. Define molecules.
3. What are catalysts and why are they important to nail chemistry?
4. A _____ is anything which dissolves another substance called a _____.
5. True or False? Primers can eat the nail plate. Explain your answer.
6. Define monomers.
7. What are the two main differences between irritations and allergic reactions?
8. What six things can you avoid or do to ensure that clients never suffer from product allergy?
9. Only _____ and _____ skin contact can cause a client to become allergic to products.
10. In your own words explain what Paracelsus discovered about toxic substances. How can you use this knowledge to work safely?

chapter 6
ANATOMY AND PHYSIOLOGY

LEARNING OBJECTIVES

After you have studied this chapter, you should be able to:

1. Explain how an understanding of anatomy and physiology will help you become a better nail technician.
2. Describe the purpose of cells within the human body.
3. Describe cell metabolism and explain the difference between the two phases of metabolism.
4. Name the different types of body tissue and explain the function of each type.
5. Name the most important organs of the body and explain the function of each organ.
6. Name the systems that make up the human body and explain the function of each system.
7. List the ways in which muscles are stimulated.
8. Name the types of muscles that are affected by massage.
9. Name the divisions of the nervous system and explain the function of each division.
10. Identify the chief functions of the blood.

INTRODUCTION

Although you may have groaned when you saw a chapter on anatomy and physiology, these are important subjects in a practice of nail technology. A basic understanding of the structure of the human body and the functions it performs will give you a scientific background for many of the nail services you will learn about. This background will help you decide which service is best for a client's nail or skin condition, and how to adjust and control the service for the best results.

Very generally, anatomy is the study of the structure of the body and what it is made of—for example, bones, muscles, and skin. Histology is the study of the small, individual structures of the body, such as hair, nails, sweat glands, and oil glands.

Although the names of bones, muscles, arteries, veins, and nerves are seldom used in the nail salon, an understanding of body structures will help make you more proficient in performing many services, such as hand and arm massage. Your study of anatomy and physiology will include cells, tissues, organs, and systems of the human body.

CELLS

Cells are the basic units of all living things, including bacteria, plants, and animals. The human body is made up entirely of cells, fluids, and cellular products. As the basic functional units of all living, things, the cells carry on all of our life processes. Cells also have the ability to reproduce, providing new cells that enable us to grow and that replace worn or injured tissues.

Cells are made up of **protoplasm** (**PROH**-toh-plaz-em), a colorless, jellylike substance that contains food elements such as protein, fat, carbohydrates, and mineral salts.

The **protoplasm** of the cells includes the **nucleus** (**NOO**-klee-us), cytoplasm (**SEYE**-toh-plaz-em), centrosome (**SEN**-tro-sohm), and cell membrane.

The **nucleus** is made of dense protoplasm and is found in the center of the cell within the nuclear membrane. It plays an important role in cell reproduction.

Cytoplasm is found outside of the nucleus and contains food materials necessary for the growth, reproduction, and self-repair of the cell.

The **centrosome**, a small, round body in the cytoplasm, affects the reproduction of the cell.

The **cell membrane** encloses the cytoplasm. It controls the transportation of substances in and out of the cells. (Fig. 6.1)

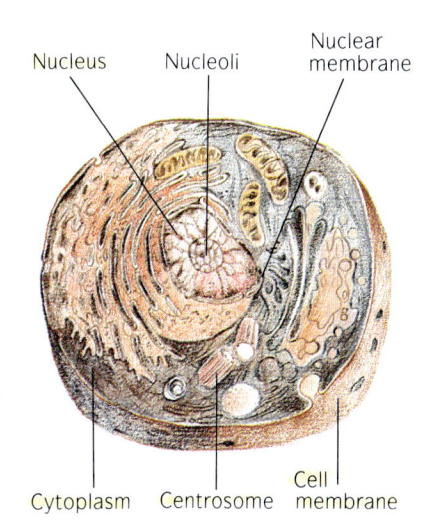

6.1 - Cells consist of protoplasm and contain essential elements.

CELL GROWTH

As long as the cell receives an adequate supply of food, oxygen, and water, eliminates waste products, and is maintained at the proper temperature, it will continue to grow and thrive. However, if these conditions do not exist and toxins (poisons) or pressure are present, then the growth and health of the cells are impaired. Most of our body cells are capable of growing and repairing themselves during their life cycle. Cells also reproduce themselves through a process of division known as mitosis. (Fig. 6.2)

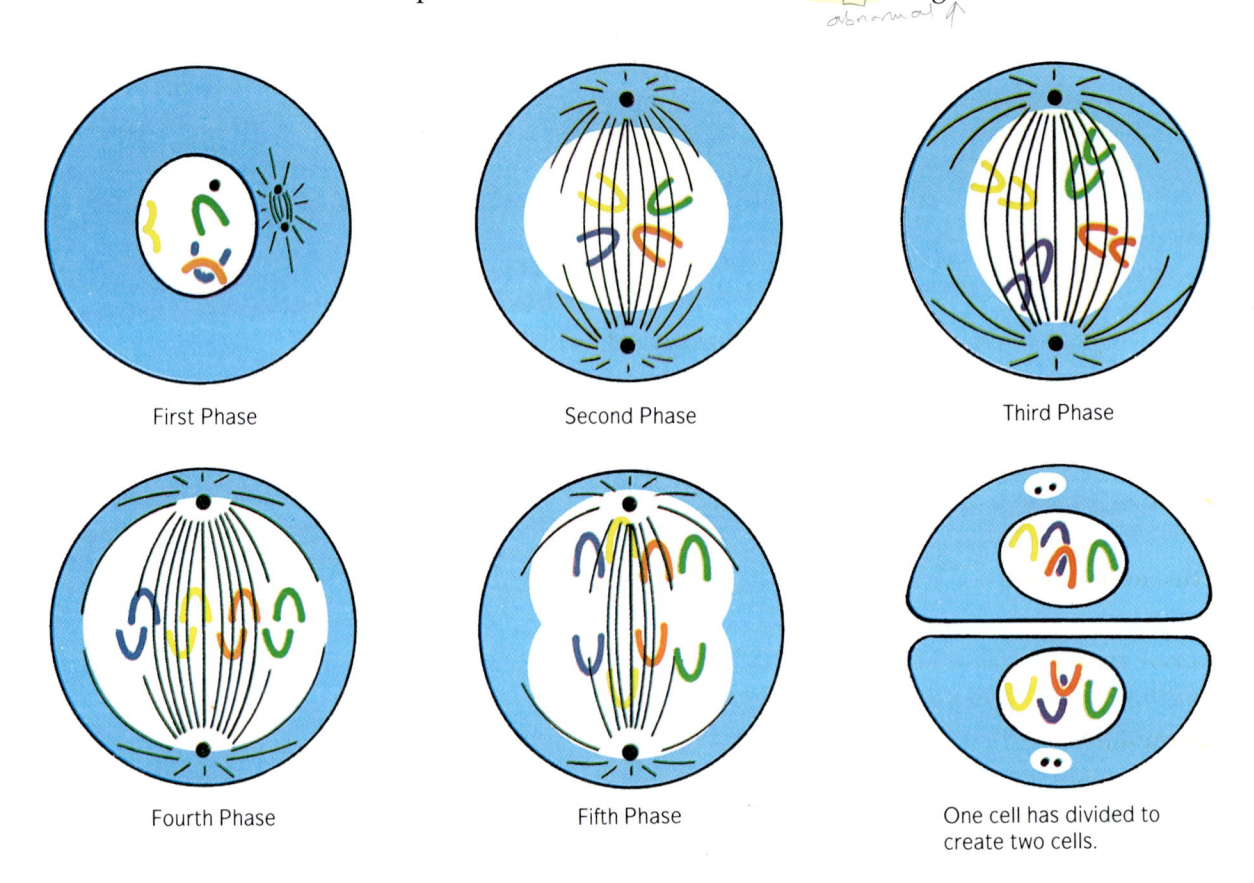

First Phase

Second Phase

Third Phase

Fourth Phase

Fifth Phase

One cell has divided to create two cells.

6.2 — Mitosis—indirect division of the human cell

CELL METABOLISM

Metabolism (meh-**TAB**-o-liz-em) is a complex chemical process whereby the body cells are nourished and supplied with the energy needed to carry on their many activities. There are two phases of metabolism:

1. **Anabolism** (ah-**NAB**-o-liz-em) is the process of building up larger molecules from smaller ones. During this process the body stores water, food, and oxygen for the time when these substances are needed for cell growth and repair.

CHAPTER 6　ANATOMY AND PHYSIOLOGY　◆　67

2. **Catabolism** (kah-**TAB**-o-liz-em) is the breaking down of larger substances or molecules into smaller ones. This process releases energy that can be stored by special molecules for use in muscle contraction, secretion, or heat production.

Anabolism and catabolism are carried out at the same time and happen continuously. Their activities are closely regulated so that the breaking down, energy-releasing reactions are balanced with the building-up, energy-consuming reactions. Therefore, **homeostasis** (ho-me-oh-**STAY**-sus) (the maintenance of normal, internal stability in the body) is achieved. However, if we use less energy than we manufacture, we may notice a weight gain. The molecules of energy that are not used may turn to fat. To get rid of built-up fat, we must use more energy by exercising or take in less energy by eating less.

TISSUES

Tissues are composed of groups of cells of the same kind. Each tissue has a specific function and can be recognized by its characteristic appearance. Body tissues are classified as follows:

1. **Connective tissue** serves to support, protect, and bind together tissues of the body. Bone, cartilage, ligament, tendon, fascia (which separates muscles), and fat tissue are examples of connective tissue.
2. **Muscular tissue** contracts and moves various parts of the body.
3. **Nerve tissue** carries messages to and from the brain, and controls and coordinates all body functions.
4. **Epithelial** (ep-i-**THE**-le-al) **tissue** is a protective covering on body surfaces, such as the skin, mucous membranes, linings of the ear, digestive and respiratory organs, and glands.
5. **Liquid tissue** carries food, waste products, and hormones by means of the blood and lymph.

ORGANS

Organs are structures designed to accomplish a specific function. The most important organs of the body are described below.

The **brain** controls the body.
The **heart** circulates the blood.
The **lungs** supply oxygen to the blood.
The **liver** removes toxic products of digestion.
The **kidneys** excrete water and other waste products.
The **stomach** and **intestines** digest food.

SYSTEMS

Systems are groups of organs that cooperate for a common purpose, namely the welfare of the entire body. The human body is made up of ten important systems.

The **integumentary** (in-**TEG**-yoo-men-ta-ree) **system**, is made up of the skin and its various accessory organs, such as the oil and sweat glands, sensory receptors, hair, and nails. This system is composed of two distinct layers, the dermis and epidermis. It functions as a protective covering and contains sensory receptors that give us our sense of touch. This system also plays an important role in regulating the temperature of the body.

The **skeletal system** is the physical foundation or framework of the body. The bones of the skeletal system serve as a means of protection, support, and locomotion (movement).

The **muscular system** covers, shapes, and supports the skeleton. Its function is to produce all the movements of the body.

The **nervous system** controls and coordinates the functions of all the other systems of the body.

The **circulatory** (**SUR**-kyoo-lay-tohr-ee) **system** supplies blood throughout the body.

The **endocrine** (**EN**-doh-krin) **system** is made up of ductless glands that secrete hormones into the bloodstream.

The **excretory** (**EK**-skre-tohr-ee) **system** eliminates waste from the body.

The **respiratory** (**RES**-pi-rah-toh-ree) **system** supplies oxygen to the body.

The **digestive system** changes food into substances that can be used by the cells of the body.

The **reproductive system** enables human beings to reproduce.

THE SKELETAL SYSTEM

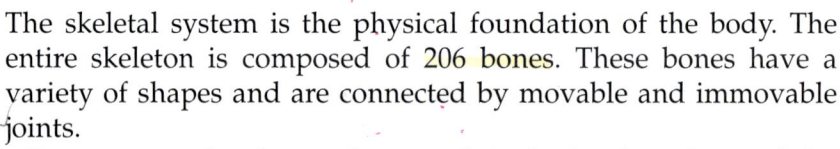

The skeletal system is the physical foundation of the body. The entire skeleton is composed of 206 bones. These bones have a variety of shapes and are connected by movable and immovable joints.

Bone, except for the tooth enamel, is the hardest tissue of the body. It is composed of connective tissues consisting of about one-third animal (organic) matter, such as cells and blood, and two-thirds mineral (inorganic) matter, mainly calcium carbonate and calcium phosphate. The scientific study of bones, their structure, and functions is called *osteology* (os-tee-**OL**-oh-jee). The technical term for bone is **os**.

The following are primary functions of the bones:

1. Give shape and support to the body.

2. Protect various internal structures and organs.

CHAPTER 6   ANATOMY AND PHYSIOLOGY   ◆   69

3. Serve as attachments for muscles and act as levers to produce body movements.

4. Produce various blood cells in the red bone marrow.

5. Store various minerals, such as calcium, phosphorus, magnesium, and sodium.

STRUCTURE OF BONE

Bone is white on the outside and deep red on the inside. Bone marrow is a soft, fatty, dark red substance filling the cavities of the bones. The **periosteum** (pe-ree-**OS**-tee-um) is a pink fibrous membrane that covers and protects the bone, and serves as an attachment for tendons, ligaments, blood vessels, and nerves. The blood vessels that enter the bone through the periosteum provide nutrition for the bones.

The structures attached to the bone include:

Cartilage (**CAR**-tih-ledj) is a tough elastic substance similar to bone but it has no mineral content. Cartilage cushions bones at the joints and gives shape to some external features such as the nose and ears.

Ligaments (**LIG**-e-mentz) are bands or sheets of fibrous tissue that support the bones at the joints.

Synovial (sy-**NOV**-ee-al) **fluid** is the lubrication that prevents friction at the joints where bones meet. This slippery fluid also furnishes nourishment to the cartilage.

JOINTS

The various bones of the body meet at junctions called **joints**, which can move in many ways. At **pivot** (**PIH**-vut) **joints** like the neck, one bone turns on another bone. At **hinge** (**HINJ**) **joints**, which are found in the elbow and knee, two or more bones connect like a door. At a **ball-and-socket joint** such as the hip or shoulder, one bone is rounded and fits into the socket, or hollow part, of another bone. In **gliding joints**, which are found in the ankle and wrist, two bones glide over each other.

BONES OF THE ARM AND HAND

The **scapula** (**SKAP**-yoo-lah) and the **clavicle** (**KLAV**-i-kul) form the shoulder. The clavicle is also known as the collar bone.

The **humerus** (**HYOO**-mo-rus) is the uppermost and largest bone of the arm.

The **ulna** (**UL**-nah) is the large bone on the small-finger side of the forearm.

The **radius** (**RAY**-dee-us) is the small bone in the forearm on the same side as your thumb. (Fig. 6.3)

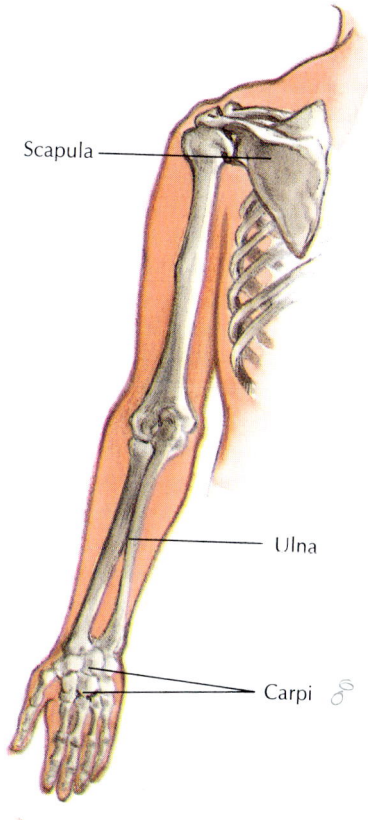

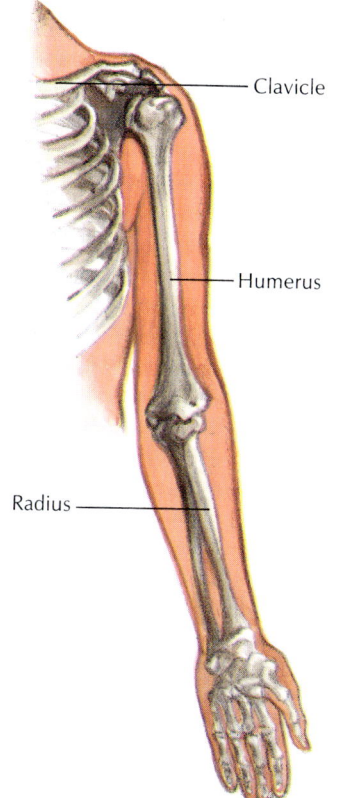

6.3 - Bones of the arm

The **carpus** (KAHR-pus) or wrist, is a flexible joint composed of eight small, irregular bones held together by ligaments.

The five **metacarpals** (met-a-KAHR-puls), the bones of the palm of the hand, are long and slender.

The **digits** or **fingers** consist of three **phalanges** (fl-LAN-jeez) in each finger and two in the thumb, totaling fourteen bones. (Fig. 6.4)

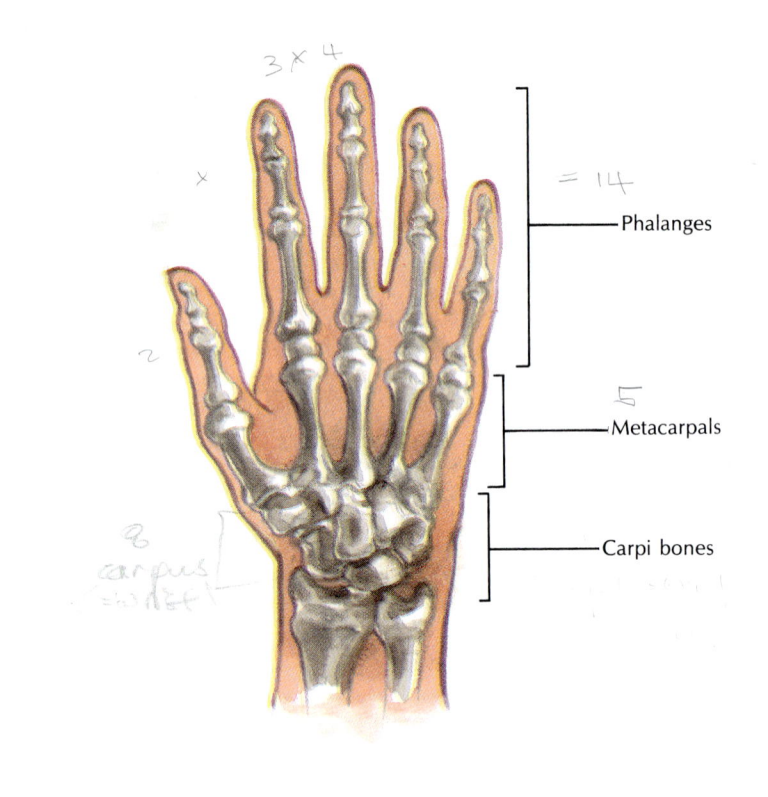

6.4 — Bones of the hand and wrist

BONES OF THE LEG AND FOOT

The **femur** (FEE-mur) is a heavy, long bone that forms the leg above the knee.

The **tibia** (TIB-ee-ah) is the larger of the two bones that form the leg below the knee.

The **fibula** (FIB-ya-lah) is the smaller of the two bones that form the leg below the knee.

The **patella** (pah-TEL-lah), also called the accessory bone, forms the knee cap. (Fig. 6.5)

The ankle is made up of seven **tarsal** (TAR-sul) bones. The **calcaneous** (kal-KAY-nee-us), or heel, is considered to be part of the ankle.

The five **metatarsals** (met-ah-TAHR-suls) of the foot are long and slender like the metacarpal bones of the hand.

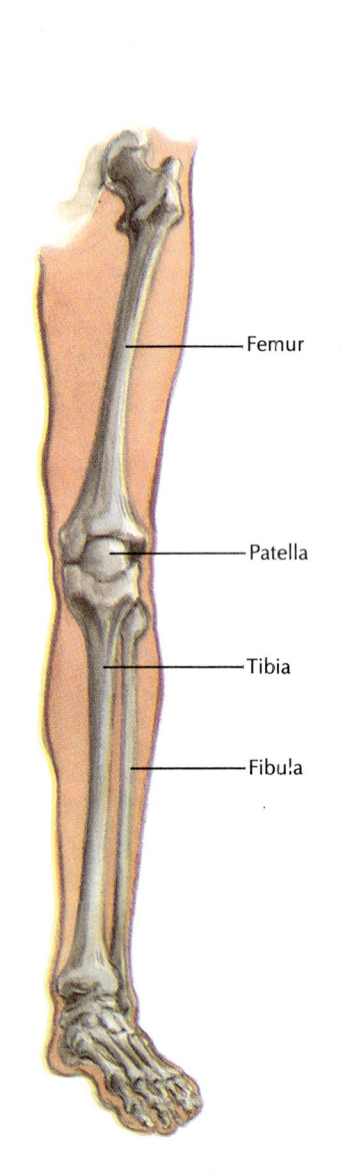

6.5 — Bones of the leg

CHAPTER 6   ANATOMY AND PHYSIOLOGY ◆ 71

The bones of the toes are called **phalanges** and are similar to the finger bones. There are three phalanges in each toe, except for the big toe, which has only two. (Fig. 6.6)

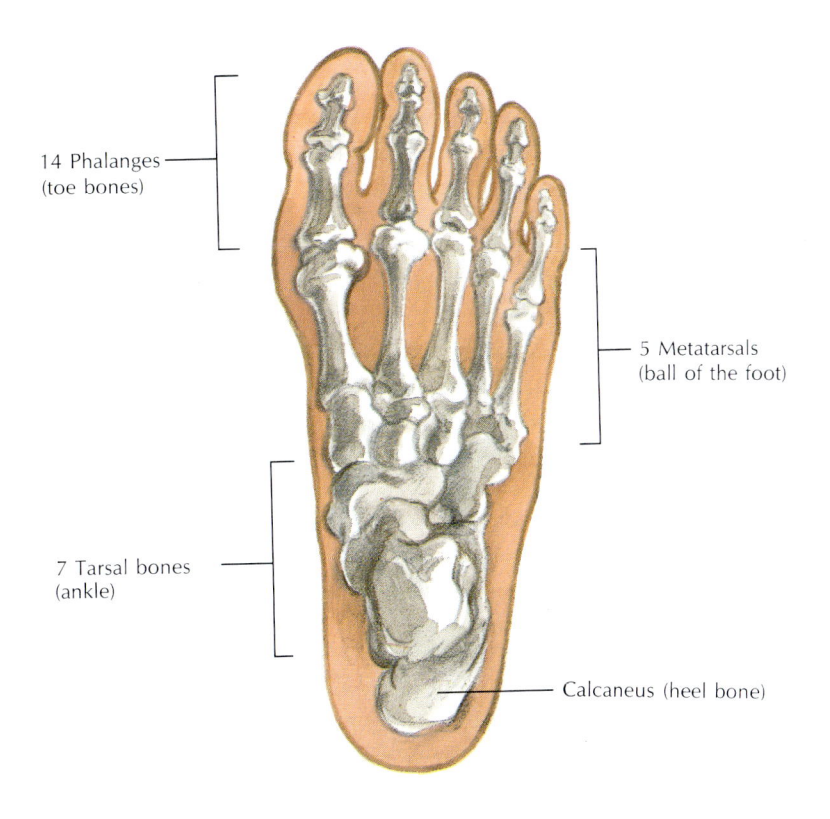

14 Phalanges (toe bones)

5 Metatarsals (ball of the foot)

7 Tarsal bones (ankle)

Calcaneus (heel bone)

6.6 — Bones of the foot and ankle

THE MUSCULAR SYSTEM

The **muscular** (MUS-kyoo-lahr) **system** covers, shapes, and supports the skeleton. Its function is to produce all movements of the body. **Myology** (meye-OL-oh-jee) is the study of the structure, functions, and diseases of the muscles.

The muscular system consists of over 500 muscles, large and small, comprising 40 to 50 percent of the weight of the human body.

Muscles are fibrous tissues that have the ability to stretch and contract according to our movements. Different types of movements —for example, stretching and bending—depend on muscles performing in specific ways.

There are three kinds of muscular tissue:

1. **Striated** (STRY-ate-id) muscles are voluntary muscles that you can move whenever you want. Muscles of the face, arm, and leg are striated muscles. The word striated means striped. (Fig. 6.7)

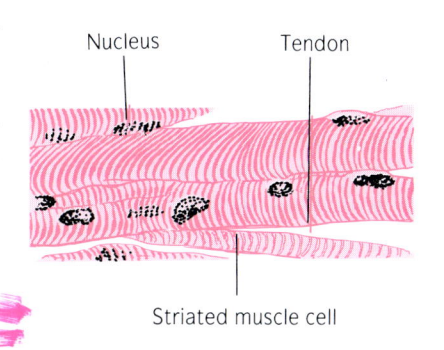

Nucleus   Tendon

Striated muscle cell

6.7 — Striated muscle cells

2. **Non-striated** muscles are involuntary. Muscles of the stomach and intestines are non-striated. These muscles function automatically. Non-striated means smooth or not striped. (Fig. 6.8)

3. **Cardiac** (**CAR**-dee-ak) muscle is heart muscle, which is not found anywhere else in the body. (Fig. 6.9)

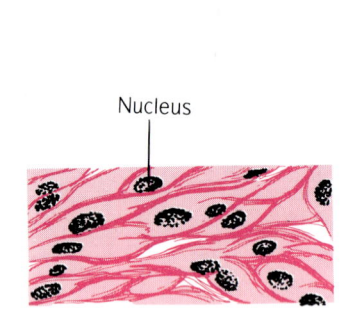

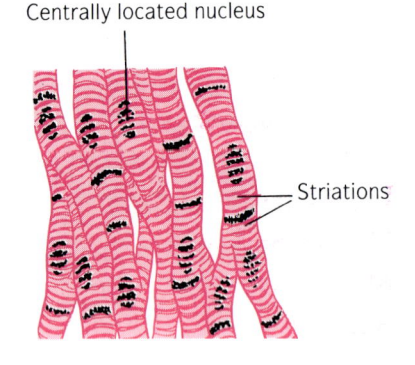

6.8 — Non-striated muscle

6.9 — Cardiac muscle cells

MUSCLE PARTS

There are three parts to a muscle: the origin, the insertion, and the belly. The **origin** is the part that does not move. It is attached to the skeleton, and is usually part of the skeletal muscles. The **insertion**

The Consultation

A good consultation is the beginning of a beautiful client-professional relationship. Take time out to talk with a new client about her nailcare goals—is she trying to grow her short nails long, to switch from extensions to natural nails, or simply to have better groomed hands? Understanding her goals helps you know how to proceed to meet her expectations. The initial consultation is also the time to look for an existing medical problem, such as a severe case of eczema, a fungal infection or any other disorder. If you encounter such a problem, don't try to solve it yourself. Suggest that she see her physician who will give her the names of dermatologists who can help. Tell her that healthy nails sometimes require the help of a medical expert and that you look forward to working on her once the problem clears up. She'll be so impressed with your professional concern that she'll be sure to return once the condition is treated.

CHAPTER 6 ANATOMY AND PHYSIOLOGY ◆ 73

is the part that moves, and the **belly** is the middle part. During a contraction, when the muscle shortens, one of the attachments usually remains fixed and the other moves. Muscles are joined together by **sinews** (**SIN**-yooz) or **tendons** (**TEN**-dunz) which look like white glistening cords.

STIMULATION OF MUSCLES

Muscle tissue can be stimulated in any of the following ways:

Massage—hand massage and electric vibrator.
Electric current—applied to the muscle area to produce visible muscle contractions.
Light rays—infrared rays and ultraviolet rays.
Heat rays—heating lamps and heating caps.
Moist heat—steamers or moderately warm steam towels.
Nerve impulses—through the nervous system.
Chemicals—certain acids and salts.

MUSCLES AFFECTED BY MASSAGE

As a nail technician, you are concerned with the voluntary muscles of the hands, arms, legs, and feet. It is essential to know where these muscles are located and what they control. Pressure in massage is usually directed from the insertion to the origin.

Muscles of the Shoulder and Upper Arm

The **deltoid** (**DEL**-toid) is a large, thick triangular muscle that covers the shoulder and lifts and turns the arm.
  Biceps (**BEYE**-seps) is the muscle on the front of the upper arm that lifts the forearm, flexes the elbow and turns the palm up. It has two heads or points of attachment.
  Triceps (**TREYE**-seps) are muscles that cover the entire back of the upper arm and extend the forearm forward. They have three heads or points of attachment.

Muscles of the Forearm

The **forearm** contains a series of muscles and strong tendons.
  The **pronator** (**PRO**-nay-tor) turns the hands inward, so the palm faces downward.
  Supinator (**SUE**-pi-nay-tor) turns the hand outward so the palm faces upward.
  Flexors (**FLEKS**-ors) bend to the wrist, draw the hand upward, and close the fingers toward the forearm.
  Extensor (eck-**STEN**-sur) straightens the wrist, hand, and fingers to form a straight line. (Fig. 6.10)

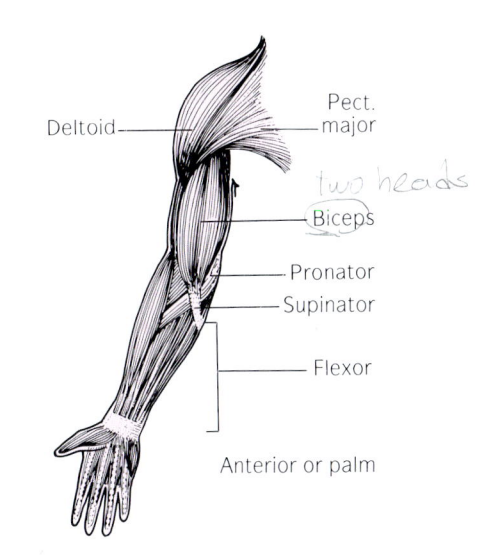

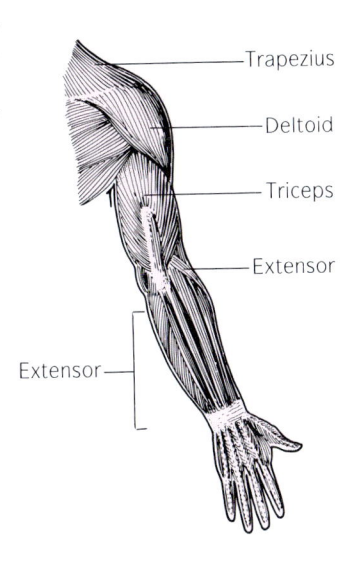

6.10 — Muscles of the arm

74 ◆ PART 2 THE SCIENCE OF NAIL TECHNOLOGY

Abductors (separate fingers)

Adductors (draw fingers together)

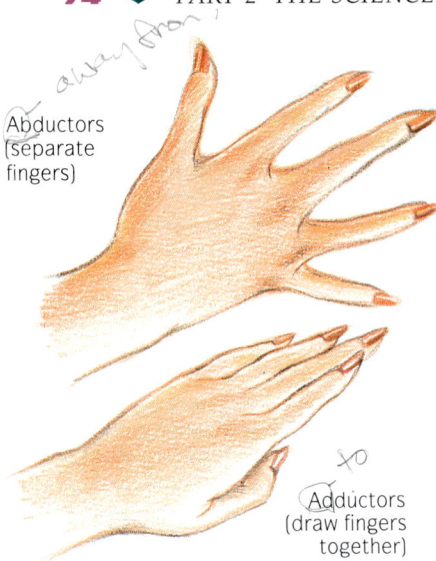

6.11 — Muscles of the hand

Muscles of the Hand

The hand has many small muscles that overlap from joint to joint, giving flexibility and strength. When the hands are properly cared for, these muscles will remain supple and graceful. They close and open the hands and fingers.

Abductors (ab-**DUK**-tohrs) separate the fingers and **adductors** (a-**DUK**-tohrs) draw the fingers together. Both of these muscles are located at the base of the thumbs and fingers. (Fig. 6.11)

Opponent muscles are located in the palm of the hand and act to bring the thumb toward the fingers, allowing the grasping action of the hands.

Muscles of the Lower Leg and Foot

As a nail technician, you will use your knowledge of the muscles of the foot and leg during a pedicure. The muscles of the foot are small and provide proper support and cushioning for the foot and leg. (Fig. 6.12)

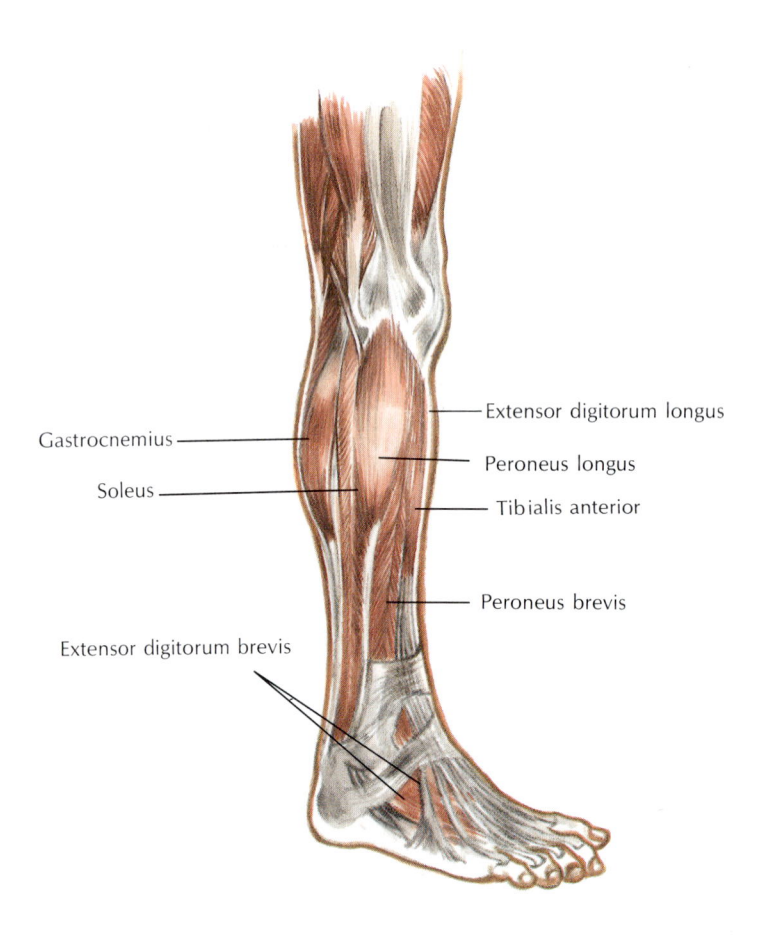

Gastrocnemius
Soleus
Extensor digitorum longus
Peroneus longus
Tibialis anterior
Peroneus brevis
Extensor digitorum brevis

6.12 — Muscles of the lower leg and foot

The **extensor digitorum longus** (eck-STEN-sur dij-it-TOHR-um LONG-us) bends the foot up and extends the toes.

The **tibialis anterior** (tib-ee-AHL-is an-TEHR-ee-ohr) covers the front of the skin. It bends the foot upward and inward.

The **peroneus longus** (per-oh-NEE-us LONG-us) covers the outer side of the calf and inverts the foot and turns it outward.

The **peroneus brevis** (**BREV**-us) originates on the lower surface of the fibula. It bends the foot down and out.

The **gastrocnemius** (gas-truc-NEEM-e-us) is attached to the lower rear surface of the heel and pulls the foot down.

The **soleus** (SO-lee-us) originates at the upper portion of the fibula and bends the foot down.

The muscles of the feet include the **extensor digitorum brevis** (ek-STEN-sur dij-it-TOHR-um BREV-us), **abductor hallucis** (ab-DUK-tohr ha-LU-sis), **flexor digitorum brevis** (FLEKS-or dij-it-TOHR-um BREV-us) and the **abductor.** The foot muscles move the toes and help maintain balance while walking and standing. (Fig. 6.13)

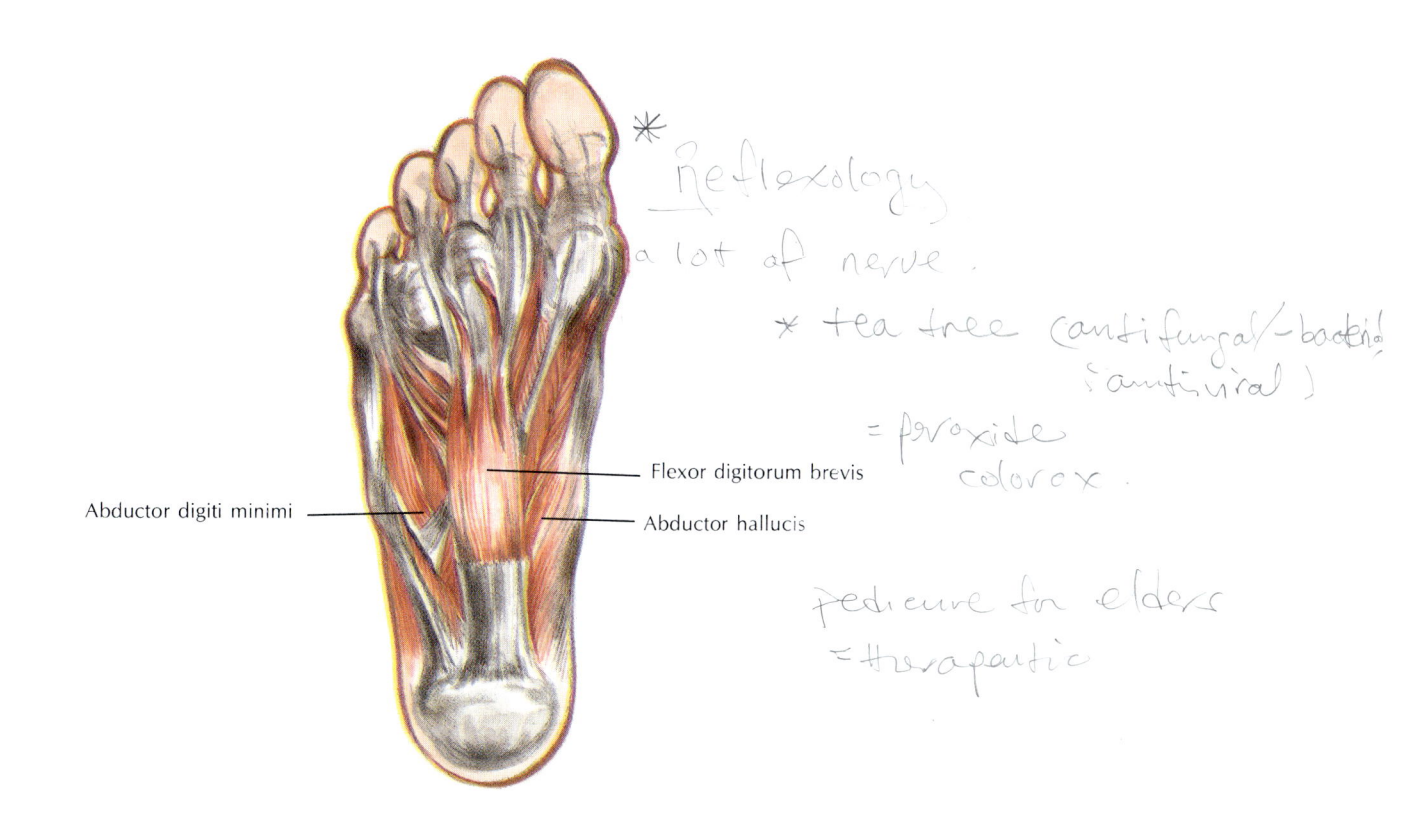

Abductor digiti minimi

Flexor digitorum brevis

Abductor hallucis

6.13 — Muscles of the foot (bottom)

THE NERVOUS SYSTEM

Neurology is the branch of medicine that deals with the nervous system and its disorders. The *nervous system* is one of the most important systems of the body. It controls and coordinates the functions of all the other systems and makes them work in harmony. Every square inch of the human body is supplied with fine fibers called **nerves**. As a nail technician, you should study the nervous system in order to understand the effect massage has on the nerves of the feet, legs, hands, arms, and the whole body.

The nervous system is composed of three divisions: the central nervous system, the peripheral system, and the autonomic nervous system.

1. The *cerebro-spinal* (ser-EE-broh SPEYE-nahl) or **central nervous system** consists of the brain and spinal cord and has the following functions.
    a) Controls consciousness and all mental activities.
    b) Controls functions of the five senses: seeing, smelling, tasting, feeling, and hearing.
    c) Controls voluntary muscle actions, such as all body movements and facial expression.

2. The *peripheral* (pe-RIF-er-al) *system* is made up of the sensory and motor nerve fibers that extend from the brain and spinal cord and are distributed to all parts of the body. Its function is to carry messages to and from the central nervous system.

3. The *autonomic* (aw-toh-NAHM-ik) *nervous system* is the portion of the nervous system that functions without conscious effort and regulates the activities of the smooth muscles, glands, blood vessels, and heart. The system has two divisions, the **sympathetic** and **parasympathetic systems,** which act in direct opposition to each other. They regulate such things as heart rate, blood pressure, breathing rate, and body temperature to aid the body in the maintenance of homeostasis, or normal internal stability. The sympathetic division is primarily activated during stressful, energy-demanding, or emergency situations; the parasympathetic division is most active in ordinary restful energy-conserving situations.

THE BRAIN AND SPINAL CORD

The brain is the largest mass of nerve tissue in the body and is contained in the cranium. The weight of the average brain is 44 to 48 ounces (1232 to 1344 g). It is considered to be the central processing unit of the body, sending and receiving digital messages. Twelve pairs of cranial nerves originate in the brain and reach various parts of the head, face, and neck.

The spinal cord is composed of masses of nerve cells, with fibers running upward and downward. It originates in the brain, extends the length of the trunk, and is enclosed and protected by the spinal column. Thirty-one pairs of spinal nerves, extending from the spinal cord, are distributed to the muscles and skin of the trunk and limbs. Some of the spinal nerves supply the internal organs controlled by the sympathetic nervous system.

NERVE CELLS AND NERVES

A *neuron* (**NOOR**-on) or *nerve cell* is the primary structural unit of the nervous system. It is composed of a cell body, **dendrites** (**DEN**-dreyets), which receive messages from other neurons, and an **axon** (**AK**-son) and axon terminal, which send messages to other neurons, glands, or muscles. (Fig. 6.14)

Nerves are long, white cords made up of fibers that carry messages to and from various parts of the body. Nerves have their origin in the brain and spinal cord, and distribute branches to all parts of the body.

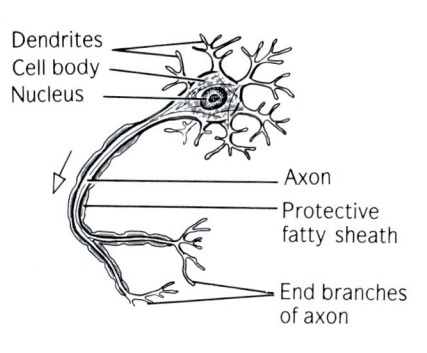

6.14 — A neuron or nerve cell

Types of Nerves

Sensory nerves, also called **afferent** (**AF**-fer-ent) **nerves**, carry impulses or messages from sense organs to the brain, where sensations of touch, cold, heat, sight, hearing, taste, smell, pain, and pressure are experienced.

Motor nerves, also called **efferent** (**EF**-fer-ent) **nerves**, carry impulses from the brain to the muscles. The transmitted impulses produce movement.

Mixed nerves contain both sensory and motor fibers and have the ability to both send and receive messages.

Sensory nerve endings, called **receptors**, are located near the surface of the skin. Impulses pass from the sensory nerves to the brain and back over the motor nerves to the muscles. A complete circuit is established and movements of the muscles result.

A *reflex* is an automatic response to a stimulus that involves the transmission of an impulse from a sensory receptor along an afferent nerve to the spinal cord, and a responsive impulse along an efferent neuron to a muscle, causing a reaction. An example of a reflex is the quick removal of the hand from a hot object. A reflex action does not have to be learned.

Nerves of the Arm and Hand

The **ulnar** (**UL**-ner) **nerve** and its branches supply the small finger side of the arm and the palm of the hand.

The **radial** (**RAY**-dee-al) **nerve** and its branches supply the thumb side of the arm and the back of the hand.

78 ◆ PART 2 THE SCIENCE OF NAIL TECHNOLOGY

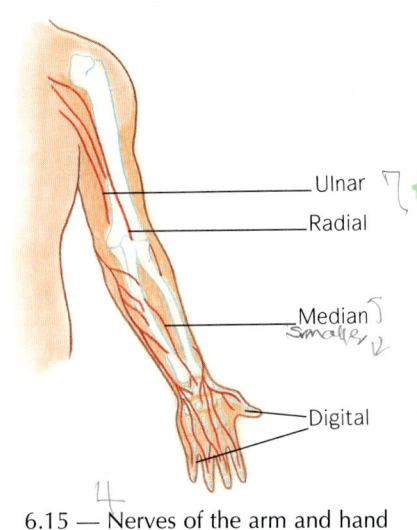

The **median** (**MEE**-di-an) **nerve** is a smaller nerve than the ulnar and radial nerves. With its branches, it supplies the arm and hand.

The **digital** (**DIJ**-it-al) **nerve** and its branches supply all fingers of the hand. (Fig. 6.15)

Nerves of the Lower Leg and Foot

The **tibial** (**TIB**-ee-al) **nerve**, located in the thigh, passes behind the knee. It subdivides and supplies impulses to the knee, the muscles of the calf, the skin of the leg, and the sole, heel, and underside of the toes.

The **common peroneal** (per-oh-**NEE**-al) **nerve,** a division of the sciatic nerve, is located behind the knee and has two parts. The **deep peroneal nerve** passes down the back of the leg. The **superficial peroneal** nerve passes downward in front of the fibula and supplies impulses to the skin of the foot and toes.

The **saphenous** (sa-**FEEN**-us) **nerve** supplies impulses to the skin of the inner side of the leg and foot.

The **sural nerve** supplies impulses to the outer side and back of the foot and leg.

The **dorsal** (**DOOR**-sal) **nerve** supplies impulses to the top of the foot. (Fig. 6.16)

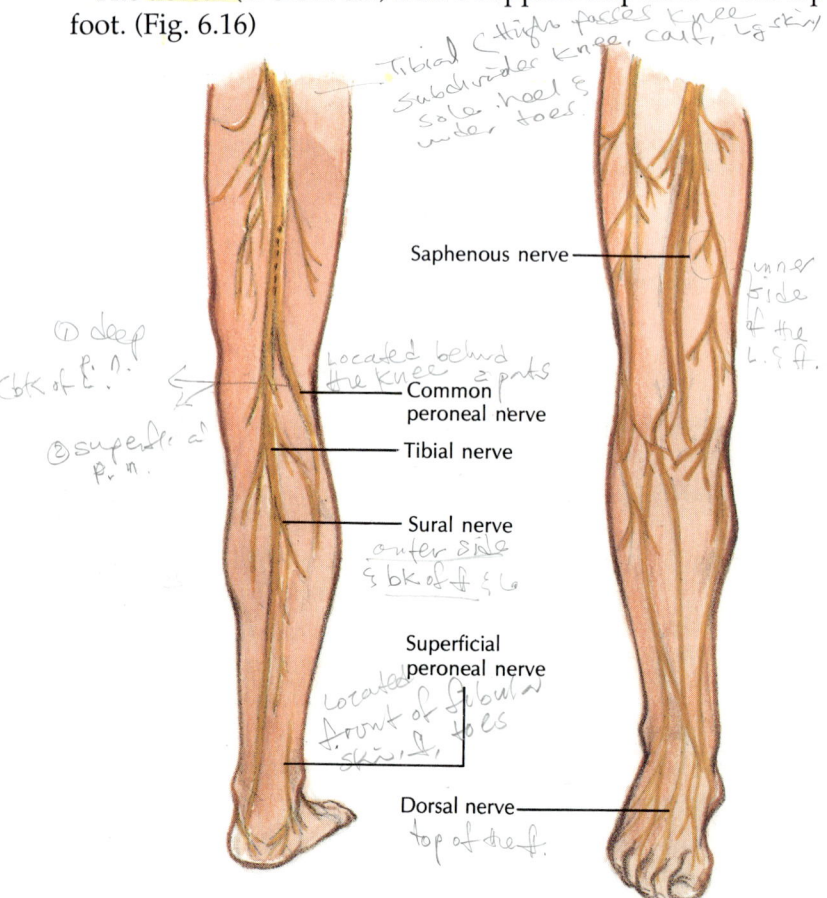

6.15 — Nerves of the arm and hand

6.16 — Nerves of the lower leg and foot

CHAPTER 6　ANATOMY AND PHYSIOLOGY　◆　79

THE CIRCULATORY SYSTEM

The *circulatory* (**SUR**-kyoo-lah-tohr-ee), or **vascular** (**VAS**-kyoo-lahr) **system** is vital to the maintenance of good health. It controls the steady circulation of the blood through the body by means of the heart and the blood vessels (the arteries, veins, and capillaries).

The *blood-vascular system consists* of the heart and blood vessels and circulates the blood. The *lymph* (**LIMF**)-*vascular* or **lymphatic** (lim-**FAT**-ik) **system** consists of lymph glands and vessels through which a slightly yellow fluid called lymph circulates. These two systems are intimately linked with each other. Lymph is derived from the blood and flows gradually back into the bloodstream.

THE HEART

The heart is a muscular, cone-shaped organ about the size of a closed fist. It is located in the chest cavity, and is enclosed in a membrane, the **pericardium** (per-i-**KAHR**-dee-um). It is an efficient pump that keeps the blood moving within the circulatory system. At the normal resting rate, the heart beats about 72 to 80 times a minute. The **vagus** (**VAY**-gus) (tenth cranial nerve) and nerves from the autonomic nervous system regulate the heartbeat. (Fig. 6.17)

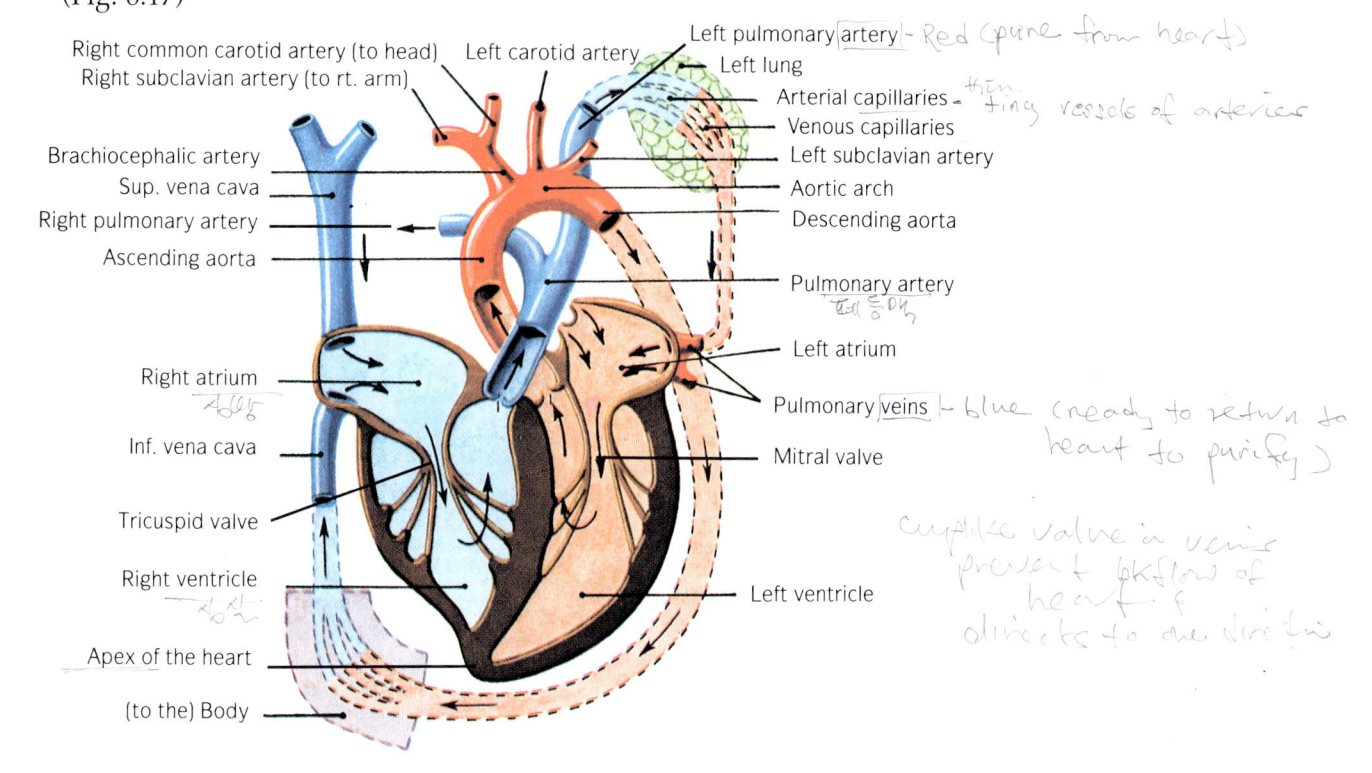

6.17 — Diagram of the heart

The interior of the heart contains four chambers and four cavities. The upper, thin-walled chambers are the **right atrium** (**AY**-tree-um) and **left atrium**. The lower, thick-walled chambers are the right **ventricle** (**VEN**-tri-kel) and **left ventricle. Valves** allow the blood to flow in only one direction. With each contraction and relaxation of the heart, the blood flows in, travels from the **atria** (both right atrium and left atrium) to the ventricles, and is then driven out, to be distributed all over the body. Another name for the atrium is **auricle** (**OR**-ik-kel).

Blood Vessels

Blood vessels, which include *arteries, capillaries,* and *veins,* are tubelike in construction. They transport blood to and from the heart and to various tissues of the body.

Arteries are thick-walled muscular and elastic tubes that carry oxygen-filled blood from the heart to the capillaries throughout the body.

Capillaries are tiny, thin-walled blood vessels that connect the smaller arteries to the veins. Through their walls, the tissues receive nourishment and eliminate waste products.

Veins carry blood that lacks oxygen from the capillaries back to the heart. They are thin-walled blood vessels that are less elastic than arteries. They contain cuplike valves to prevent backflow. Veins are located closer to the outer surface of the body than arteries are. (Fig. 6.18)

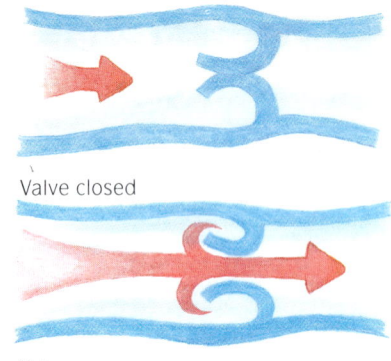

Valve closed

Valve open

6.18 — Cross-sections of a vein

THE BLOOD

Blood is a nutritive fluid that moves throughout the circulatory system. It is a red, salty fluid with a consistency similar to that of tomato juice. Blood has a normal temperature of 98.6 degrees Fahrenheit (37 degrees Celsius), and it makes up about one-twentieth of the weight of the body. Approximately 8 to 10 pints of blood fill the blood vessels of an adult. Blood is bright red in color in the arteries, except for in the pulmonary artery, and dark red in the veins (except for in the pulmonary vein). This change in color is due to the exchange of carbon dioxide for oxygen as the blood passes through the lungs and the exchange of oxygen for carbon dioxide as the blood circulates throughout the body.

Circulation of the Blood

The blood is in constant circulation from the moment it leaves the heart until it returns. There are two systems that control this circulation:

The *pulmonary* (**PUL**-mo-ner-ee) *circulation* is the blood circulation that goes from the heart to the lungs to be purified.

The *systemic*, or *general, circulation* is the blood circulation from the heart throughout the body and back again to the heart.

Composition of the Blood

The blood is composed of red and white corpuscles, platelets, and plasma. (Figs. 6.19, 6.20)

The function of **red corpuscles** (KOR-pus-els) (red blood cells), or **erythrocytes** (ih-RITH-ruh-syts) is to carry oxygen to the cells. **White corpuscles** (white blood cells), or **leucocytes** (LOO-ko-seyets), perform the function of destroying disease-causing germs.

Blood platelets (PLAY-tel-lets), or **thrombocytes** (throm-BOH-syts) are much smaller than the red blood cells. They play an important part in the clotting of the blood. (Fig. 6.21)

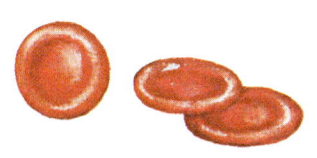

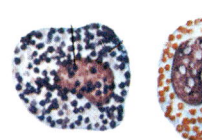

6.19 — Red corpuscles

6.20 — White corpuscles

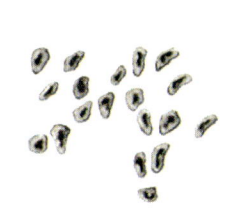

6.21 — Platelets

Plasma is the fluid part of the blood, in which the red and white blood cells and blood platelets flow. It is straw-like in color and is about nine-tenths water. It carries food and secretions to the cells and carbon dioxide from the cells.

Chief Functions of the Blood

The primary functions of the blood are described below:

1. Carries water, oxygen, food, and secretions to all cells of the body.

2. Carries away carbon dioxide and waste products to be eliminated through the lungs, skin, kidneys, and large intestine.

3. Helps to equalize the body temperature, thus protecting the body from extreme heat and cold.

4. Aids in protecting the body from harmful bacteria and infections through the action of the white blood cells.

5. Clots, thereby closing tiny, injured blood vessels and preventing the loss of blood.

Blood Supply for the Arm and Hand

The **ulnar** (UL-ner) and **radial** (RAY-dee-ul) arteries are the main blood supply for the arm and hand.

The ulnar artery and its numerous branches supply the little-finger side of the arm and the palm of the hand. The radial artery and its branches supply the thumb side of the arm and the back of the hand.

The important veins are located almost parallel with the arteries and take the same names as the arteries. While the arteries are found deep in the tissues, the veins lie nearer to the surface of the arms, hands, legs, and feet. (Fig. 6.22)

Blood Supply to the Lower Leg and Foot

There are several major arteries that supply blood to the lower leg and foot. The **popliteal** (pop-lih-**TEE**-ul) **artery** divides into two separate arteries known as the **anterior tibial** (**TIB**-ee-al) and the **posterior tibial**. The **anterior tibial** goes to the foot and becomes the **dorsalis pedis** which supplies the foot with blood.

As in the arm and hand, the important veins of the lower leg and foot are almost parallel with the arteries and take the same names. (Fig. 6.23)

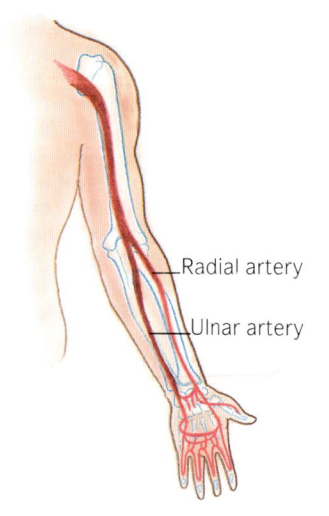

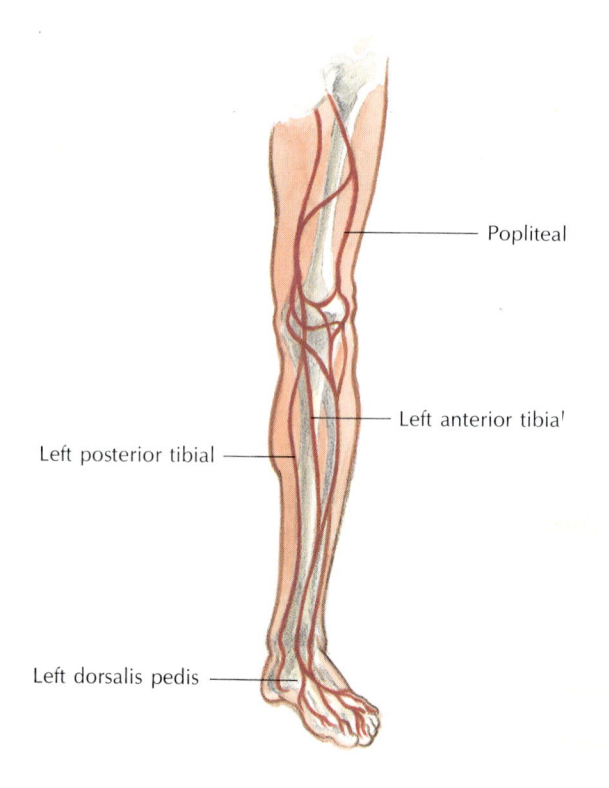

6.22 - Arteries of the hand and arm

6.23 — Arteries of the lower leg and foot

The Lymph-Vascular System

The **lymph-vascular system**, also called the **lymphatic system**, acts as an aid to the blood system, and consists of lymph spaces, lymph vessels, and lymph glands.

Lymph is a slightly yellow, watery fluid that is made from the plasma of the blood. It is created when the plasma filters through the capillary walls into the tissue spaces. The tissue found in the tissue spaces bathes all cells and trades its nutritive materials to the cells in return for the waste products of metabolism. This fluid is absorbed into the lymphatics or lymph capillaries to become lymph and is then filtered and detoxified as it passes through the lymph nodes. It is eventually reintroduced into the blood circulation.

The following are the primary functions of lymph:

1. Reaches the parts of the body not reached by blood and carries on an interchange with the blood.
2. Carries nourishment from the blood to the body cells.
3. Acts as a bodily defense against invading bacteria and toxins.
4. Removes waste material from the body cells to the blood.
5. Provides a suitable fluid environment for the cells.

THE ENDOCRINE SYSTEM

The *endocrine* (EN-doh-krin) *system* is made up of ductless glands that secrete substances into the bloodstream. A **gland** is a specialized organ that secretes substances. Glands convert certain elements from the blood into new compounds that the body needs. The **endocrine glands** secrete **hormones,** chemicals that affect metabolism and other body processes, directly into the bloodstream. The endocrine system works with the nervous system to regulate and integrate the various organs and systems of the body.

THE EXCRETORY SYSTEM

The *excretory* (EK-skr-tohr-ee) *system,* including the kidneys, liver, skin, intestines, and lungs, purifies the body by eliminating waste matter.

Each of the following plays a part in the excretory system:

1. **Kidneys** excrete urine.
2. The **liver** discharges bile.
3. The **skin** eliminates perspiration.
4. The **large intestine** evacuates decomposed and undigested food.
5 The **lungs** exhale carbon dioxide.

Metabolism of the cells of the body forms various toxic substances which, if retained, might poison the body.

THE RESPIRATORY SYSTEM

The *respiratory system* is situated within the chest cavity, which is protected on both sides by the ribs. The **diaphragm** is a muscular partition that controls breathing, and separates the chest from the **abdominal** region.

The **lungs** are spongy tissues composed of microscopic cells that take in air. These tiny air cells are enclosed in a skin-like tissue. Behind this, the fine capillaries of the vascular system are found.

When we breathe, an exchange of gases takes place. When we **inhale,** oxygen is absorbed into the blood. Carbon dioxide is expelled when we **exhale.** Oxygen is more essential than either food or water. Although a person may live more than 60 days without food, and a few days without water, if deprived of oxygen, he or she will die in a few minutes.

Breathing through your nose is healthier than breathing through your mouth because the air is warmed by the surface capillaries and the bacteria in the air are caught by the hairs that line the mucous membranes of the nasal passages.

Your rate of breathing depends on your level of activity. Muscular activities and energy expenditures increase the body's demands for oxygen. As a result, the rate of breathing is increased. You require about three times more oxygen when walking than when standing.

THE DIGESTIVE SYSTEM

Digestion is the process of converting food into a form that can be used by the body. The **digestive system** changes food into soluble form, suitable for use by the cells of the body. Digestion begins in the mouth and is completed in the small intestine. From the mouth, the food passes down the **pharynx** (FAR-ingks) and the **esophagus** (i-SOF-a-gus), or food pipe, and into the stomach. The food is completely digested in the stomach and small intestine and is assimilated or absorbed into the bloodstream. The large intestine (colon) stores the refuse for elimination through the rectum. The complete digestive process of food takes about 9 hours.

Enzymes, which are present in the digestive secretions, are responsible for the chemical changes in food. **Digestive enzymes** are chemicals that change certain kinds of food into a form capable of being used by the body. Intense emotions, excitement, and fatigue seriously disturb digestion. On the other hand, happiness and relaxation promote good digestion.

REVIEW QUESTIONS

1. How can an understanding of anatomy and physiology help you become a better nail technician?

2. What is the purpose of cells within the human body?

3. What is cell metabolism?

4. Name the five types of body tissue and explain the function of each.

5. What are the five most important organs of the body? Explain the function of each.

6. List the ten systems that make up the human body. What is the function of each system?

7. What are four ways in which muscles are stimulated?

8. What are four types of muscles that are affected by massage?

9. What are the three divisions of the nervous system? What is the function of each division?

10. What are the chief functions of the blood?

Chapter 7

THE NAIL AND ITS DISORDERS

LEARNING OBJECTIVES

After you have studied this chapter, you should be able to:

1. Identify the parts of the nail.
2. Define the term nail disorder.
3. Cite the golden rule for dealing with nail disorders.
4. Identify the nail disorders that can be serviced by a nail technician.
5. Identify the nail disorders that cannot be serviced by a nail technician.

CHAPTER 7   THE NAIL AND ITS DISORDERS   ◆   87

INTRODUCTION

To give your clients professional and responsible service and care, you need to learn about the structure and function of the nails. You also must be able to know when it is safe to work on a client and when they need to see a dermatologist, a medical doctor who is a skin specialist.

Nails are an interesting and surprising part of the human body. They are small mirrors of the general health of the body. Healthy nails are smooth, shiny, and translucent pink. Systemic problems in the body can show in the nails as nail disorders or poor nail growth. The technical term for nail is *onyx* (**ON**-iks). Nails are a part of the skin and are made of the same protein, **keratin** (**KER**-a-tin), as skin and hair. Nails are composed of the hardest keratin. Hair is made of a hard keratin, but not as hard as the keratin in nails, and skin is made of soft keratin. The purpose of nails is to protect the ends of fingers and toes and to help the fingers grasp small objects. Adult fingernails grow at an average rate of 1/8 inch a month; toenails grow more slowly.

Ordinarily, nails replace themselves every four months and grow more quickly in summer than in the winter. The nail grows fastest on the middle finger and slowest on the thumb.

PARTS OF THE NAIL

The entire nail structure consists of parts of the actual nail and structures of skin beneath and surrounding the nail.

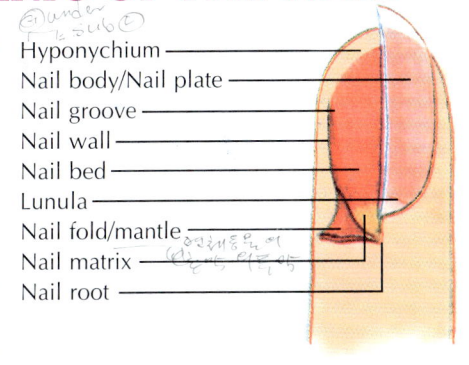

PARTS OF THE NAIL

The actual nail consists of the nail body, nail root, and free edge. The **nail body** or **plate** is the main part or plate of nail that is attached to the skin at the tip of the finger. Although the nail plate appears to be one piece, it is actually constructed of layers. (Fig. 7.1)

The **nail root** is where the nail growth begins. It is embedded underneath the skin at the base of the nail.

The **free edge** is the end of the nail that extends beyond the fingertip.

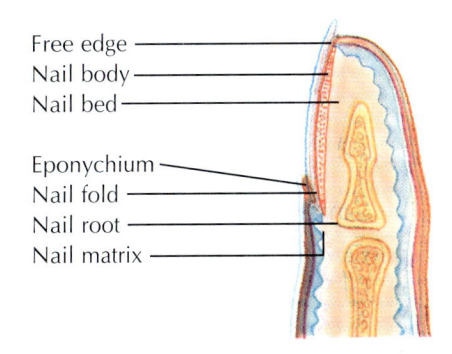

STRUCTURES BENEATH THE NAIL

The structures beneath the nail include the nail bed, matrix, and lunula. The **nail bed** is the portion of skin beneath the nail body that the nail plate rests upon. The nail bed is supplied with blood vessels that provide the nourishment necessary for nail growth. The nail bed also contains nerves. (Fig. 7.2)

Hyponychium
Nail body/Nail plate
Nail groove
Nail wall
Nail bed
Lunula
Nail fold/mantle
Nail matrix
Nail root

7.1 – Diagram of the nail

Free edge
Nail body
Nail bed

Eponychium
Nail fold
Nail root
Nail matrix

7.2 – Cross section of the nail

The *matrix* (**MAY**-triks) contains nerves together with lymph and blood vessels that produce nail cells and control the rate of growth of the nail. It is located under the nail root. The matrix is a very sensitive part of the nail and if injured will produce nails with irregular growth and disorders. Be careful not to apply excessive pressure to this area during a manicure.

The *lunula* is the light-colored half-moon shape at the base of the nail. This is where the matrix connects with the nail bed.

SKIN SURROUNDING THE NAIL

The skin surrounding the nail includes the cuticle, nail fold, nail grooves, nail wall, eponychium, perionychium, and hyponychium.

The *cuticle* (**KYOO**-ti-kel) is the overlapping skin around the nail. A normal cuticle should be loose and pliable.

The *nail fold* or *mantle* (**MAN**-tel) is the deep fold of skin at the base of the nail where the nail root is embedded.

The *nail grooves* are slits or tracks in the nail bed at the sides of the nail on which the nail grows.

The *nail wall* is the skin on the sides of the nail above the grooves.

The *eponychium* (ep-o-**NIK**-ee-um) is the thin line of skin at the base of the nail that extends from the nail wall to the nail plate.

The *perionychium* (**PER**-i-o-nik-ee-um) is the part of the skin that surrounds the entire nail area.

The *hyponychium* (heye-poh-**NIK**-ee-um) is the part of the skin under the free edge of the nail.

NAIL DISORDERS

A *nail disorder* is a condition caused by injury to the nail or disease or imbalance in the body. Most, if not all, of your clients have had some type of common nail disorder and may have one when they are scheduled for a manicure. As a nail technician, you learn to recognize the symptoms of nail disorders so you can make a responsible decision about whether you should perform a service on your client.

You may be able to help your clients with nail disorders in one of two ways. You can tell clients that they may have a disorder and refer them to a physician. In other cases you can cosmetically improve a nail disorder and improve the overall beauty of your clients' nails.

It is your responsibility to know when it is safe to work on your clients' nails. You must learn to recognize the symptoms of nail disorders that cannot be worked on. In addition, you must know when to treat nails with extra care and when you can perform a

CHAPTER 7　THE NAIL AND ITS DISORDERS　◆　**89**

service to cosmetically improve a disorder. Use the "golden rule" to make a responsible decision about the health of your clients' nails.

"**The golden rule**" is that, if the nail or skin to be worked on is infected, inflamed, broken, or swollen, a nail technician should not service the client. Instead refer the client to a doctor. An *inflammation* (in-flam-**MAY**-shun) is red and sore. An *infection* (in-**FEK**-shun) will have evidence of pus. Inflammation and infection are not the same thing, although they often occur at the same time. *Broken* skin or nail tissue is a cut or tear that exposes deeper layers of these structures. *Raised* or *swollen* skin will appear fatter than normal skin and rise above the normal level.

The lists below contain the names of nail disorders and a short description of each one. The first list contains the names of nail disorders that nail technicians can work on if there is not evidence of infection, inflammation, broken tissue, or swelling. The list also suggests services you might perform. The second list contains descriptions of nail disorders that are too serious for a nail technician to work on and that must be referred to a physician.

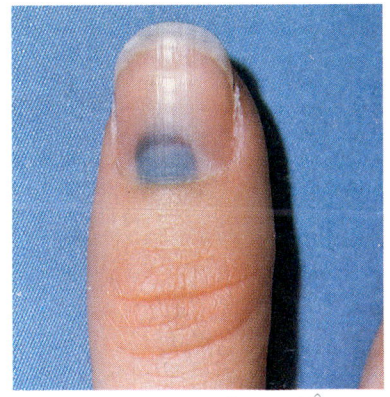

7.3 — Bruised nail

NAIL DISORDERS THAT CAN BE SERVICED BY A NAIL TECHNICIAN

Bruised nails is a condition in which a clot of blood forms under the nail plate. The clot is caused by injury to the nail bed. It can vary in color from maroon to black. In some cases, a bruised nail will fall off during the healing process. Applying artificial nail services to a bruised nail is not recommended. (Fig. 7.3)

Discolored nails is a condition in which the nails turn a variety of colors including yellow, blue, blue-grey, green, red, and purple. Discoloration can be caused by poor blood circulation, a heart condition, or topical or oral medications. It may also indicate the presence of a systemic disorder. Artificial tips or wraps or an application of colored nail polish can hide this condition.

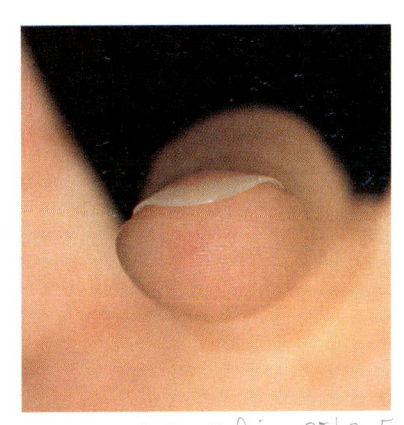

Eggshell nails are thin, white, and curved over the free edge. The condition is caused by improper diet, internal disease, medication, or nervous disorders. Be very careful when manicuring these nails because they are fragile and can break easily. Use the fine side of an emery board to file gently and do not use pressure with a metal pusher at the base of the nail. (Figs. 7.4, 7.5)

Furrows, also known as corrugations, are long ridges that run either lengthwise or across the nail. Some lengthwise ridges are normal in adult nails, and they increase with age. Lengthwise ridges can also be caused by conditions such as psoriasis, poor circulation, and frostbite. Ridges that run across the nail can be caused by conditions such as high fever, pregnancy, measles in childhood, and a zinc deficiency in the body. If ridges are not deep and the nail is not broken, you can correct the appearance of this disorder.

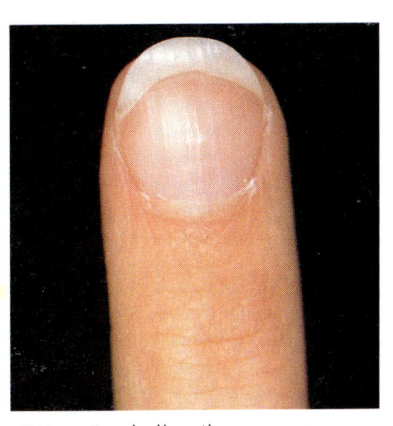

7.4 — Eggshell nail

7.5 — Eggshell nail

90 ◆ PART 2 THE SCIENCE OF NAIL TECHNOLOGY

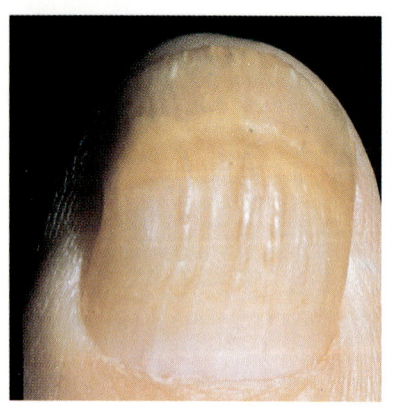

7.6 — Furrows or corrugations

Since these nails are exceedingly fragile, great care must be exercised when giving a manicure. Avoid the use of the metal pusher; use a cotton-tipped orange-wood stick around the cuticle. Carefully buff the nails with pumice powder to remove or shorten the ridges. The remaining ridges can be filled with ridge filler and covered with colored polish to give a smooth, healthy look to the nail. (Fig. 7.6)

Hangnails, also known as *agnails*, is a common condition in which the cuticle around the nail splits. Hangnails are caused by dry cuticles or cuticles that have been cut too close to the nail. This disorder can be improved by softening the cuticles with oil and trimming the cuticles with nippers. Though this is a simple and common disorder, hangnails can become infected if not serviced properly. (Fig. 7.7)

Leukonychia (loo-ko-**NIK**-ee-ah) is a condition in which white spots appear on the nails. It is caused by air bubbles, a bruise, or other injury to the nail. Leukonychia cannot be corrected, but it will grow out. (Fig. 7.8)

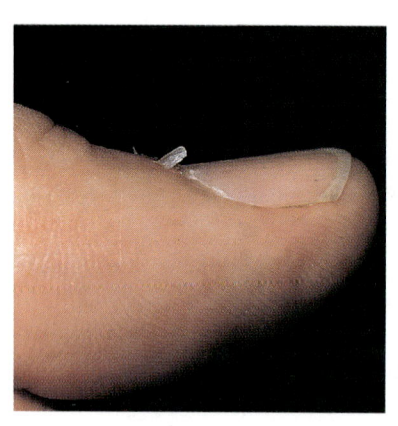

7.7 — Hangnail

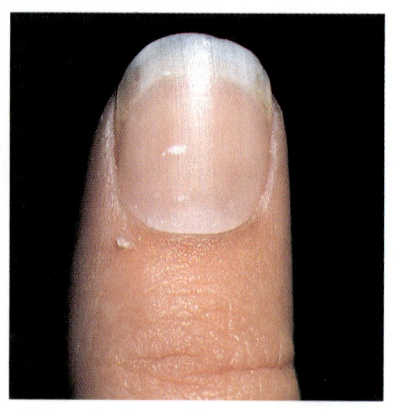

7.8 — Leukonychia

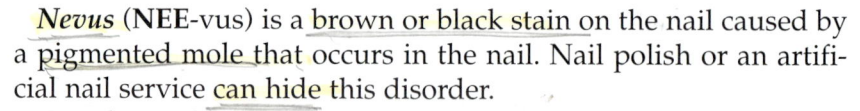

Nevus (**NEE**-vus) is a brown or black stain on the nail caused by a pigmented mole that occurs in the nail. Nail polish or an artificial nail service can hide this disorder.

Onychatrophia (on-i-kah-**TROH**-fee-ah), also known as atrophy, describes the wasting away of the nail. The nail loses its shine, shrinks, and falls off. Onychatrophia can be caused by injury to the nail matrix or by internal disease. Handle this condition with extreme care. File the nail with the fine side of the emery board and do not use a metal pusher or strong soaps or washing powders. If the condition is caused by internal disease and the disease is cured, new nails may grow back. (Fig. 7.9)

Onychauxis (on-i-**KIK**-sis) or *hypertrophy* (hy-**PER**-troh-fee) shows the opposite symptoms of onychatrophia. Onychauxis is the overgrowth of nails. Nails with this disorder are abnormally thick. The condition is usually caused by internal imbalance, local

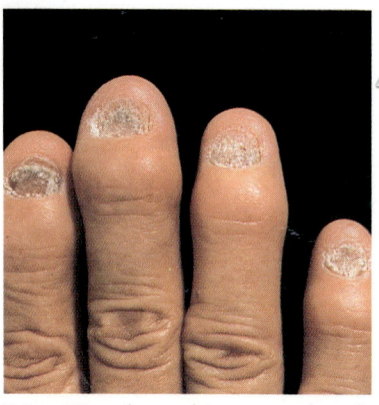

7.9 — Onychatrophia or atrophy of the nail

CHAPTER 7   THE NAIL AND ITS DISORDERS   ◆   91

infection, or heredity. File the nail smooth and buff it with pumice powder. (Figs. 7.10, 7.11)

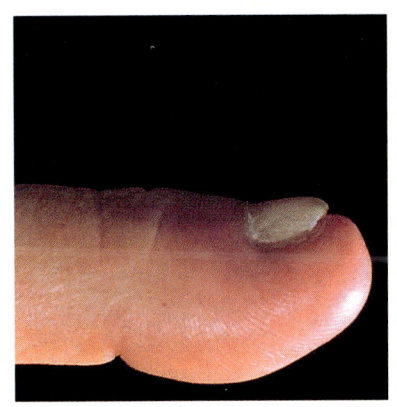

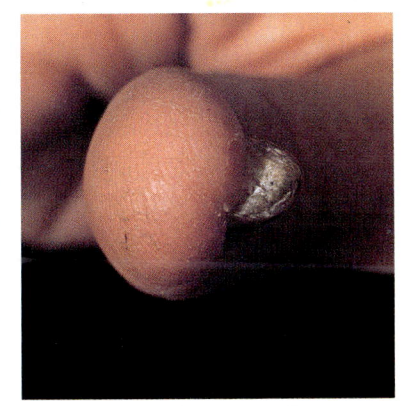

7.10 — Onychauxis

7.11 — Onychauxis (end view)

Onychocryptosis (on-i-koh-krip-**TOH**-sis) or ***ingrown nails*** is a familiar condition of the fingers and toes in which the nail grows into the sides of the tissue around the nail. Improper filing of the nail and poor-fitting shoes are causes of this disorder. If the tissue around the nail is not infected or if the nail is not too deeply imbedded in the flesh, you can trim the corner of the nail in a curved shape to relieve the pressure on the nail groove. If the nail has grown very deeply into the groove, refer the client to a physician. (Fig. 7.12)

Onychophagy (on-i-**KOH**-fa-jee) is the medical term for nails that have been bitten enough to become deformed. This condition can be improved greatly by professional manicuring techniques. Give frequent manicures, using the techniques described in the manicuring chapters of this book. As those chapters suggest, any of the artificial tips and wraps can hide and beautify deformed nails. (Fig. 7.13)

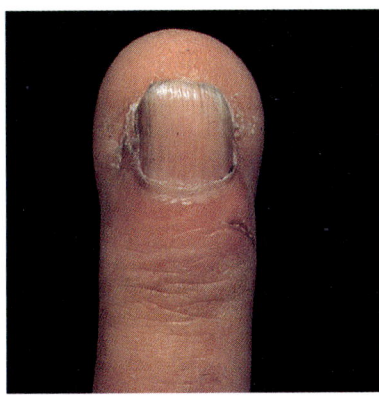

7.12 — Onychocryptosis or ingrown nail

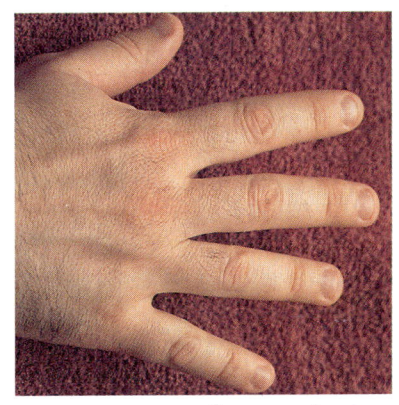

7.13 — Bitten nails or onychophagy

92 ◆ PART 2   THE SCIENCE OF NAIL TECHNOLOGY

Onychophosis (on-ih-**KOH**-foh-sis) refers to a growth of horny epithelium in the nail bed.

Onychophyma (on-ih-koh-**FEE**-mah) more commonly referred to as onychauxis, denoted a swelling of the nail.

Onychorrhexis (on-i-kohr-**REK**-sis) refers to split or brittle nails that also have a series of lengthwise ridges. It can be caused by injury to the fingers, excessive use of cuticle solvents, nail polish removers, and careless, rough filing. Nail services can be performed only if the nail is not split below the free edge. This condition may be corrected by softening the nails with a reconditioning treatment and discontinuing the use of harsh soaps, polish removers, or improper filing. (Fig. 7.14)

Onychosis (on-ih-**KOH**-sis) is a technical term applied to nail disease.

Pterygium (te-**RIJ**-ee-um) describes the common condition of the forward growth of the cuticle on the nail. The cuticle sticks to the nail and, if not treated, will grow over the nail to the free edge.

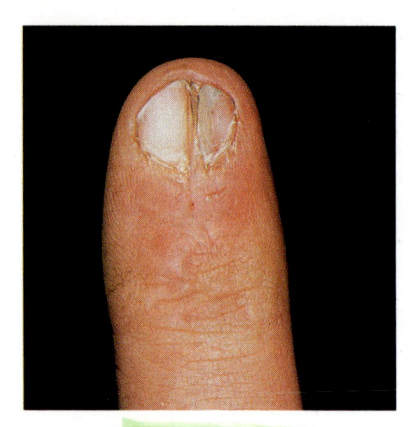

7.14 — Onychorrhexis

The Power of Diversity

Just as a successful hairstylist must offer a spectrum of hair services to be successful, so must a nail professional. Although many technicians may rely on only one system — natural, acrylic, fiberglass or gel wraps — it's important to learn as many systems as possible. This way you'll be covered if someone develops an allergy or a customer insists on a specific type of tip. For help, visit nail shows, read nail magazines and enroll regularly in continuing education classes.

CHAPTER 7 THE NAIL AND ITS DISORDERS ◆ 93

This condition can easily be treated by a reconditioning hot oil manicure, which will soften the cuticle so it can be pushed back by a metal pusher and then removed. (Fig. 7.15)

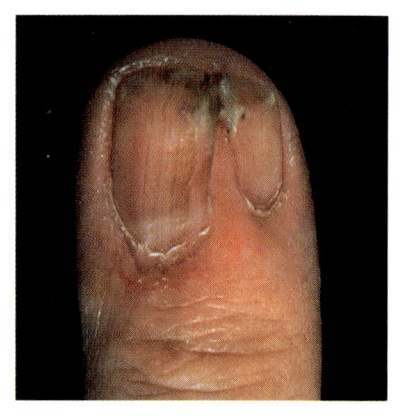

7.15 — Pterygium

NAIL DISORDERS THAT CANNOT BE SERVICED BY A NAIL TECHNICIAN

Mold is a fungus infection of the nail that is usually caused when moisture seeps between an artificial nail and the free edge of the nail, but can also affect a natural nail. Mold starts with a yellow-green color and darkens to black if not treated by a doctor. A client with mold must be referred to a doctor. (Fig. 7.16)

Onychia (on-**NIK**-ee-ah) is an inflammation somewhere in the nail. The tissue at the base of the nail may be red and swollen and pus may form. It is often caused by improperly sanitized manicuring implements. (Fig. 7.17)

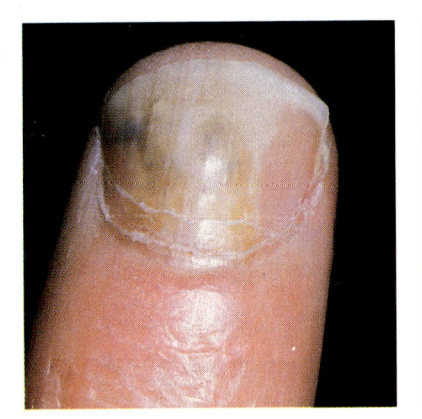

7.16 — Mold

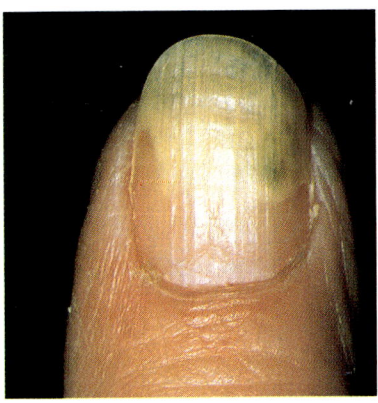

7.17 — Onychia

Onychogryposis (on-i-koh-greye-**POH**-sis) is a condition in which the nail curvature is increased and enlarged. The nail becomes thicker and curves, sometimes extending over the tip of the finger or toe. This condition results in inflammation and pain if the nail grows into the skin. The cause of this disorder is unknown.

Onychomycosis (oni-koh-meye-**KOH**-sis), *tinea unguium* (**TIN**-ee-ah **UN**-gwee-um), of the nails, is an infectious disease caused by a fungus (vegetable parasite). A common form is whitish patches

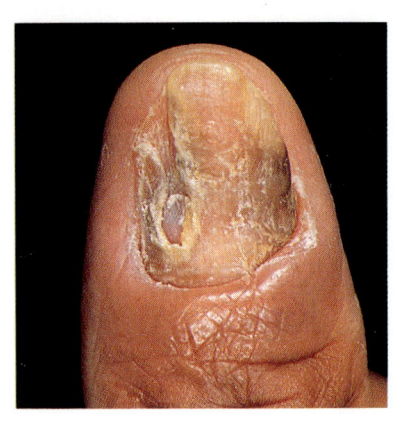

94 ◆ PART 2 THE SCIENCE OF NAIL TECHNOLOGY

that can be scraped off the surface. A second form is long, yellowish streaks within the nail substance. The disease invades the free edge and spreads toward the root. The infected portion is thick and discolored. In a third form, the deeper layers of the nail are invaded, causing the superficial layers to appear irregularly thin. These infected layers peel off and expose the diseased parts of the nail bed. (Fig. 7.18)

7.18 — Onychomycosis

Onycholysis (on-i-**KOL**-i-sis) is a condition in which the nail loosens from the nail bed, beginning usually at the free edge and continuing to the lunula, but does not come off. It is caused by an internal disorder, trauma, infection, or certain drug treatments. It can occur on the nails of the hands or feet. (Figs. 7.19, 7.20)

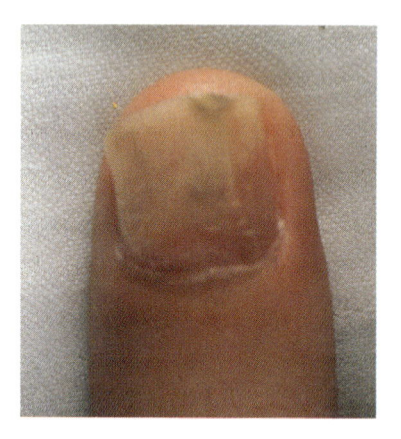

7.19 — Onycholysis (caused by trauma)

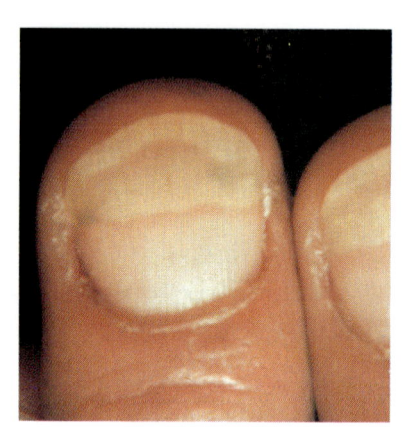

7.20 — Onycholysis

Onychoptosis (on-i-kop-**TOH**-sis) is a condition in which part or all of the nail sheds periodically and falls off the finger. It is a condition that can affect one or more nails. It can occur during or after certain diseases of the body, such as syphilis, as a result of a fever and system upsets, as a reaction to prescription drugs, or as a result of trauma.

Paronychia (par-oh-**NIK**-ee-ah) is a bacterial inflammation of the tissue around the nail. The symptoms are redness, swelling, and tenderness of the tissue surrounding the nail.

Paronychia can occur at the base of the nail, around the entire nail plate, or on the fingertip. Paronychia around the entire nail is sometimes referred to as runaround. Chronic paronychia occurs continually over a long period of time and causes damage to the

CHAPTER 7   THE NAIL AND ITS DISORDERS ◆ 95

nail plate. Paronychia can be caused by the use of unsanitary implements or by aggressive pushing or cutting of the cuticle. (Figs. 7.21, 7.22, 7.23)

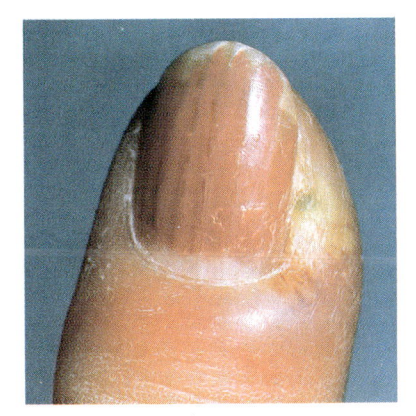

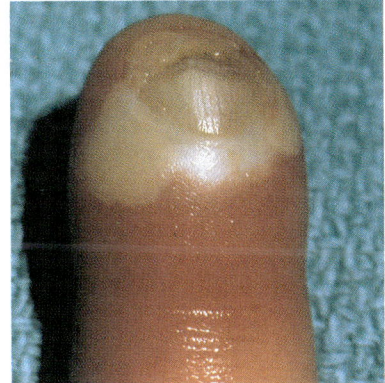

7.21 — Paronychia

7.22 — Paronychia (runaround)

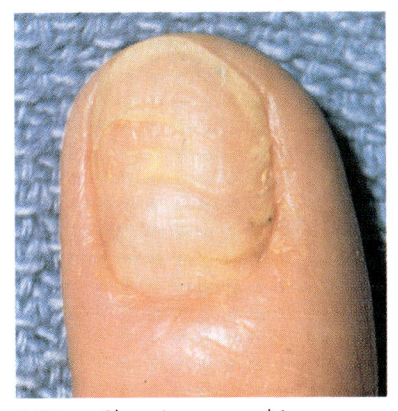

7.23 — Chronic paronychia

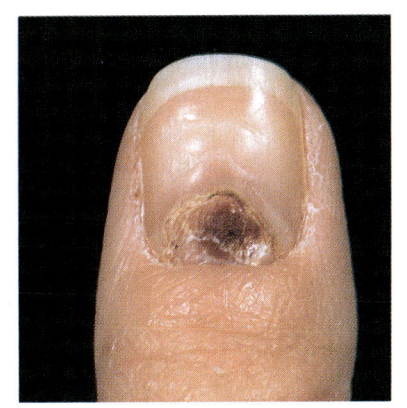

7.24 — Pyogenic granuloma

Pyogenic granuloma is a severe inflammation of the nail in which a lump of red tissue grows up from the nail bed to the nail plate. (Fig. 7.24)

REVIEW QUESTIONS

1. What are the three parts that make up the nail?
2. Define nail disorder.
3. What is the golden rule for dealing with nail disorders?
4. List five nail disorders that can be serviced by a nail technician.
5. List five nail disorders that cannot be serviced by a nail technician.

Chapter 8

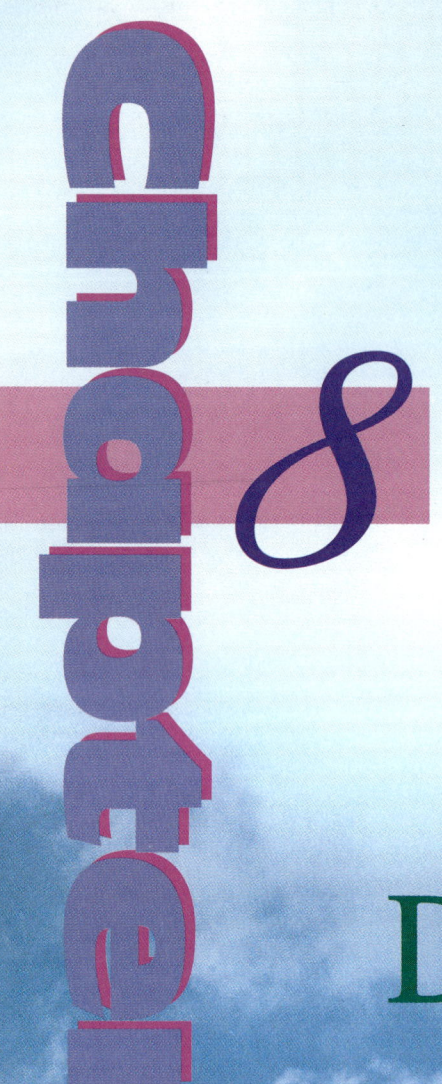

THE SKIN AND ITS DISORDERS

LEARNING OBJECTIVES

After you have studied this chapter, you should be able to:

1. Describe the characteristics of healthy skin.
2. List the functions of the skin.
3. Describe the epidermis and dermis.
4. Explain how the skin is nourished.
5. Describe the function of sweat glands.
6. Define lesion.
7. Describe the characteristics of eczema and psoriasis.

INTRODUCTION

As a nail technician you must have a basic understanding of the skin and its disorders in order to serve your clients responsibly and professionally. You will have the opportunity to improve the appearance of the skin on the hands and feet and therefore to enhance your client's appearance. The finished nails will look their best when set off by beautiful, healthy skin. In addition, it is your responsibility to know when you cannot work on a client or must not use certain products on your client due to a skin condition. Knowledge of the skin will help you avoid the spread of infectious disease and aggravation of skin conditions or sensitivities. Before you can judge whether a particular service or product is appropriate for your client's skin, you must have a general understanding of what the skin is and how it functions. Because the nails are an appendage of the skin, problems with the skin can cause nail problems.

HEALTHY SKIN

To be a nail technician, you must learn about **dermatology** (der-mah-**TOL**-o-jee), the study of healthy skin and skin disorders. Healthy skin is slightly moist and acid, soft and flexible. Unless the skin is aged, healthy skin has **elasticity** that allows it to regain its shape immediately after being pulled away from the bone. Healthy skin is free of blemishes and disease and its texture is smooth and fine-grained. The skin on the human body varies in thickness. It is thinnest on the eyelids and thickest on the palms of the hands and soles of the feet.

FUNCTION OF THE SKIN

The skin performs eight jobs for the body. They include protection, the prevention of fluid loss, response to external stimuli, heat regulation, secretion, excretion, absorption, and respiration.

1. **Protection.** The skin covers every part of the body and protects it from injury and invasion by bacteria.

2. **Prevention of fluid loss.** The skin seals blood and other bodily fluids inside the body.

3. **Response to *external stimuli.*** The skin contains nerve endings that respond to stimuli from outside the body, such as heat,

cold, touch, pressure, pain. This sensitivity helps the body find the most comfortable environment.

4. **Heat regulation.** The skin keeps the body's internal temperature at 98.6 degrees Fahrenheit (37 degrees Celsius). When the temperature outside the body changes, the blood and sweat glands of the skin heat or cool the body to maintain its temperature.

5. **Secretion.** The oil (sebaceous) glands secrete **sebum**, a fatty, oily substance that maintains the skin's moisture level by slowing the evaporation of moisture from the skin and preventing excess water from penetrating the skin.

6. **Excretion.** The sweat (sudoriferous) glands excrete salt and other waste chemicals from the body through the pores of the skin (perspiration).

7. **Absorption.** The skin absorbs small amounts of chemicals, drugs, and cosmetics through the pores.

8. **Respiration.** The skin breathes through the pores. Oxygen is absorbed and carbon dioxide is discharged.

STRUCTURE OF THE SKIN

The skin has two layers or parts. The outer layer is called the epidermis; the deep layer under the epidermis is called the dermis. (Figs. 8.1, 8.2)

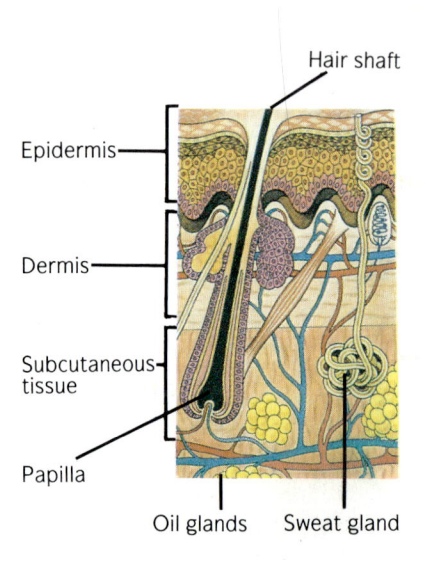

8.1 — A microscopic section of the skin

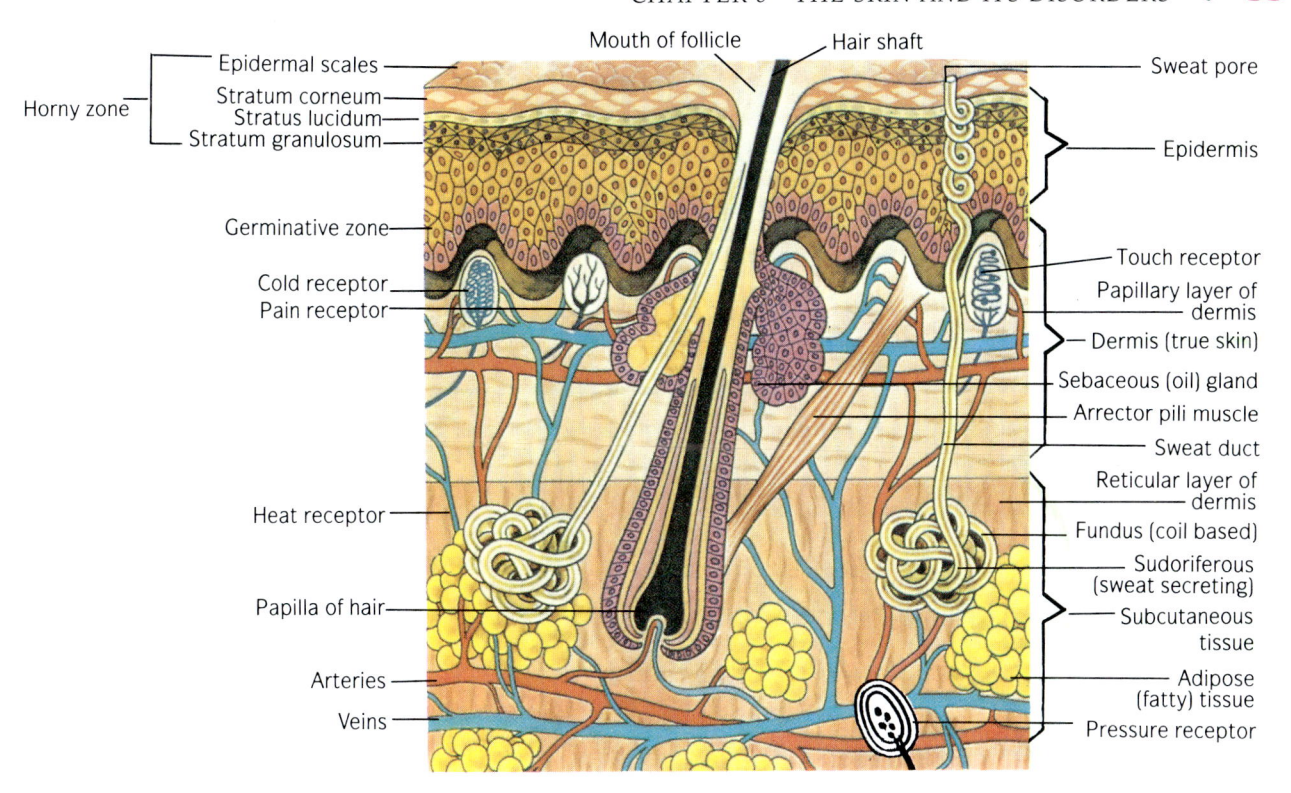

8.2 — Diagram of the skin

Epidermis

The *epidermis* (ep-i-**DUR**-mis), also called the *cuticle* or *scarf skin,* is the outermost protective covering of the skin. It contains no blood vessels, but contains many small nerve endings. The epidermis is made of the following four layers:

The *stratum corneum* (**STRAT**-um **KOHR**-nee-um), also called the *horny layer,* which consists of tightly packed, scalelike cells that are continually shed and replaced. These cells form keratin, the substance that makes up skin, nails, and hair. The keratin also acts as a waterproof coating for the skin.

The *stratum lucidum* (**STRAT**-um **LOO**-si-dum) is a small layer of clear cells that light can pass through.

The *stratum granulosum* (**STRAT**-um gran-yoo-**LOH**-sum) consists of cells that look like granules. These cells change into keratin near the surface of the skin.

The *stratum germinativum* (**STRAT**-um jur-mi-nah-**TIV**-um), formerly known as the *stratum mucosum* (**STRAT**-um myoo-**KOH**-sum), can also be referred to as the basal of Malpighian layer. This layer is composed of several layers of differently shaped cells. The deepest layer is responsible for supplying new cells to make up for the ones that are continually worn away. It also contains a dark skin pigment, called *melanin* (**MEL**-a-nin), which determines skin color and protects the sensitive cells below from the destructive effects of excessive ultraviolet rays from the sun or an ultraviolet lamp.

The Dermis

The **dermis** is the deep layer of the skin and is also called the "true skin," **derma, corium,** or **cutis.** Blood vessels and lymph vessels, nerves, sweat glands, and oil glands are contained in this layer in an elastic network made up of collagen. The dermis contains three separate layers.

The *papillary* (**PA**-pil-ah-ry) *layer* lies directly under the epidermis and contains the *papillae* (pa-**PIL**-e), little cone-like projections that extend upward into the epidermis. Some of the papillae contain looped capillaries, and small blood vessels; others contain nerve endings, called tachle corpuscles. This layer also contains some of the melanin pigment.

The *reticular* (re-**TIK**-u-lar) *layer* contains fat cells, blood and lymph vessels, sweat and oil glands, hair follicles, and the arrector pili.

The *subcutaneous* (sub-kyoo-**TAY**-nee-us) *tissue* is made up of fatty tissue known as *adipose* (**AD**-i-pohs). This tissue gives smoothness and shape to the body, contains a store of fat to be burned for energy, and acts as a protective cushion for the outer skin. It varies in thickness according to the age, sex, and general health of the individual.

NOURISHMENT OF THE SKIN

The skin is nourished by blood and lymph. See Chapter 6 for more information about blood and lymph. One-half to two-thirds of the total blood supply of the body is distributed to the skin. The blood and lymph supply essential nourishment for growth and repair of skin, hair, and nails. The subcutaneous layer of the skin contains arteries and lymphatic vessels that send small branches to provide nourishment to hair papillae, hair follicles, and skin glands. The skin also contains numerous capillaries.

NERVES OF THE SKIN

A *nerve* is made of cordlike fibers and sends messages from the body organs to the central nervous system which consists of the brain and the spinal cord. The skin contains the surface endings of many nerve fibers.

These nerve endings are called *tactile corpuscles* (**TAK**-til **KOR**-puh-sils) and they perform the following functions:

Motor nerves move the blood vessels and the *arrector pili* (a-**REK**-tohr **PIGH**-ligh) muscles that are attached to the hair follicles. These muscles can cause goose bumps.

Sensory nerves, which are found in the papillary layer of the dermis, give the skin a sense of touch. They allow you to react to heat,

CHAPTER 8　THE SKIN AND ITS DISORDERS　◆　**101**

cold, touch, pressure, and pain. Sensory nerve endings are most abundant in the fingertips. Complex sensations, such as vibrations, seem to depend on the sensitivity of a combination of these nerve endings. (Fig. 8.3)

Secretory (se-**KREET**-e-ree) *nerves* are the nerves of the sweat and oil glands.

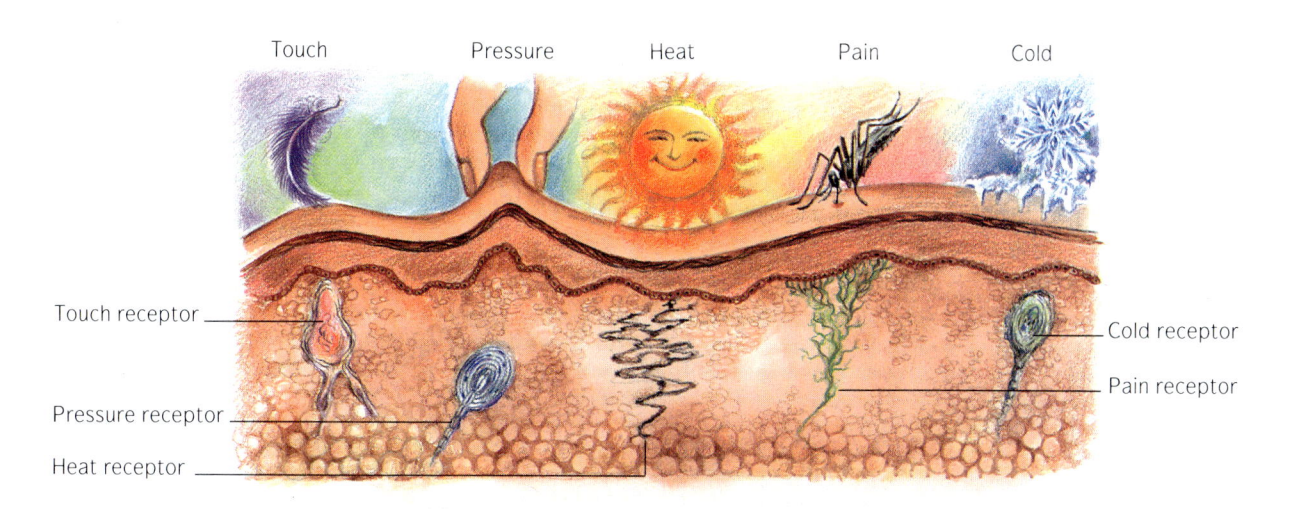

8.3 — Sensory nerves of the skin

GLANDS OF THE SKIN

The skin contains two types of duct glands that extract materials from the blood and turn them into different substances. These new substances are secreted for use by the body or excreted from the body.

The *sudoriferous* (su-dohr-**IF**-er-us) *glands,* or *sweat glands,* regulate body temperature and eliminate waste products through perspiration. Though the nervous system controls the excretion of sweat, activity is greatly increased by heat, exercise, emotions, and certain drugs. One to two pints of liquids containing salts are normally eliminated daily through the sweat pores in the skin. (Fig. 8.4)

Sweat glands consist of a coiled base, called a *fundus* (**FUN**-dus) and a tubelike duct that ends at the skin surface to form a *sweat pore.* A sweat pore is a small opening in the skin surface from which the sweat gland eliminates waste. Most parts of the body have sweat glands. The palms of the hands, soles of the feet, forehead, and armpits have the greatest number of sweat glands.

The *sebaceous* (si-**BAY**-shus) or *oil glands* secrete an oily substance, called sebum, as you learned earlier in this chapter.

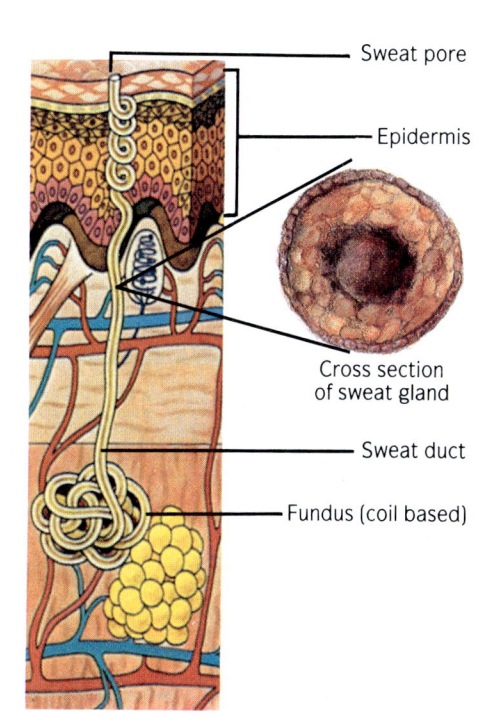

8.4 — Sudoriferous or sweat glands

Sebum lubricates the skin and softens the hair. All parts of the body except the palms of the hands and soles of the feet have oil glands. The oil glands consist of little sacs with ducts that open into the other follicles. When the oil gland produces sebum in the sac, it flows through the oil duct into the hair follicle. If the sebum hardens and the duct becomes clogged, a **blackhead,** or comedone, forms. Cleansing skin regularly will prevent the oil ducts from clogging. (Fig. 8.5)

ELASTICITY OF THE SKIN

The *elastic tissue* in the papillary layer of the dermis gives the skin its ability to return to its original shape after it has been stretched. As a person ages, the papillary tissue begins to lose its elastic nature. The skin begins to sag or wrinkle because it no longer can return to its original shape.

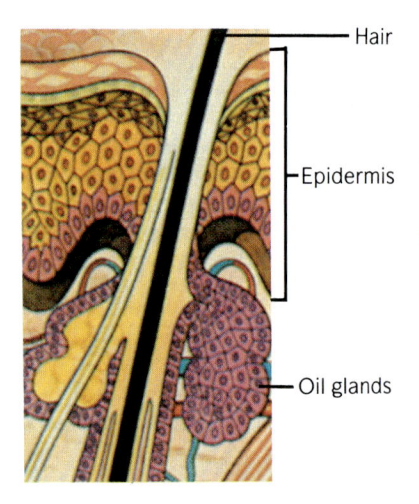

8.5 — Sebaceous or oil glands

SKIN DISORDERS

As a nail technician, you need to learn about skin disorders so you can decide when it is safe and appropriate to work on a client. Your goal is to prevent the spread of an infectious disease and to avoid worsening a condition your client already has. You will observe the skin of a client during the consultation and use your special knowledge to make an informed decision about servicing your client. While only a medical doctor is qualified to make a diagnosis, you should learn to recognize the symptoms that indicate that a disorder is present. It is difficult to recognize some skin disorders in practice, so you must use the following "golden rule" when making your decision.

The golden rule of skin disorders is that if the area of skin to be worked on is infected, inflamed, broken, or raised, a nail technician should not service the client. The client should be referred to a dermatologist. **Inflamed skin** is red, sore, and swollen. Inflamed skin is not the same as infected skin. **Infected skin** will have evidence of pus. **Broken skin** occurs when the epidermis is cut or torn, exposing the deeper layers of skin. **Raised skin** is a symptom of a variety of skin conditions, some of which are lesions, and will be described below. If the skin is raised at all, do not work on it; refer your client to a physician.

LESIONS OF THE SKIN

A *lesion* (**LEE**-zhun) is a structural change in tissue caused by injury and disease. There are two main types: primary and secondary. Primary lesions are the original lesions manifesting a disease. Secondary lesions are those that develop in the later stages of the disease. While studying the different skin lesions, remember that you will always use your "golden rule" to decide whether or not it is safe to work on your client. The symptoms or signs of diseases of the skin are divided into two groups:

1. *Subjective symptoms* are those that can be felt, such as itching, burning, or pain.

2. *Objective symptoms* are those that are visible, such as pimples, postules, or inflammation. (Fig. 8.6)

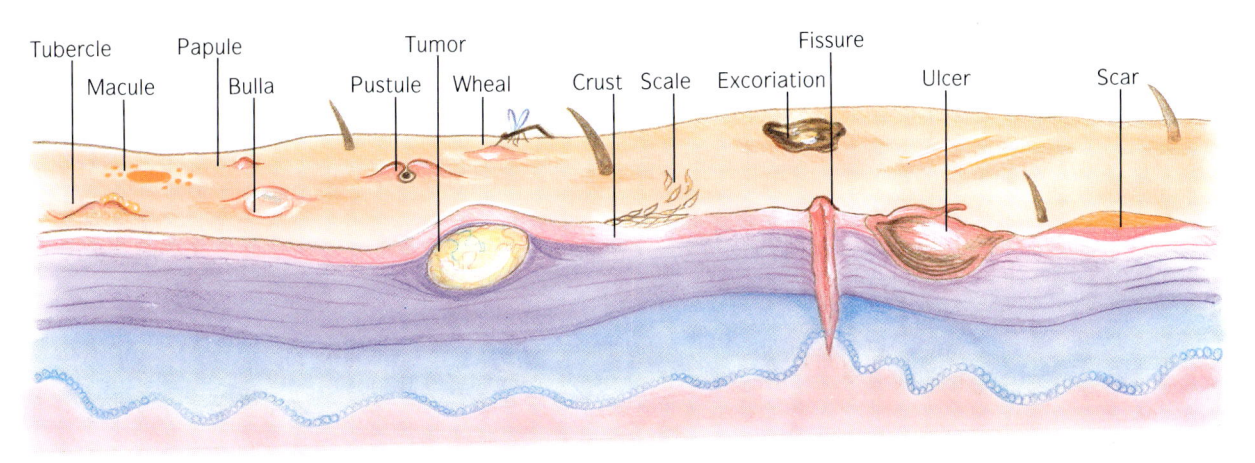

8.6 —Lesions of the skin

A *bulla* (**BYOO**-lah) is a blister containing watery fluid.

A *crust* is an accumulation of serum and pus mixed with epidermal flakes. An example of crust is a scab on a sore.

A *cyst* (**SIST**) is a semisolid or fluid lump above and below the skin surface.

Excoriation (ed-skohr-i-**AY**-shun) is a sore or abrasion caused by scratching or scraping.

A *fissure* (**FISH**-ur) is a crack in the skin that penetrates the dermis. Chapped hands or lips are an example.

A *macule* (**MAK**-ul) is a small, discolored spot or patch on the surface of the skin. Some macules are safe and some are not.

A *papule* (**PAP**-yool) is a small pimple that does not contain fluid, but can develop pus.

A *pustule* (**PUS**-chool) is a lump on the skin with an inflamed base and a head containing pus.

Scales are produced during the shedding of the epidermis. Severe dandruff is an example of scales.

A *scar* is a light-colored, slightly raised mark on the skin formed after an injury or lesion of the skin has healed.

A *stain* is an abnormal discoloration that remains after moles, freckles, or liver spots disappear, or after certain diseases.

A *tubercle* (**TOO**-ber-kyool) is a solid lump larger than a papule. It varies in size from a pea to a hickory nut.

A *tumor* is an abnormal cell mass that varies in size, shape, and color. *Nodules* are small tumors.

An *ulcer* (**UL**-ser) is an open lesion on the skin or mucous membrane of the body. Ulcers are accompanied by pus and loss of skin depth.

A *vesicle* (**VES**-i-kell) is a blister containing clear fluid. Poison ivy is an example of a condition that produces vesicles.

Wheals (**HWEELS**) or *hives* are swollen, itchy bumps on the skin that last for several hours. They are often caused by insect bites or by allergic reactions.

INFLAMMATIONS OF THE SKIN

There are several types of **inflammations** of the skin, also known as dermatitis. If inflammation, infection, or raised or broken skin is present, do not work on the inflamed area. Be very cautious when working on a client who suffers from these disorders because the skin is sensitive and the condition can be aggravated by the use of chemicals.

Eczema (**EK**-se-mah) is a chronic, long-lasting disorder of unknown cause. It is characterized by itching, burning, and the formation of scales and oozing blisters.

Psoriasis (so-**REYE**-a-sis) is a chronic inflammation with round, dry patches covered with coarse silvery scales. It is usually found on the scalp, elbows, knees, chest, and lower back; rarely on the face.

Offer Spa-Style Services

Spa-style services give clients a chance to get away from it all without even leaving the nail station—plus, they help you stand apart from the competition. Here are a few to consider:

- Aromatherapy. Add a quick massage with soothing aromatic oils to your regular nail services for a relaxing, restoring treat.
- Paraffin manicure and pedicure. Dry skin becomes soft and supple when paraffin—which encourages skin to absorb moisture—is painted on moisturized hands and feet.
- Reflexology pedicure. Consider taking a continuing education class to learn massage techniques. As a part of a pedicure, reflexology massage relieves tension and helps clients relax.
- Ageless manicure. To keep hands looking young, treat them with glycolic acid. A member of the alpha-hydroxy family, it's famous for its line-softening and age spot-lightening abilities.

INFECTIONS OF THE SKIN

You cannot perform nail services on a customer who has either a fungus infection or a viral infection of the skin. Clients with either type of infection should be referred to a physician.

Athlete's foot, also known as *tinea pedis* (**TIN**-ee-ah **PEH**-dus) or ringworm of the foot, is a fungus infection of the foot. The symptoms are small, pink spots or blisters and itching around the toes and on the sole of one or both feet. In extreme cases the nail can become infected. Athlete's foot is highly contagious and should not be touched by a nail technician. (Fig. 8.7)

Herpes simplex is a skin infection common in dental staff and others involved with care of the mouth. It may start as painful paronychia (see Chapter 6). This is a serious viral infection that may occur periodically. (Fig. 8.8)

Ringworm (tinea) of the hand is a highly contagious disease caused by a fungus. The principal symptoms are red lesions occurring in patches or rings over the hands. Itching may be slight or severe. (Fig. 8.9)

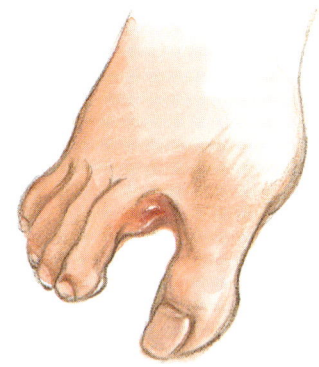

8.7 — Athlete's foot

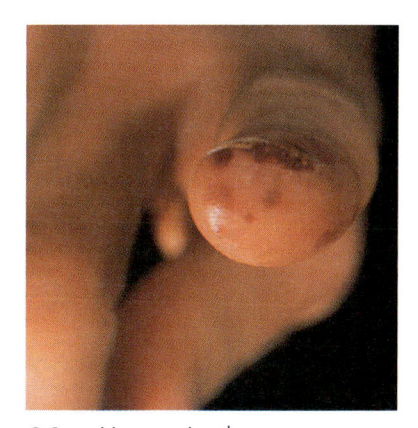

8.8 — Herpes simplex

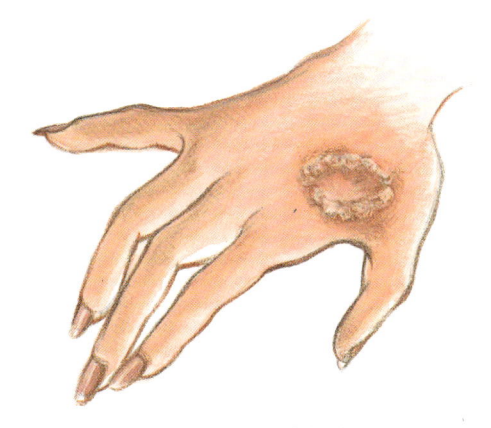

8.9 — Ringworm of the hand

PIGMENTATION OF THE SKIN

The color of the skin is determined in part by the blood supply to the skin, but mostly by melanin, or coloring matter. Abnormal pigmentary conditions may be caused by internal or external factors. Certain medications are also known to cause pigmentary irregularities. Clients with these irregularities can receive nail services.

Albinism (**AL**-bi-niz-em) is a congenital absence of melanin pigment in the body, including the skin, hair, and eyes. The hair is silky white. The skin is pinkish white and does not tan. The eyes are pink and the skin ages early. Albinism is a form of *leucoderma* (loo-ko-**DER**-ma), a general term for the abnormal lack of pigmentation.

Chloasma (kloh-**AZ**-mah) are brown spots on the skin, especially the face and hands. Chloasma are also called "liver spots" or "moth patches."

Lentigines (len-ti-**JEE**-neez), or *freckles,* are small brown or yellow spots.

A *birthmark* or *nevus* (**NEE**-vus) is a malformation of the skin due to abnormal pigmentation or dilated capillaries. The condition may be inherited.

A *tan* is the darkening of the skin caused by exposure to the ultraviolet rays of the sun.

Vitiligo (vit-l-**EYE**-go) is an acquired form of leucoderma that affects the skin or hair. People with vitiligo must be protected from the sun.

HYPERTROPHIES (NEW GROWTHS) OF THE SKIN

A *keratoma,* or *callus,* is an acquired superficial, round and thickened patch of epidermis due to pressure or friction on the hands and feet. If the thickening grows inward it is called a corn.

A *mole* is a small, brown spot on the skin. Moles are believed to be inherited. They range in color from pale tan to brown or bluish black. Some moles are small and flat and look like freckles. Others are raised and darker than freckles in color. Moles often have hairs growing out of them. **Do not touch or remove hair from moles.**

Melanotic sarcoma is a fatal skin cancer that begins with the growth of a mole. A physician should be consulted immediately if there is any change in a mole.

REVIEW QUESTIONS

1. What are the characteristics of healthy skin?
2. What are five functions of the skin?
3. Describe the epidermis and dermis.
4. How is the skin nourished?
5. What are the functions of sweat glands?
6. Name five types of lesions.
7. What are the characteristics of eczema and psoriasis?

Chapter 9

CLIENT CONSULTATION

LEARNING OBJECTIVES

After you have studied this chapter, you should be able to:

1. Explain the purpose of a client consultation.
2. Describe the appearance of healthy nails.
3. Explain why knowing a client's lifestyle is helpful in making decisions about products and services.
4. Determine when it is necessary to refer a client to a physician.
5. Describe the information that should be gathered on the client health/record card.

INTRODUCTION

Before you perform a service on a client, you should take time to talk with that client and complete a client health/record card and a client service record. During this conversation, called the **client consultation,** you will discuss the client's general health, the health of his or her nails and skin, the client's lifestyle and needs, and the nail services that you can perform. You will use your knowledge of skin, nails, and each type of nail service to help your client select the most appropriate service. If the client has a nail or skin disorder that prevents you from performing a service, you should refer that client to his or her physician and offer to perform a service as soon as the disorder has been treated. A good client consultation is the difference between being a professional and just "doing nails."

DETERMINING THE CONDITION OF NAILS AND SKIN

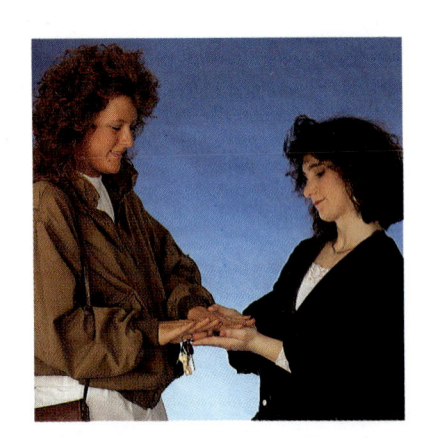

9.1 — Are your client's nails and skin healthy?

Are your client's nails and skin healthy? Look at the nails and skin of the hands or feet (depending on the service). Examine them for disorders. Generally, if there is no inflammation, infection, swelling, or broken skin it is okay to work on that client. It may be necessary to refer a client to his or her physician if you find a problem. It is important to handle this situation very delicately. (Fig. 9.1)

If you need to refer a client to a physician, you must act responsibly and tactfully. Explain to your client that you think there may be a problem and to be safe you will not perform a service until the client has visited a doctor. Never attempt to diagnose the problem because you could cause unnecessary stress for your client. While it may be difficult to turn a client away, you must do so. Performing a service on an infected nail could cause great pain to your client, for which you would be blamed. In addition, your client will be impressed with your professionalism and concern for health and safety.

Does your client have allergies? You should always try to avoid using products that can cause an allergic reaction. If your client does have a reaction to a product, be sure to make a note on his or her client health/record card that includes both the product and the type of reaction.

DETERMINING YOUR CLIENT'S NEEDS

What nail service does the client want? If your client asks for a specific nail service, discuss the procedure used to create that service, the benefits, and proper maintenance. Make sure that your client's expectations are realistic. Keep this desired service in mind as you discuss the client's lifestyle. You may know of a nail service that is better suited to the client's needs.

What kind of lifestyle does the client have? What kind of job does your client have? What hobbies? Are your client's hands often in water? Does your client walk a lot? By learning the answers to these types of questions, you will be able to decide such things as the best length for your client/s nails or how much callus to remove from the feet. Is the client a gardener, model, guitar player, or runner? A gardener might need short nails because it would be difficult to remove dirt from under a long nail. Dirt that cannot be removed can lead to infection or a painful break. A guitar player may need short nails on the left hand and want longer nails on the right hand. He or she also needs calluses on the fingertips of the left hand. A model needs beautiful nails and skin. (Fig. 9.2) A runner may have calluses on the feet that protect the feet during running. You must always consider your client's personality styles and activities when choosing a nail service. (Fig. 9.3) In each of these cases the wrong service could make a client unhappy and even cause pain. You're the professional; it's your job to make the client happy. If your client gets a service and is not happy with it, he or she may not return. If you offer a different service than was originally requested and explain why you feel that service is better suited for the client, you will have that client for life.

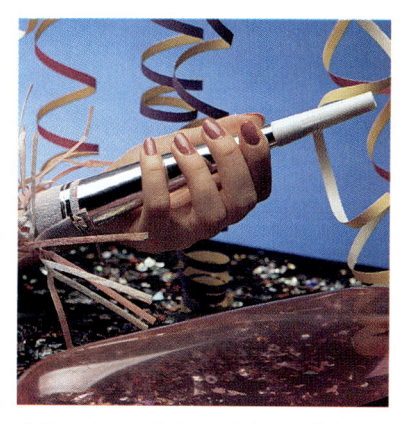

9.2 — A model needs beautiful nails.

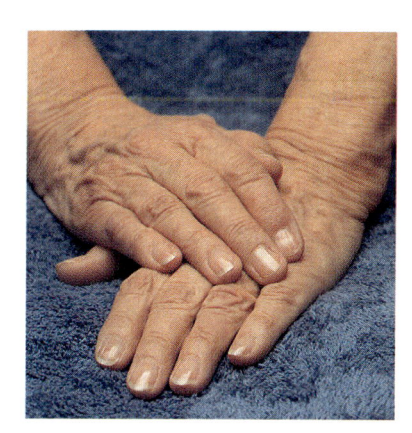

9.3 — Many people prefer natural looking nails.

MEETING YOUR CLIENT'S NEEDS

What is the client's final decision about nail services? After talking with your client about his or her needs, expectations, and nail health you will either confirm the client's service choice or recommend another service. At this time, explain why this service is best for the client, what you will do during the procedure, and what results the client can expect. For example, you would not want your client to believe that nail wraps stayed on forever and needed no maintenance. The client would be very disappointed, despite having a very professional service, when the wrap began to grow out. This is the appropriate time to explain any safety precautions you will take during the procedure. For example, if you are going to apply acrylic nails, you should explain why you will wear safety goggles while applying primer. It is also a good idea to offer your client the same protection. (Fig. 9.4)

After you have completed this process with your client you will start the procedure. You and your client can be sure that it is the appropriate service. Time and money are being spent wisely. The nail service will not conflict with the client's lifestyle and should meet all expectations; your client will also know that you are concerned about health and safety. Your client will leave your salon as a satisfied client and will also return to you again and again as a steady client!

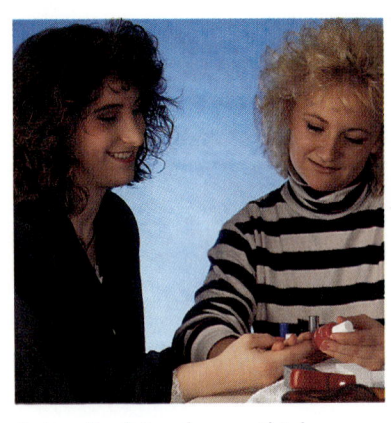

9.4 — Explain why you think a particular service is best for your client.

Reward Repeat Performances

In today's competitive business climate, your customers' loyalty determines your ultimate success. For this reason, it's crucial to show clients you appreciate their repeat business. One easy way to express your appreciation is with cards sent on special occasions, such as birthdays or anniversaries. Reward your patron's loyalty by including a gift certificate for 10 percent off the next service. Also consider sending "advance notice" flyers or a regular newsletter informing your clients of upcoming promotions, new products or additions to your service menu. Because everyone loves a party, you may even try hosting a once- or twice-yearly thank-you night: Invite twenty of your long-time regulars and treat them to refreshments and goody bags of trial-sized products.

COMPLETING THE CLIENT HEALTH/RECORD CARD

Client health/record cards will vary from one salon to another. These cards should be kept in a convenient location where they can provide ready reference for every nail technician in the salon. If the salon is computerized, health/record information can be kept on computer and accessed by making a few simple keystrokes.

CLIENT HEALTH/RECORD CARD

Name: _____

Home address: _____ Work address: _____

Home telephone: _____ Work telephone: _____

Best hours for appointment are: _____

CLIENT PROFILE

1. What type of work do you do?

2. Do you have any hobbies that require you to work with your hands?

3. Do you participate in sports activities? If so, what type?

4. Do you wear rubber gloves when doing housework?

5. How much time do you spend each week caring for your own nails?

6. How frequently do you have professional nail services?

MEDICAL RECORD

Do you have: NO   YES

Arthritis   _____   _____

Cancer   _____   _____

Diabetes   _____   _____

Heart problems   _____   _____

High blood pressure   _____   _____

If you answered yes to any of the above questions, what kind, if any, of medication do you take?

Have you ever had a stroke? If so, how long ago?

Are there any other medical conditions or medications that we should be aware of?

CLIENT SERVICE RECORD

Name: _____

Home address: _____ Work address: _____

_____ _____

Best hours for appointment are: _____

DATE	SERVICE PERFORMED	OBSERVATIONS	PRICE

DATE	RETAIL PRODUCTS SOLD	PRICE

What future nail services were discussed?

_____

_____

_____

Client health/record cards usually include three valuable types of information:

General information asks for the client's name, address, telephone number, and preferred appointment hours.

The **client profile** asks for information about the type of work and leisure activities the client participates in.

The **medical record** asks for information about the client's general health. This information will help you determine whether it is safe to perform nail services or hand and foot massage on the client.

MAINTAINING THE CLIENT SERVICE RECORD

Each time a client receives a service in the salon, an entry should be made in the client service record. This record is usually kept on an index card and includes information about services performed, retail products sold, and future nail services discussed.

The client service record is a valuable record for the salon to maintain in case a client comes in for a nail service when his or her usual nail technician is not available.

Both the client health/record card and the client service record are client consultation tools that tell your clients that you are professional. As a professional you care about health, safety, and the quality of the services your clients receive.

REVIEW QUESTIONS

1. What is the purpose of a client consultation?
2. What are the characteristics of healthy nails?
3. How would your services differ for a runner or a guitar player?
4. Under what circumstances would you refer a client to a physician?
5. What are the three types of information on the client health/record card?

Part 3

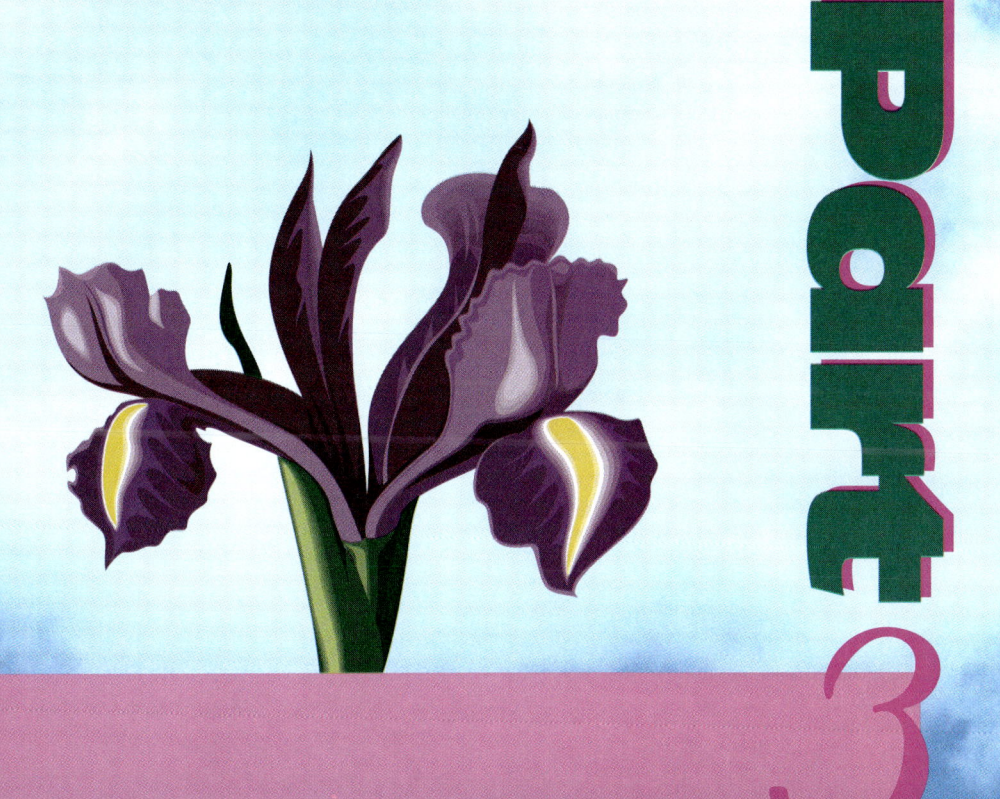

BASIC PROCEDURES

- *CHAPTER 10* - Manicuring
- *CHAPTER 11* - Pedicuring

Chapter 10
MANICURING

LEARNING OBJECTIVES

After you have studied this chapter, you should be able to:

1. Identify the equipment, implements, materials, and cosmetics needed for a manicure and explain what they are used for.
2. Describe the basic table set-up.
3. Describe the four basic nail shapes.
4. List the steps in the pre-service procedure for a water manicure.
5. Demonstrate the proper procedure and precautions for a water manicure.
6. List the steps in the post-service procedure for a water manicure.
7. Describe the five types of polish application.
8. Demonstrate the proper procedure and precautions for the reconditioning hot oil manicure.
9. Describe the steps in a man's manicure.
10. Demonstrate your ability to perform hand and arm massage properly.

INTRODUCTION

The information and procedures you learn in this chapter will give you the basic skills to be a professional nail technician. When you master these skills and use them with your clients, you will gain the confidence and efficiency needed to develop a loyal clientele. The first step of this learning process is to become acquainted with the tools of your trade. The four types of nail technology tools are:

1. Equipment
2. Implements
3. Materials
4. Nail Cosmetics

NAIL TECHNOLOGY SUPPLIES

EQUIPMENT

Permanent items used in nail technology are called equipment. They can be used for all your services and do not have to be replaced until they wear out.

Manicure table with adjustable lamp. Most standard manicuring tables will include a drawer (for storing sanitized implements and cosmetics) and will have an attached, adjustable lamp. The lamp should have a 40 watt bulb. The heat from a higher wattage bulb will interfere with manicuring and sculptured nail procedures. A lower wattage bulb will not be able to warm a client's nails in a room that is highly air conditioned. The warmth from the bulb will help you maintain product consistency.

Client's chair and nail technician's chair or stool.

Fingerbowl. A plastic, china, or glass bowl that can be specially shaped for soaking the client's fingers in warm water and antibacterial soap. (Fig. 10.1)

Disinfection container. A receptacle large enough to hold the disinfectant solution in which objects to be sanitized are immersed. A cover is provided with most disinfection containers to prevent contamination of the solution when it is not in use. (Fig. 10.2)

Client's cushion. The cushion can be 8 by 12 inches and especially made for manicuring; a towel that is folded to cushion size can also be used. The cushion or folded towel should be covered with a clean, sanitized towel before each appointment.

Sanitized wipe container. This container will hold clean, absorbent cotton or lint-free wipes.

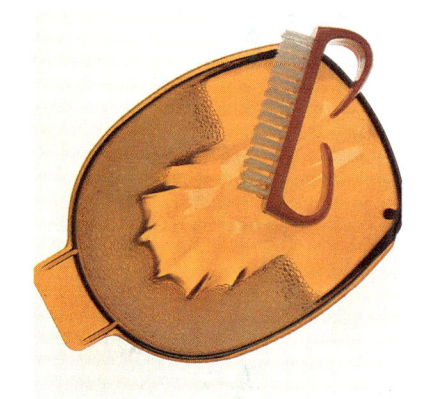

10.1 — Fingerbowl filled with warm water and antibacterial soap and nail brush

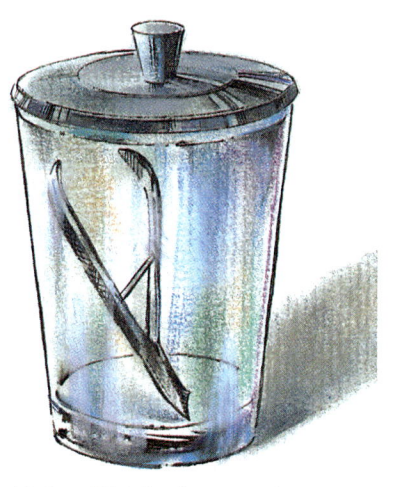

10.2 — Disinfection container

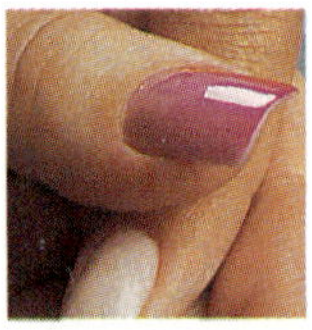

Sanitation Caution

If you drop an orangewood stick on the floor, it must be discarded. It is a disposable implement that cannot be sanitized or reused.

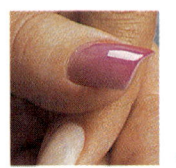

Sanitation Caution

The cotton on your orangewood stick needs to be changed after each use.

Supply tray. The tray holds cosmetics such as polishes, polish removers, and creams.

Electric nail dryer. A nail dryer is an optional item used to shorten the length of time necessary for the client's nails to dry.

IMPLEMENTS

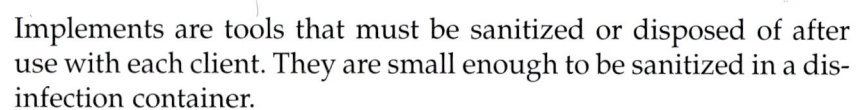

Implements are tools that must be sanitized or disposed of after use with each client. They are small enough to be sanitized in a disinfection container.

Orangewood stick. Use the orangewood stick to loosen cuticle around the base of a nail or to clean under the free edge. Hold the stick as you would a pencil. When you use it to apply cosmetics, wrap a small piece of cotton around the end. An orangewood stick cannot be sanitized, so you must either give it to your client or break it in half and discard it after use. (Fig. 10.3)

Steel Pusher. The steel pusher, also called a cuticle pusher, is used to push back excess cuticle growth. Hold the steel pusher the way you hold a pencil. The spoon end is used to loosen and push back cuticle. If you have rough or sharp edges on your pusher, use an emery board to dull them. This prevents digging into the nail plate. (Fig. 10.4)

Metal nail file. A metal nail file is used to shape the free edge of hard or sculptured nails. Most professional nail technicians use 7"–8" nail files because some states do not allow shorter files to be used. Since a nail file is metal and reusable, it must be disinfected after each use. When using a nail file, hold it with your thumb on one side and the handle and four fingers on the other side. (Fig. 10.5)

STATE REGULATION ALERT

Some states do not permit nail technicians to use metal nail files. Be guided by your instructor.

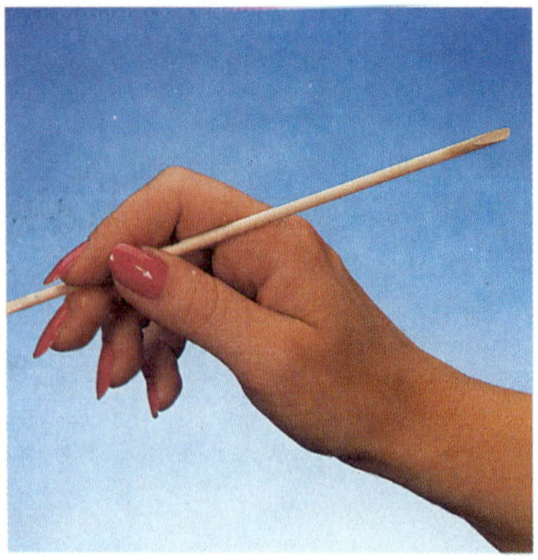

10.3 — Orangewood stick

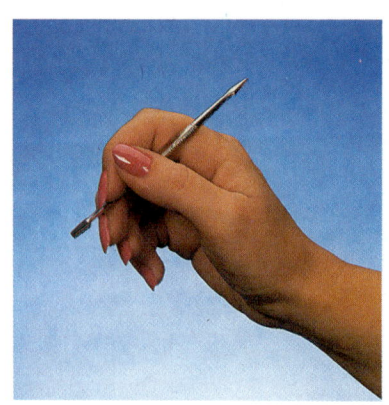

10.4 — Steel pusher

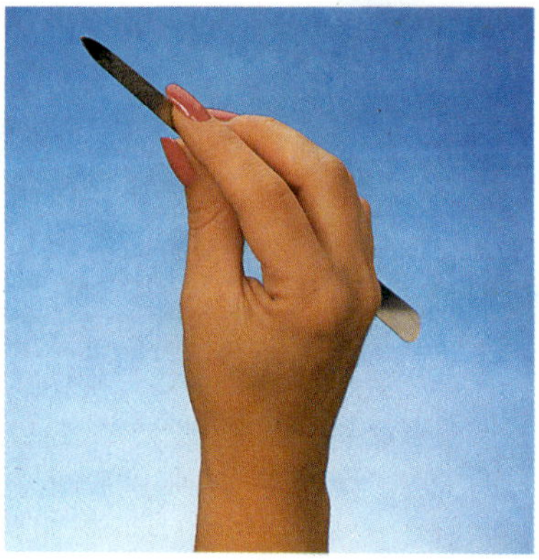

10.5 — Metal nail file

Emery board. Many nail technicians prefer an emery board to a nail file. It is also a good choice for filing soft or fragile nails, because it is not as coarse as a nail file. An emery board has two sides, a coarse-grained side and a fine-grained side. The coarse side is used to shape the free edge of the nail, and the fine side is used to bevel the nail or smooth the free edge. Hold the emery board the way you hold a nail file, with the wider end in your hand so you can file with the narrow end. To bevel, hold the emery board at a 45 degree angle and file, using light pressure, on the top or underside of the nail. Most professional nail technicians use 7"–8" emery boards because some states do not allow the use of smaller ones. The emery board cannot be sanitized, so you must either give it to your client or break it in half and discard it after use. It is not a good idea to save an emery board in a plastic bag for each client. Bacteria can grow on the unsanitized implement before your client's next appointment. (Fig. 10.6)

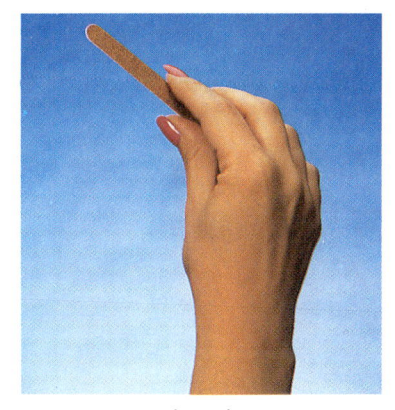

Cuticle nipper. A cuticle nipper is used to trim away excess cuticle at the base of the nail. To use the nippers, hold them in the palm of your hand with the blades facing the cuticle. Place your thumb on one handle and three fingers on the other handle, with your index finger on the screw to help guide the blade around cuticle. (Fig. 10.7)

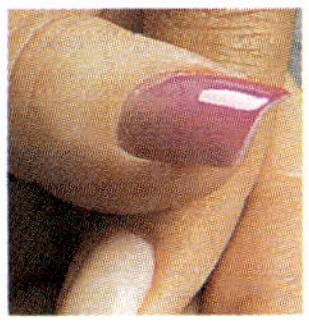

10.6 — Emery board

Sanitation Caution

If you drop an emery board on the floor during a procedure, it must be discarded. This is a disposable item and cannot be reused or sanitized.

STATE REGULATION ALERT

Some states do not permit nail technicians to clip cuticles. Be guided by your instructor.

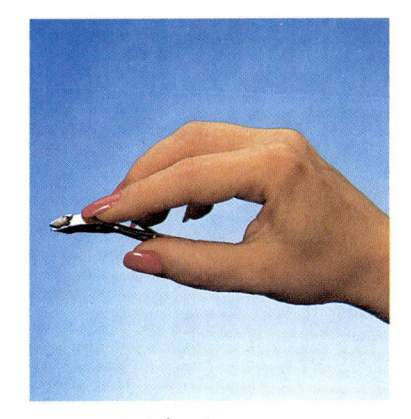

Tweezers. Tweezers are used to lift small bits of cuticle from the nail.

Nail Brush. A nail brush is used to clean fingernails and remove bits of cuticle with warm soapy water. Hold the nail brush with the bristles turned down and away from you. Place your thumb on the handle side of the brush that is facing you and your fingers on the other side.

Chamois buffer. The chamois (**SHAM**-ee) buffer is used to add shine to the nail and to smooth out corrugations or wavy ridges on nails. There are two types of chamois buffer. The first has an open handle; the second has a closed handle on the top. To use the open-handled buffer, place your fingers around the handle with your thumb on the side of the handle to help guide it. To use the closed-handled type, rest your thumb along the edge of the buffer

10.7 — Cuticle nippers

120 ◆ PART 3 BASIC PROCEDURES

to guide and support your use of this implement. Another way to hold a closed-handled chamois buffer is to place the middle and ring fingers through the closed-handled buffer if it has an open slot. Be guided by your instructor on how to hold the chamois buffer. (Figs. 10.8, 10.9)

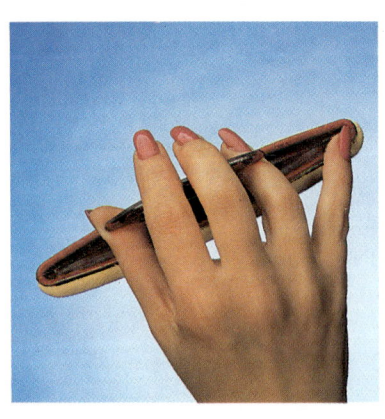

10.8 — Holding a nail buffer

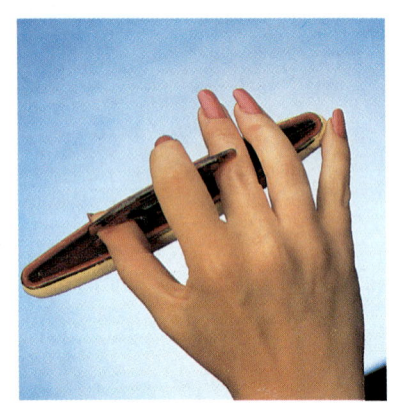

10.9 — Alternative way to hold a nail buffer

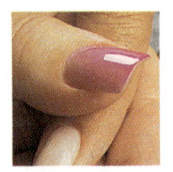

STATE REGULATION ALERT
Some states do not permit the use of a chamois buffer. Be guided by your instructor.

Fingernail clippers. Fingernail clippers are used to shorten nails. If your client's nails are very long, clipping cuts filing time.

Sanitation for Implements

It is a good idea to have two complete sets of metal implements, so you will always have a completely sanitized set for each client, with no waiting between appointments. If you have only one set of implements, remember that it takes twenty minutes to sanitize implements after each use. A few sanitation hints are given below. For a complete discussion of sanitation, see pages 25-36.

- Wash all implements thoroughly with soap and warm water and rinse off all traces of soap with plain water. Dry thoroughly with a sanitized towel.
- Metal implements should be immersed in a disinfection container that is filled with an approved disinfectant. Follow manufacturer's instructions for the required sanitation time. Rinse the implements, then dry them with a sanitized towel when you remove them from the disinfection container.
- Follow your state regulations for storage of sanitized manicuring implements. The regulations will tell you to store them in sealed containers, sealed plastic bags, or in a cabinet sanitizer until they are ready for use.

Sanitation Caution

Your chamois buffer must be designed so the chamois can be changed for each client. Be sure to discard the used chamois after each use.

STATE REGULATION ALERT
In some states, it is a violation of sanitary codes to have metal implements on your table when not in use. Be guided by your instructor about proper storage.

MATERIALS

Materials are supplies that are used during a manicure and need to be replaced for each client.

Disposable towels or terry cloth towels. A fresh, sanitized terry towel is used to cover the client's cushion before each manicure. Another fresh towel should be used to dry the client's hands after soaking in the fingerbowl. Other terry or lint-free disposable towels are used to wipe spills that may occur around the fingerbowl.

Cotton or cotton balls. Cotton is used to remove polish, wrap the end of the orangewood stick, an apply nail cosmetics. Some nail technicians prefer to use small fiber-free squares to remove polish because they don't leave cotton fibers on the nails that might interfere with polish application.

Plastic spatula. The spatula is used to remove nail cosmetics from their containers. Always use your plastic spatula, not your fingers, to remove cosmetics. A closed container of nail cosmetics is a perfect place for bacteria from your fingers to grow.

Plastic bags. Tape or clip a bag to the side of the manicuring table to hold the used materials you discard during a service. Line all trash cans with plastic bags. Be sure to have a generous supply of bags so you can change them regularly during the day.

Powdered alum or styptic powder. Powdered alum, or styptic (**STIP**-tik) powder, is used to contract the skin to stop minor bleeding that may occur during a manicure. To use, blot cut with powdered alum on a cotton-tipped orangewood stick.

STATE REGULATION ALERT

Styptic pencils are not permitted for use in most states because they are unsanitary.

NAIL COSMETICS

As a professional nail technician, you need to know how to use each nail cosmetic and what ingredients it contains. You need to know how to apply each cosmetic and when to avoid using a product because of a client's allergies or sensitivities. In this section you will learn what some of the basic nail cosmetics are, what each product does, and the basic ingredients each contains.

Antibacterial soap. This soap is mixed with warm water and used in the fingerbowl. It contains a soap or detergent and an antibacterial agent to sanitize the client's hands. It comes in four forms: flaked, beaded, cake, and liquid.

Polish remover. Polish remover is used to dissolve and remove nail polish. It usually contains organic solvents and acetone. Sometimes, oil is added to offset the drying effect of the acetone. Use non-acetone polish remover for clients who have artificial nails, because acetone will weaken or dissolve tips, wrap glues, and sculptured nail compound.

Cuticle cream. Cuticle cream is used to lubricate and soften dry cuticles and brittle nails. It contains fats and waxes, such as lanolin, cocoa butter, petroleum, and beeswax.

Cuticle oil. Cuticle oil keeps the cuticle soft and helps to prevent hangnails or rough cuticles. It gives an added touch to the finish of a manicure. Cuticle oil contains ingredients such as vegetable oil, vitamin E, mineral oil, jojoba, and palm nut oil. Suggest that your clients use it as bedtime to keep their cuticles soft.

Cuticle solvent or cuticle remover. Cuticle solvent makes cuticles easier to remove and minimizes clipping. It contains 2-5 percent sodium or potassium hydroxide plus glycerin.

Nail bleach. Apply nail bleach to nail plate and under free edge to remove yellow stains. It contains hydrogen peroxide. If nail bleach cannot be purchased, use 20 volume (6 percent) hydrogen peroxide.

Nail whitener. Nail whiteners are applied under the free edge of a nail to make the nail appear white. They contain zinc oxide or titanium dioxide. Nail whiteners are available in a paste, cream, coated string, and pencil form.

Safety Caution

Care must be taken not to get nail bleach on cuticles or skin because it can cause irritation.

STATE REGULATION ALERT

Nail white pencils are not permitted in most states because they are unsanitary.

Dry nail polish. Dry nail polish, or **pumice** (**PUM**-is) powder is used with the chamois buffer to add shine to the nail. Some clients prefer it to liquid clear polish. Dry nail polish contains mild abrasives (ah-**BRAY**-sihvs), which are used for smoothing or sanding, such as tin oxide, talc, silica, and kaolin. Dry nail polish is available in powder and cream form.

Colored polish, liquid enamel, or lacquer (**LAK**-er). Colored polish is used to add color and gloss to the nail. It is usually applied in two coats. Colored polish contains a solution of nitrocellulose in a volatile solvent, such as amyl acetate and evaporates easily. Manufacturers add castor oil to prevent the polish from drying too rapidly.

Base coat. The base coat is colorless and is applied to the natural nail before the application of colored polish. It prevents red or dark polish from yellowing or staining the nail plate. Base coat is the first polish you apply in the polish procedure, unless you are using a nail strengthener. It contains more resin than colored polish to maintain a tacky surface so the colored polish will adhere better. It contains ethyl acetate, a solvent, isopropyl alcohol, butyl acetate, nitrocellulose, resin, and sometimes formaldehyde.

Nail strengthener/hardener. Nail strengthener is applied to the natural nail before the base coat. It prevents splitting and peeling of the nail. There are three types of nail strengthener:

Protein hardener is a combination of clear polish and protein, such as collagen.

Nylon fiber is a combination of clear polish with nylon fibers. It is applied first vertically and then horizontally on the nail plate. It can be hard to cover because the fibers on the nail are visible.

Formaldehyde strengthener contains 5 percent formaldehyde.

Top coat or sealer. The top coat, a colorless polish, is applied over colored polish to prevent chipping and add a shine to the finished nail. It contains nitrocellulose, toluene (**TOL**-yoo-een), a solvent, isopropyl alcohol, and polyester resins.

Liquid nail dry. Liquid "nail dry" is used to prevent smudging of the polish. It promotes rapid drying so that the polish is not tacky and prevents the polish from dulling. It has an alcohol base and is available in brush-on or spray.

Hand cream and hand lotion. Hand lotion and hand cream add a finishing touch to a manicure. Since they soften and smooth the hands, they make the finished manicure as beautiful as possible. Hand cream helps the skin retain moisture, so hands are not dry, cracked, and wrinkled. Hand cream is thicker than hand lotion and is made of emollients and humectants, such as glycerin, cocoa butter, lecithin, and gums. Hand lotion has a thinner consistency than hand cream because it contains more oil. In addition to oil, hand lotion contains stearic acid, water, mucilage of quince seed as a healing agent, lanolin, glycerin, and gum. Hand cream or hand lotion can be used as oil in a reconditioning hot oil manicure.

Nail conditioner contains moisturizers, and should be applied at night before bedtime to help prevent brittle nails and dry cuticles.

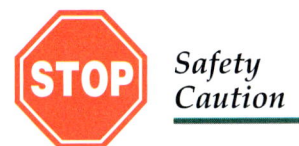

Safety Caution

All nail polishes are flammable.

PROCEDURE FOR BASIC TABLE SET-UP

It is important that your manicure table is sanitary and properly equipped with implements, materials, and cosmetics. Anything you need during a service should be at your fingertips. Having an orderly table will give you and your client confidence during the manicure. The actual placement of supplies on the manicuring table is a suggestion. Since regulations regarding table set-up vary from state to state, be guided by your instructor. To set up your table, use the following procedure.

0. tape plastic bag

1. Wipe manicure table with approved disinfectant.

2. Wrap your client's cushion with a clean, sanitized towel, either terry cloth or disposable. Put it in the middle of the table so the cushion is towards the client and the end of towel is towards you.

3. Fill the disinfection container with an approved hospital-grade disinfectant 20 minutes before your first manicure of the day. Put all metal implements into the disinfection container. Place the disinfection container to your right if you are right-handed, or to your left if you are left-handed.

4. Put the cosmetics (except polish) on the right side of the table behind your disinfection container (if left-handed, place on left).

5. Put emery boards on chamois buffer on the table to your right (if left-handed, to the left).

6. Put fingerbowl and brush in the middle or to the left, towards the client. The fingerbowl or hot oil heater should not be moved from side to side of the manicure table. It should stay where you put it for the duration of your manicure. If you're doing a reconditioning hot oil manicure, replace fingerbowl and brush with electric hot oil heater.

7. Tape or clip a plastic bag to right side of table (if left-handed, tape to left side). This is used for depositing used materials during your manicure.

8. Put polishes to the left (if left-handed, place on right).

9. Your drawer can be used to keep the following items: extra cotton or cotton balls in their original container or in a fresh plastic bag; pumice stone or powder; extra chamois for buffer; instant nail dry or other supplies. Be sure to wipe drawer with

an approved hospital-grade disinfectant before putting supplies in it. Never place used materials in your drawer. Only completely sanitized implements (sealed in air-tight containers) and extra materials or cosmetics should be placed in this drawer. Always keep it clean and sanitary. (Fig. 10.10)

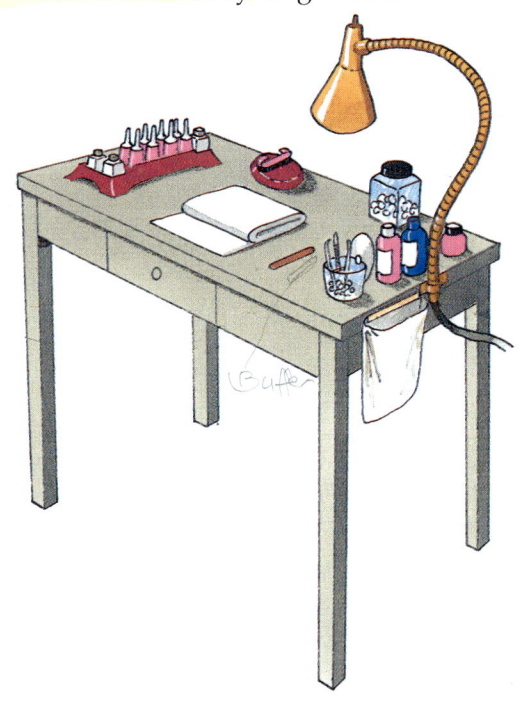

10.10 — Basic table set-up. Your instructor's table set-up is equally correct.

CHOOSING A NAIL SHAPE

After the client consultation, you will discuss what shape and color nails your client wants. Keep the following considerations in mind: the shape of the hands, length of fingers, shape of the cuticles, and the type of work clients do. The following are four shapes from which to choose. (Fig. 10.11)

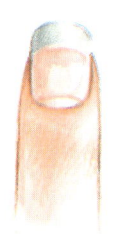

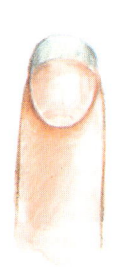

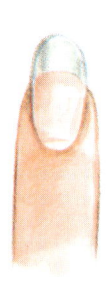

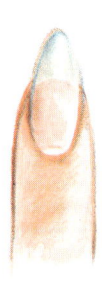

10.11 — The four basic nail shapes: rectangular, round, oval, and pointed.

- The *rectangular or square nail* should extend only slightly past the tip of the finger with the free edge rounded off. This shape is sturdy because the full width of the nail remains at the free edge. Clients who work with their hands—on a typewriter, computer, or assembly line—will need shorter, square nails.

- The *round nail* should be slightly tapered and extend just a bit past the tip of the finger. Round nails are the most common choice for male clients because of their natural shape.

- The *oval nail* is an attractive nail shape for most women's hands. It is a square nail with slightly rounded corners. Professional clients who have their hands on display (professional business people, teachers, or salespeople, for example) may want longer oval nails.

- The *pointed nail* is suited to thin hands with narrow nail beds. The nail is tapered somewhat longer than usual to enhance the slender appearance of the hand; however, these nails are weak and break easily.

WATER MANICURE

As a professional nail technician, you will follow a three-part procedure for all services you perform. First, in the Pre-Service, you will sanitize, greet your client, and do a client consultation. Next you will do the steps in the actual Procedure. Then, in the Post-Service, you will schedule another appointment for your client, sell the retail products you have suggested during the service, and sanitize.

WATER MANICURE PRE-SERVICE

1. **Do your Pre-Service Sanitation Procedure.** (This procedure is described on pages 32-33.)

2. **Set up your standard manicuring table.**

3. **Greet client.** (Fig. 10.12)

4. **Wash client's hands.** Have client wash hands with antibacterial soap. Thoroughly dry hands and nails with a sanitized towel.

5. **Do client consultation.** Use the client record/health card to record responses and observations. Check for nail disorders and decide if it is safe and appropriate to perform a service on this client. If the client should not receive service, explain your reasons and refer him or her to a doctor. If you plan to proceed, discuss the service your client wants.

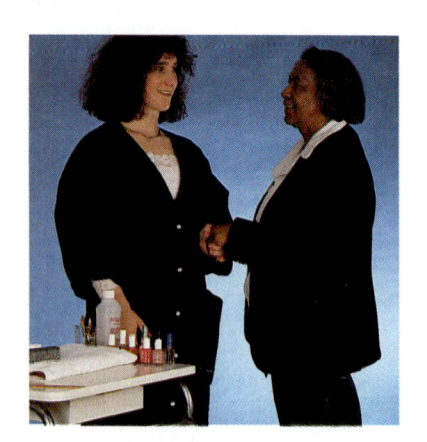

10.12 — Greet client.

CHAPTER 10   MANICURING   127

6. **Begin manicure.** Begin working with the hand that is **not** the client's favored hand. The favored hand will need to soak longer, because it is used more often. If the client is left-handed, begin with the right hand and if the client is right-handed, begin with the left hand.

WATER MANICURE PROCEDURE

During the manicure, talk with your client about the products and procedures you are using. Suggest products our client will need to maintain the manicure between salon visits. These products might include polish, lotion, top coat, and emery boards.

✤ **NOTE:** The procedure is written for a right-handed client.

1. **Remove polish.** Begin with your client's left hand, little finger. Saturate cotton with polish remover. If your client is wearing artificial nails, use non-acetone remover to avoid damaging them. Hold saturated cotton on nail while you count to ten in your mind. Wipe the old polish off the nail with a stroking motion towards the free edge. If all polish is not removed, repeat this step until all traces of polish are gone. It may be necessary to put cotton around the tip of an orangewood stick and use it to clean polish away from the cuticle area. Repeat this procedure on each finger. (Fig. 10.13)

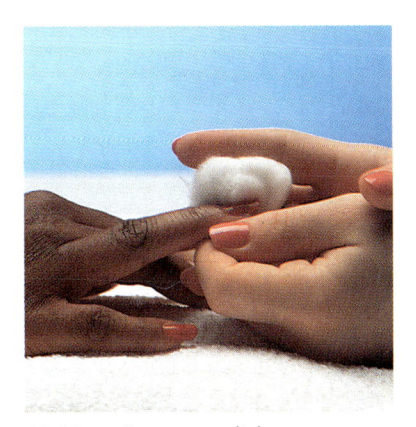

10.13 — Remove polish.

PROCEDURAL TIP

*Roll a piece of cotton between your hands before you use it. This keeps loose cotton fibers from sticking to the nail or finger. An alternative way to remove nail polish is to moisten small pieces of cotton, called pledgets (**PLEJ**-ets), with nail polish remover and put them on all the nails at the same time. Pledgets absorb and do not leave a polish smear on the cuticles.*

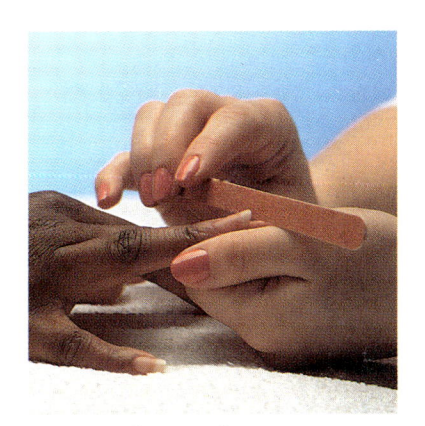

2. **Shape the nails.** Using your emery board or nail file, shape the nails as you and the client have agreed. Start with the left hand, little finger, holding it between your thumb and index finger. Use the coarse side of an emery board to shape the nail. File from the right side to the center of the free edge and from the left side to the center of the free edge. (Fig. 10.14) Do not file into the corners of the nails. (Fig. 10.15) File each hand from the little finger to the thumb.

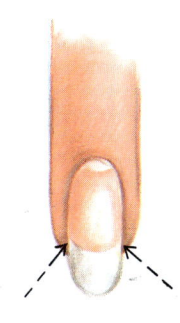

10.14 — Shape nails.

3. **Soften cuticles.** After filing left hand, put it in your soap bath to soak and soften cuticles while you file the right hand.

10.15 — Do not file into the corners of the nail.

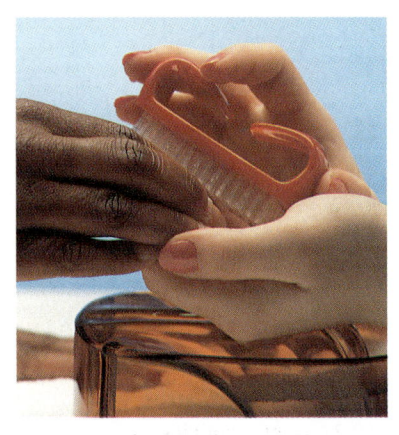

128 ◆ PART 3 BASIC PROCEDURES

4. **Clean nails.** Brushing nails and hands with a nail brush cleans fingers and pieces of cuticle from the nails. Remove the left hand from the soap bath and brush the fingers with your nail brush. Use downward strokes, starting at the first knuckle and brushing toward the free edge. (Fig. 10.16)

5. **Dry hand.** Dry the hand with the end of a fresh towel. Make sure you dry between the fingers. As you dry, gently push back the cuticle. (Fig. 10.17)

6. **Apply cuticle remover.** Use a cotton-tipped orangewood stick to apply cuticle remover to the cuticle of each nail on the hand you've just brushed. (Fig. 10.18) Saturate cotton with cuticle remover an spread generously around cuticles an dunder the free edge of each finger. This softens and removes cuticle that remains after brushing. Now, put the right hand into the soap bath to soak while you continue to work on your client's left hand. (Fig. 10.19)

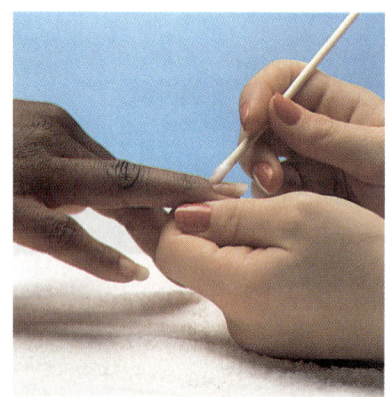

10.16 — Clean nails.

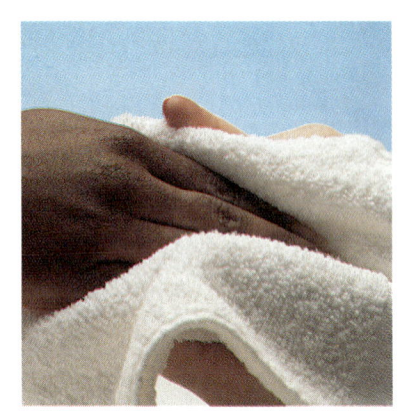

10.17 — Dry hand.

10.18 — Apply cuticle remover.

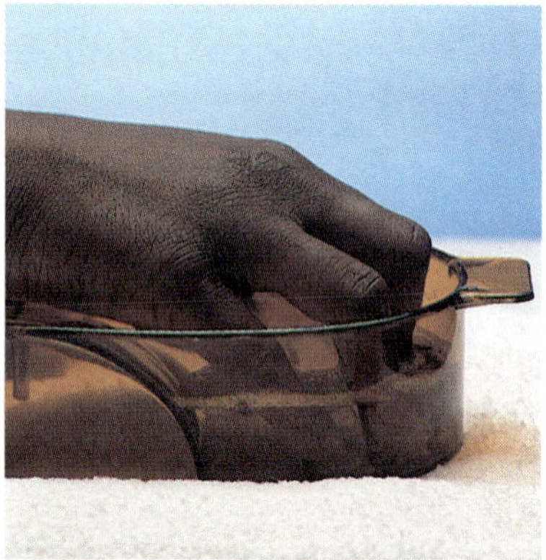

10.19 — Soak hand.

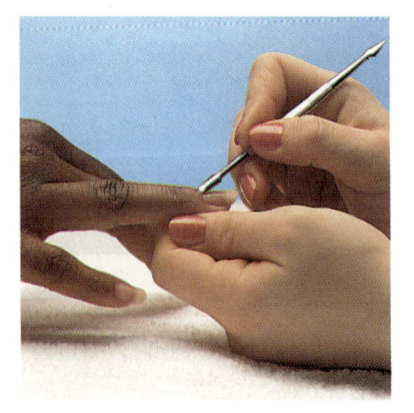

7. **Loosen cuticles.** Use your orangewood stick and/or the spoon end of your steel pusher to gently push back and lift cuticle off of the nails of the left hand. Use a circular movement to help lift cuticles that cling to the nail plate. The cuticle remover will probably remove enough cuticle so that you won't need to clip any. (Fig. 10.20)

8. **Nip cuticles.** Use your cuticle nippers to nip any ragged excess cuticle or hangnails. Try to remove cuticle in one piece. You may need to wipe away excess cuticle remover to see the cuticle

10.20 — Loosen cuticle.

clearly. Be careful not to cut into the mantle, because you will hurt your client. (Fig. 10.21)

> **STATE REGULATION ALERT**
>
> *Some states do not permit nail technicians to nip cuticles or hangnails. Be guided by your instructor.*

9. **Clean under free edge.** Clean under the free edge using a cotton-tipped orangewood stick. Remove right hand from soap bath. Hold left hand over soap bath and brush a last time to remove bits of cuticle and traces of solvent. Then let client rest the left hand on the sanitized towel. (Fig. 10.22)

10. **Repeat steps 4-9 on right hand.**

11. **Bleach nails—optional.** After the filing and cleaning steps, if the client's nails are yellow, you can bleach them with a prepared nail bleach or apply 20 volume (6 percent) hydrogen peroxide. Apply the bleaching agent to the yellowed nail with a cotton-tipped orangewood stick. Be careful not to brush bleach on your client's skin or cuticle, because it will cause irritation. Apply several times if nails are extremely yellow. You may need to bleach certain clients' nails every time you manicure them for a period of time. Since all yellow may not fade after one service, you should plan to repeat the procedure when the client gets the next manicure.

12. **Buff with chamois buffer—optional.** To buff nails, apply dry nail polish to the nail with your orangewood stick. Buff on a diagonal from the base of the nail to its free edge. (Fig. 10.23) Buff in one direction, from left to right with a downward stroke and then from right to left with a downward stroke, forming an "X" pattern. (Fig. 10.24) As you buff, lift the back

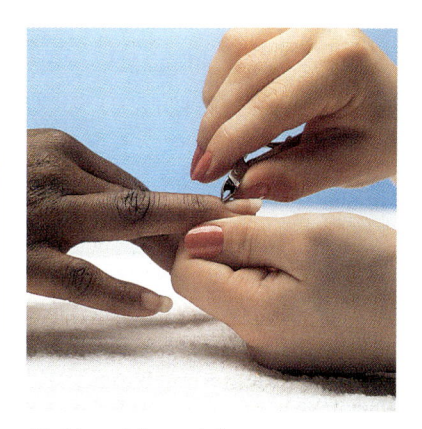

10.21 — Nip cuticles.

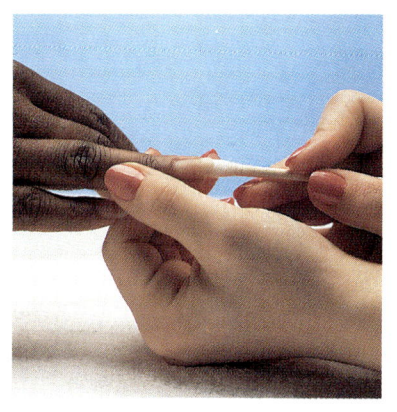

10.22 — Clean under free edge.

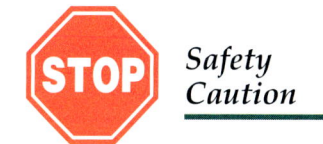

Safety Caution

When the cuticle is difficult to push back, be careful not to apply too much pressure at the base of the nail because it could damage the matrix.

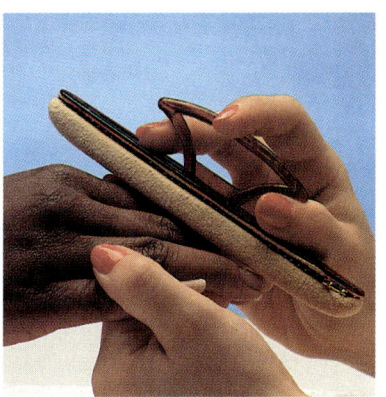

10.23 — Buff nail.

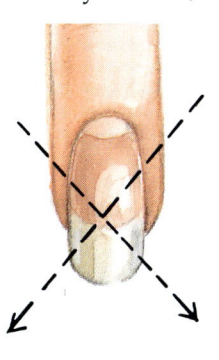

10.24 — Buff nail in an "X" pattern with downward strokes.

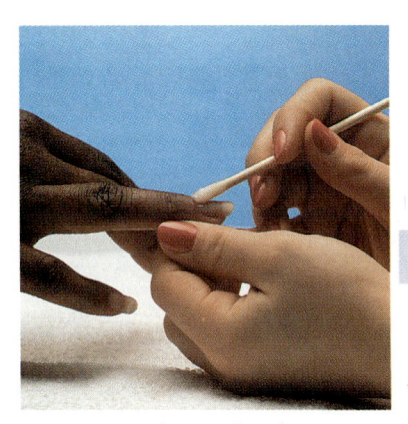

10.25 — Apply cuticle oil.

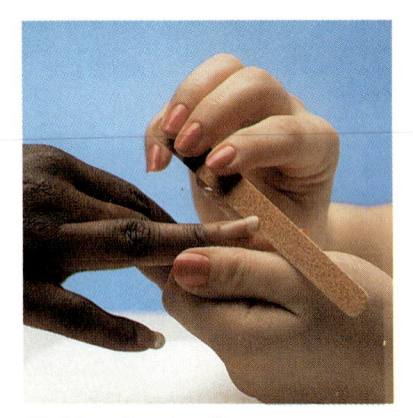

10.26 — Bevel nail.

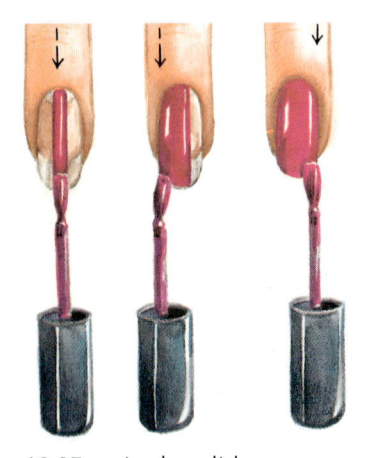

10.27 — Apply polish.

of the buffer off the nail to prevent friction that can cause your client to experience a burning sensation. After buffing, client should wash hands to remove any traces of abrasive or dry polish. The chamois buffer can also be used to smooth out wavy ridges or corrugated nails.

PROCEDURAL TIP

You may want to spray your client's nail with water before buffing to reduce the heat generated during buffing.

13. **Apply cuticle oil.** Use a cotton-tipped orangewood stick to apply cuticle oil to each nail. Start with the little finger, left hand, and rub oil into each cuticle in a circular motion. (Fig. 10.25)

14. **Bevel nails.** To bevel (BEH-vel) the underside of the free edge, hold emery board at a 45 degree angle, and file with an upward stroke. This removes any rough edges or cuticle particles. (Fig. 10.26)

15. **Apply hand lotion and massage hand and arm.** As a pleasant touch to your manicure before you apply polish, you can treat your client to a hand massage. Apply lotion or cream to the hand and arm with a sanitary spatula. (Follow the procedure for hand and arm massage on pages 140-143.)

16. **Remove traces of oil.** You must remove traces of oil from the nail so the polish will adhere better. Use a small piece of cotton saturated with alcohol or polish remover, and wipe off the nail.

17. **Choose a color.** If your client is undecided about the color of the nail polish, help her choose one. Suggest a shade that complements the skin tone. If the manicure and polish are for a special occasion, pick a color that matches the client's clothing. Generally, darker shades are appropriate for fall and winter and lighter shades are better for spring and summer. Always have a variety of nail polish colors available. Before applying polish, you may ask your client to pay for the service, put on any sweater or jacket, and get out car keys. This will avoid smudges to the fresh polish.

18. **Apply polish.** Polish is applied in four coats. The first, the base coat, is followed by two coats of color and one application of top coat. (Fig. 10.27) Roll the polish in your palms to mix. Never shake your polish. Shaking causes air bubbles to form, which will make the polish application rough.

- **Base coat.** Base coat is applied first to keep polish from staining the nails and to help colored polish adhere to the nail. The base coat will stay tacky to the touch. To apply the base coat, take the brush out of the bottle and wipe one side on the neck of the bottle. You should have a bead of polish on the end of the brush. Start in the center of the nail, position brush 1/16 inch away from the cuticle, and brush toward free edge. Using the same technique, do left side of nail, then right side. You should have enough polish on the brush to complete three strokes without having to dip the brush into the polish bottle. If you go back and dab at any spots you missed, the polish will not appear smooth on the nail. The more strokes you make, the more lines or lumps you will have on the client's nail. If you miss a small area on the first color coat, you can cover it on the second coat.

- **Colored polish.** Apply two coats of colored polish with the same technique used for the base coat. Complete your first color coat on both hands before starting the second coat. If you get polish on the cuticle, use a cotton-tipped orangewood stick saturated with polish remover to clean it off. never use a polish corrector pen because it is unsanitary.

- **Top coat.** Apply one coat of top coat to prevent chipping and to give nails a glossy look.

- **Instant nail dry—optional.** Apply instant nail dry on each nail to prevent smudging and dulling.

PROCEDURAL TIP

If you use an electric nail dryer, put one of your client's hands in the dryer while you polish the other. Put setting on cool; this helps to dry polish surface and make it less likely to smudge.

Five Types of Polish Application

You have learned how to apply polish correctly to a fingernail. You can crate the five types of polished nails listed below:

1. **Full Coverage.** Entire nail plate is polished.

2. **Free edge.** The free edge of the nail is unpolished. This helps to prevent polish from chipping.

3. **Hairline tip.** The nail plate is polished and 1/16 inch is removed from the free edge. This prevents polish from chipping.

4. **Slimline or free walls.** Leave 1/16 inch margin on each side of nail plate. This makes a wide nail appear narrow.

5. **Half moon or lunula.** A half moon shape, the lunula, at the base of the nail is unpolished. (Fig. 10.28)

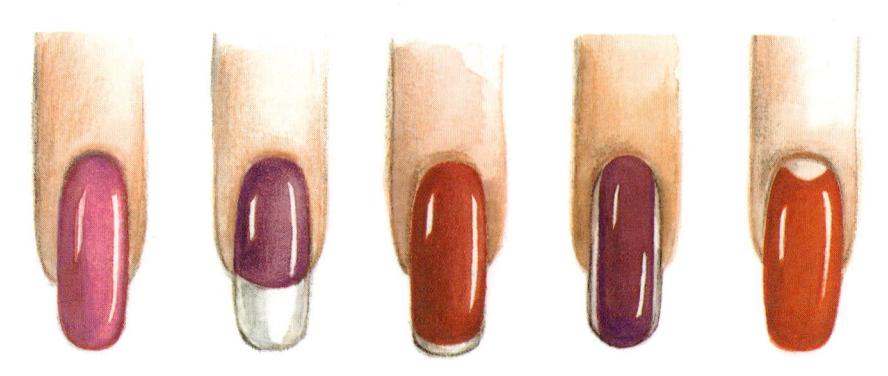

10.28 — Five polish options: full coverag;, free edge; hair line tip; slim line or free wall; half moon or lunula

> ### PROCEDURAL TIP
> If you smudge on a finished nail, apply polish remover to the smudge before you put polish on again.

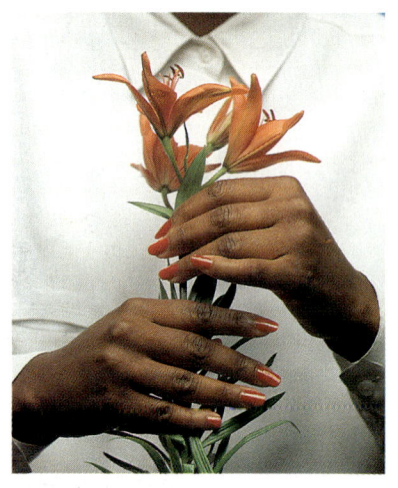

10.29 — Finished water manicure

WATER MANICURE POST-SERVICE

Your water manicure is complete. Follow the post-service procedure described below. (Fig. 10.29)

1. **Make another appointment.** Schedule another appointment with your client to maintain the manicure or to perform another service.

2. **Sell retail products.** Suggest that your client buy products you have discussed during the manicure. Polish, lotion, top coat, etc. are valuable tools for maintaining the nails between salon visits.

3. **Clean up around your table.** Take the time to restore the basic set-up of your table.

4. **Discard used materials.** Place all used materials in the plastic bag at the side of the table. If the bag is full or contains used materials from artificial nail services, discard it in a closed pail.

5. **Sanitize table and implements.** Perform the complete pre-service sanitation procedure. Implements must be sanitized for 20 minutes before they can be used on the next client.

FRENCH MANICURE

A French manicure is a clean and natural polish application that is very popular in summer months and for weddings. It is also a great base for nail art. You can create endless artistic designs with pearls, rhinestones, and silver striping tapes.

1. **Apply base coat.** Follow the water manicure procedure through the application of base coat. Apply a base coat to the nail as you learned in the water manicure. The base coat can be applied under the free edge as well.

2. **Apply white polish.** Apply white polish to the free edge by starting at one side (usually left side of nail) and sweeping across toward the center of the free edge on a diagonal line. Repeat this on the right side of the nail. This will form a "V" shape. Some clients like this look. If not, fill the open top of the "V," so that you have an even line across the free edge. White may be applied under the free edge. (Figs. 10.30, 10.31, 10.32)

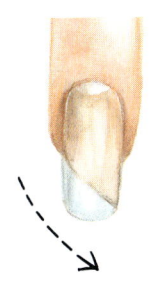

10.30 — Apply white polish on free edge from the left side of the nail to the center.

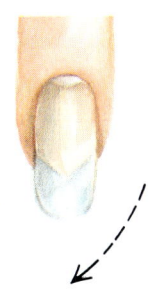

10.31 — Apply white polish on free edge from the right side of the nail to the center.

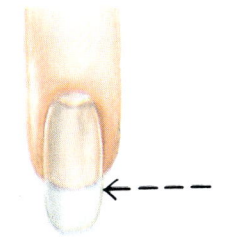

10.32 — Fill in "V" with white polish.

3. **Apply sheer pink, natural, or peach polish.** Apply a sheer pink, natural, or peach color polish from the base to the free edge. Be careful not to get any on the cuticle. Most clients will prefer a pink shade, but choose the color according to skin tone and client preference.

4. **Apply top coat.** Apply a top coat over the entire nail plate and under the free edge if you chose to put it under the free edge previously. (Fig. 10.33)

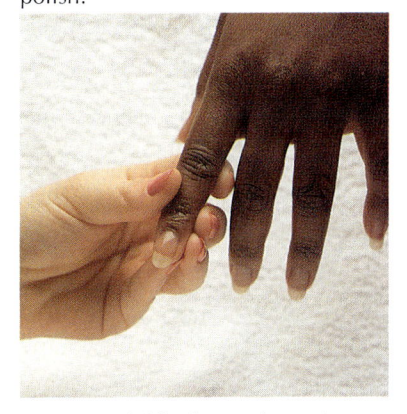

10.33 — Finished French manicure

RECONDITIONING HOT OIL MANICURE

A reconditioning hot oil manicure is of particular benefit to clients who have ridged and brittle nails or dry cuticles. It also improves the hands because it leaves the skin soft. A reconditioning hot oil manicure is recommended once a week. It will add moisture to skin and nails. The oil manicure is especially recommended for a nail biter, because it keeps rough cuticles or hangnails soft.

SUPPLIES

In addition to your standard table set-up, you will need the following items:

1. **Hot oil heater.** This electric heater is used for immersing the client's fingers in the hot oil or cream.
2. **Plastic cups to put in heater.** Most hot oil heaters are made to hold a round or kidney-shaped disposable cup that is filled with lotion, cream, or oil. This cup comes in multiple packs and should be discarded after each manicure.
3. **Oil for the heater.** Most nail technicians use an oil or cream that is specially prepared for the hot oil heater. Olive oil or hand lotion can also be used. In this procedure, all of these items are referred to as lotion.

RECONDITIONING HOT OIL MANICURE PRE-SERVICE

1. **Do your Pre-service Sanitation Procedure.**
2. **Set up table.** Set up your standard manicuring table, hot oil heater with plastic cup, and lotion.
3. **Prepare heater.** Pour lotion into a disposable cup and place it in the heater.
4. **Preheat lotion.** Preheat lotion for 10-15 minutes before seating your client to begin your manicure.
5. **Greet client.**
6. **Wash client's hands.** Have client wash hands with antibacterial soap. Dry hands thoroughly with a fresh towel.
7. **Do client consultation.**
8. **Begin manicure.** Begin working with the hand that is not the client's favored hand.

RECONDITIONING HOT OIL MANICURE PROCEDURE

During the procedure talk with your client about the products needed to maintain the manicure between salon visits.

1. **Remove old polish.**
2. **Shape nails.** Shape the nails on the hand that is not the client's favored hand.
3. **Put fingertips in hot lotion.** After shaping the nails on one hand, put it in the hot lotion and file the other hand. (Fig. 10.34)

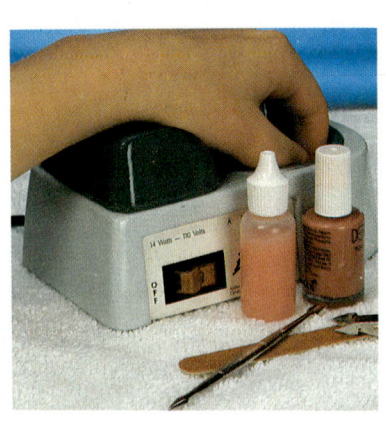

10.34 — Immerse fingertips in hot lotion.

CHAPTER 10 MANICURING ◆ 135

4. **Distribute lotion.** When you remove one hand from the lotion, place the other hand in the lotion. Spread lotion on the hand and arm to the elbow. This will give you enough lotion for the massage. If you run out of lotion, use your spatula to dip more out of the heater and apply it to the hand or arm where needed.
5. **Proceed with hand and arm massage.** Follow the procedure for hand and arm massage described on pages 141-143.
6. **Loosen cuticles.** Use orangewood stick to gently push back cuticles.
7. **Nip cuticles.** Use nippers to nip excess cuticle, if permitted in your state. Let client rest hand on sanitized towel.
8. **Repeat on other hand.** Distribute lotion on the other hand. Proceed with steps 5-7.
9. **Wipe or wash hands.** If necessary, take a warm terry towel and wipe off excess lotion, or have client wash hands.
10. **Apply cold towel.** Close pores on arm and hand with a cold towel. Wrap towel around arm and hand and gently press.
11. **Remove traces of oil.** Saturate cotton in alcohol or polish remover and wipe oil from nails.
12. **Apply polish.**
13. **Complete Manicure Post-Service.** Discard the plastic cup from the hot oil heater.
14. **Sanitize heater.** Use alcohol to prepare the hot oil heater for the next client.

MAN'S MANICURE

A man's manicure is basically the same as a woman's manicure. Table set-up will be the same, except that color polish will not be used. Some men will like a clear liquid polish, and others will prefer a dry polish with your chamois buffer. Using hand cream or lotion is optional. (Fig. 10.35)

PROCEDURE

During the procedure, talk with your client about products that will help him maintain the manicure between visits. You might suggest clear polish and hand cream.

1. **Complete Manicure Pre-Service.**
2. **Remove old polish.** If the client has clear polish from a previous manicure, it must be removed. Begin with his left hand, little finger.

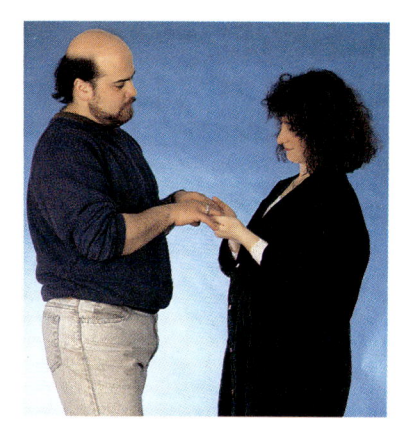

10.35 — Greet client.

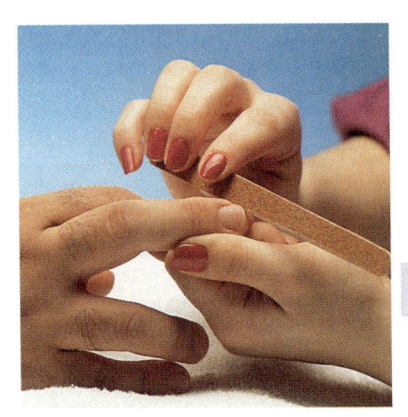

10.36 — Shape nails.

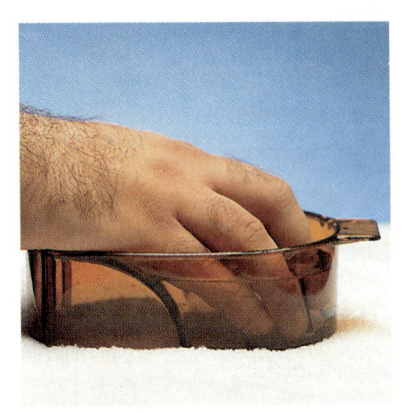

10.37 — Soften cuticles.

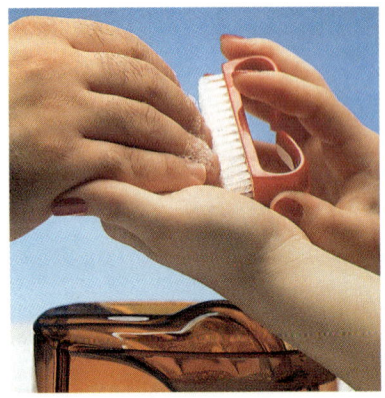

10.38 — Clean nails.

3. **Shape the nails.** Using your emery board or nail file, shape the nails. Start with the left hand, little finger, holding it between your thumb and index finger. You probably won't have much to file; most men keep their nails short. If nails are long, clip them with fingernail clippers before you file. (Fig. 10.36)

PROCEDURAL TIP

Never file nails that have been soaking. Soaking makes nails soft and easy to break or split when filed.

4. **Soften cuticles.** After filing left hand, put it in your soap bath to soak and soften cuticles while you file the right hand. (Fig. 10.37)

5. **Clean nails and hands.** Brushing hands and nails with the nail brush cleans fingers and pieces of cuticle from nails. Remove left hand from the soap bath and brush the fingers with your nail brush in downward strokes, starting at the first knuckle and brushing in one direction toward the free edge. (Fig. 10.38)

6. **Dry hand.** Dry the hand with the end of the towel that is wrapped around the cushion. Make sure you dry between the fingers. As you dry, gently push back the cuticle. (Fig. 10.39)

7. **Apply cuticle remover.** Use a cotton-tipped orangewood stick to apply cuticle remover to the back of each nail on the hand you've just brushed. Now, put the right hand into the soap bath to soak while you continue to work on your client's left hand. (Fig. 10.40)

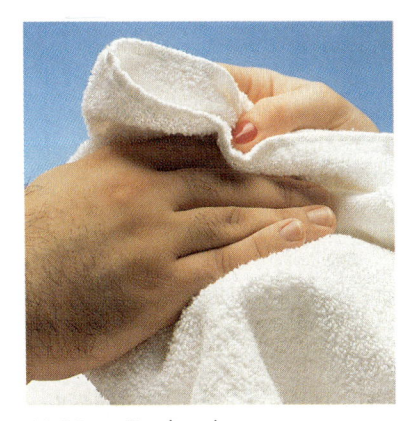

10.39 — Dry hand.

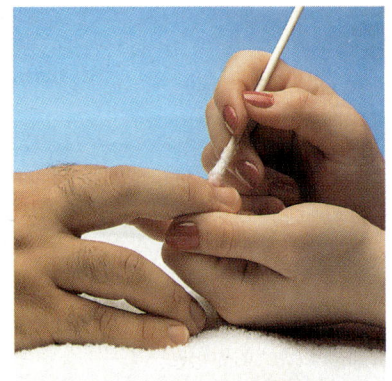

10.40 — Apply cuticle remover.

CHAPTER 10   MANICURING ◆ **137**

8. **Loosen cuticles.** Most men will need more work done on their cuticles, as they will generally have more cuticle than women. Women tend to push their own cuticles back between appointments, whereas men don't. Use pusher to gently push back and lift cuticle off of the nails of the left hand. (Fig. 10.41)

9. **Nip cuticles.** If you have to nip excess cuticle or hangnails, try to do so in one piece. (Fig. 10.42)

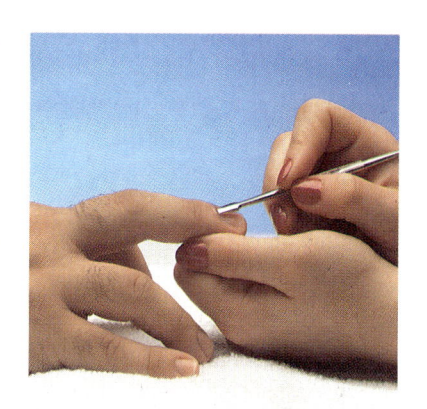

10.41 — Loosen cuticle with pusher.

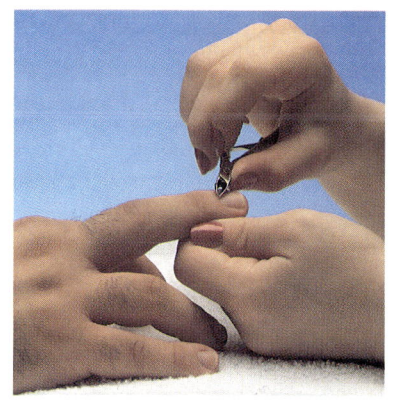

10.42 — Nip cuticles.

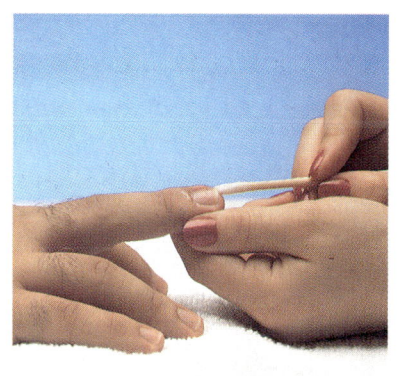

10.43 — Clean under free edge.

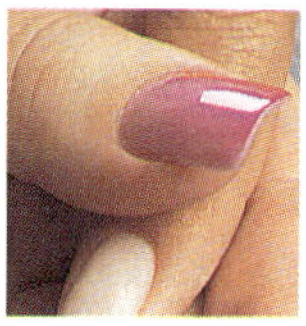

Sanitation Caution

The cotton on your orangewood stick needs to be changed after each use.

STATE REGULATION ALERT

Some states do not permit nail technicians to nip cuticles or hangnails. Be guided by your instructor.

10. **Clean under free edge.** Clean under the free edge with a cotton-tipped orangewood stick. Hold left hand over soap bath and brush a last time to remove bits of cuticle and traces of solvent that remain on the nail. Then let client put the left hand on a sanitized towel. (Fig. 10.43)

11. **Repeat steps 5-10 on right hand.**

12. **Bleach nails—optional.** If the client's nails are yellow you can bleach them with a prepared nail bleach or by applying 20 volume (6 percent) hydrogen peroxide.

13. **Buff with chamois buffer.** If you and your client wish, you can buff nails at this point. To shine nails, apply dry nail polish to the nail with your orangewood stick, buffing on a diagonal from the base of the nail to its free edge. Buff in one direction, from left to right, with a downward stroke and cross over from right to left with a downward stroke, forming an "X" pattern. As you buff, lift the back of the buffer off the nail to prevent friction that can cause your client to experience a burning sensation on the nail. After buffing, client should wash hands to

remove any traces of abrasive or dry polish. The chamois buffer can also be used to smooth out wavy ridges or corrugated nails. This is done with an abrasive, such as pumice powder, which is applied to the nail with an orangewood stick. (Fig. 10.44)

> ### STATE REGULATION ALERT
>
> *Some states do not permit the use of a chamois buffer. If they do, chamois must be changed for each client. Be guided by your instructor.*

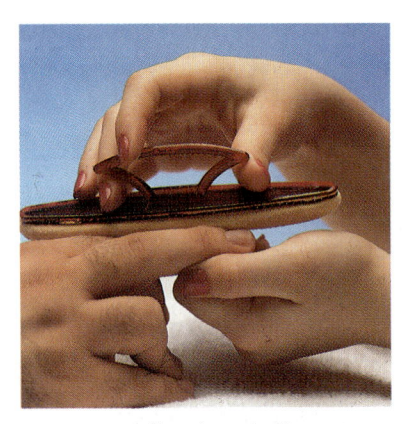

10.44 — Buff nails with chamois buffer.

14. **Apply cuticle oil.** Use a cotton-tipped orangewood stick to apply cuticle oil to each nail. Start with the little finger, left hand and rub oil into each cuticle in a circular motion. (Fig. 10.45)

15. **Bevel nails.** To bevel the underside of the free edge, hold emery board at a 45 degree angle, and file with an upward stroke. This removes any rough edges or cuticle particles.

16. **Apply hand lotion and massage hand and arm—optional.** As a pleasant touch to your manicure before you apply polish, you can treat your client to a hand lotion or hand cream massage. Apply lotion or cream to the arm and hand with a sanitary spatula. (Follow the procedure for hand and arm massage on pages 141-143.) (Fig. 10.46)

17. **Remove traces of oil.** Remove traces of oil by using a small piece of cotton that has been saturated with alcohol or polish remover. Wipe off the nail to allow polish to adhere better.

18. **Polish nails.** If your client wants polish, apply a base coat and a clear top coat. Follow with instant nail dry. (Fig. 10.47)

19. **Complete Manicure Post-Service Procedure.**

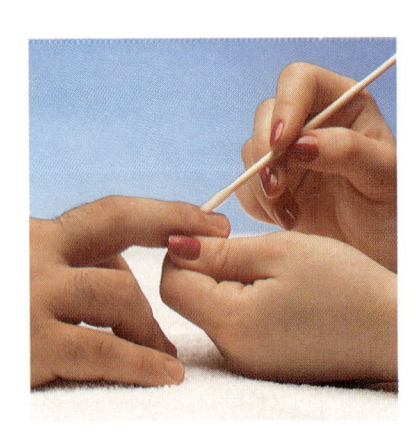

10.45 — Apply cuticle oil.

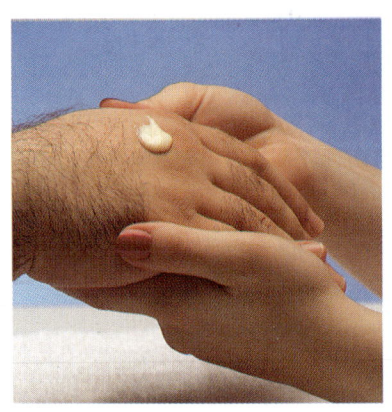

10.46 — Apply hand lotion.

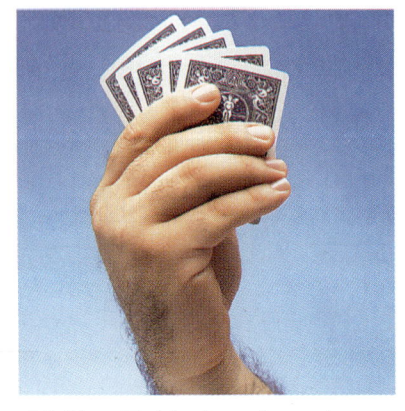

10.47 — Finished man's manicure

The Male Nail

With today's emphasis on good grooming, more and more men are interested in taking care of their nails. Unfortunately, many are unaware of their nails. Alert the male public to your nail services by advertising in the business and sports pages of local publications. Since most men are new to nail care, don't forget to include a brief written description of what the services entail and a rundown of their benefits. You may also want to distribute flyers at local gyms, athletic stores and other places where men gather. Still another option is selling gift certificates to your female clients for their boyfriends and husbands. To make men feel more at home in your chair, have men's magazines on hand and be careful that your decor is unisex. Staying open later or opening earlier makes it easier for working men and women to schedule appointments.

ELECTRIC MANICURE

The electric manicure is given with a small portable machine with a motor. The electric manicure tool looks like a portable drill. It uses a variety of attachments that include an emery wheel, cuticle pusher, brush, and nail buffing disk.

Before using an electric manicure machine, read the manufacturer's instructions carefully. State regulations on this procedure may vary.

Care should be taken with the attachments. Do not apply too much pressure at the base of the nail with the cuticle pusher and buffer. Do not hold in one spot because it will cause a burning sensation.

The emery wheel or nail shaper is like your emery board. It has a coarse side and a fine side. The cuticle pusher is like your steel pusher. It is used to push back excess cuticle. The nail brush is like the nail brush used in a water manicure. It is used to remove small bits of cuticle and to cleanse the nail. The buffing disk works like your chamois buffer. It is used to smooth corrugations and add shine to the nail. Be careful when you use the buffer because it causes a burning sensation on the nail if you apply too much pressure. Be sure to lift it frequently to prevent this or mist the nail with water before buffing.

Your electric manicure machine may include a callus remover disk. It is much coarser than the emery disk and is shaped like a cylinder. Use it around tip of finger or at the side to remove callus growth.

> **STATE REGULATION ALERT**
>
> *Some states do not permit the use of an electric manicure machine. Be guided by your instructor.*

PARAFFIN WAX

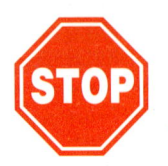

Paraffin (wax) was first used by doctors as a therapeutic treatment. It works by trapping heat and moisture in and opening up pores in the skin. The heat from the warm paraffin increases the blood supply to the skin, giving skin that was rough and dry a fresh, soft, healthy feeling.

Paraffin is a petroleum by-product that has excellent heat sealing properties. Special units are utilized to melt solid wax into a liquid that is then maintained at a temperature generally between 125 and 130 degrees Fahrenheit. Be sure to follow instructions for whichever unit you may use. Also, if you do provide this service, use equipment that is designed especially for this treatment. Do not try to heat wax in anything other than the right equipment. This service requires wax and a heater.

Paraffin treatments are ideal for the hands and feet. The treatments are especially beneficial for senior citizens and people with arthritis. However, anyone can enjoy and benefit from a foot and/or hand paraffin treatment.

If proper procedures are followed, paraffin will not affect artificial nails, wraps, tips, gels, or natural nails. Just make sure all nail repair work is completed before the paraffin treatment, not after.

Massage the hands or feet with a rich emollient and dip each hand or foot into heated paraffin wax. Repeated dipping, with a few seconds between each immersion in the wax, causes the wax to build up slowly in layers and seals the lotion. After five to seven dips, wrap the hands or feet in plastic bags, slip them into insulated mitts, and ask your client to relax. After ten minutes, peel the wax off, much like a glove or a bootie. Your client's hands or feet will look healthy and feel soft.

🛑 Safety Caution

Read and follow all operating instructions. Generally you should avoid giving paraffin treatments to anyone who has impaired circulation or skin irritations such as cuts, burns, rashes, warts, eczema, or swollen veins.

HAND AND ARM MASSAGE

Massage is a service that can be offered with any type of manicure. Massaging stimulates blood flow, and is relaxing to the client.

HAND MASSAGE TECHNIQUES

1. **Relaxer movement.** This is a form of massage known as "joint movement." At the beginning of the hand massage the client has already received hand lotion or cream. Place client's elbow on cushion. With one hand, brace client's arm. With your other hand, hold client's wrist and bend it back and forth slowly, about five to ten times, until you feel the client has relaxed. (Fig. 10.48)

2. **Joint movement on fingers.** Bring client's arm down, brace the arm with the left hand, and with your right hand start with the little finger, holding it at the base of the nail. Gently rotate fingers to form circles. Work towards the thumb, about 3-5 times on each finger. (Fig. 10.49)

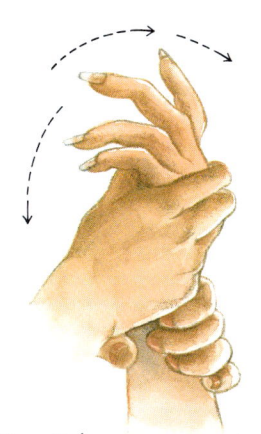

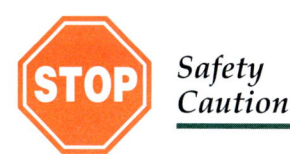

Safety Caution

DO NOT massage if client has high blood pressure, heart condition, or has had a stroke. Massage increases circulation and may be harmful to this client. Have client consult a physician first. Be very careful to avoid vigorous massage of joints if your client has arthritis. Talk with your client throughout the massage and adjust your touch to the client's needs.

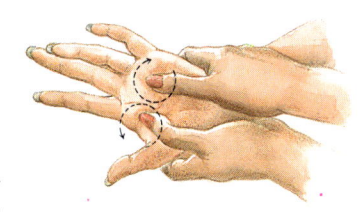

10.48 — Relaxer movement

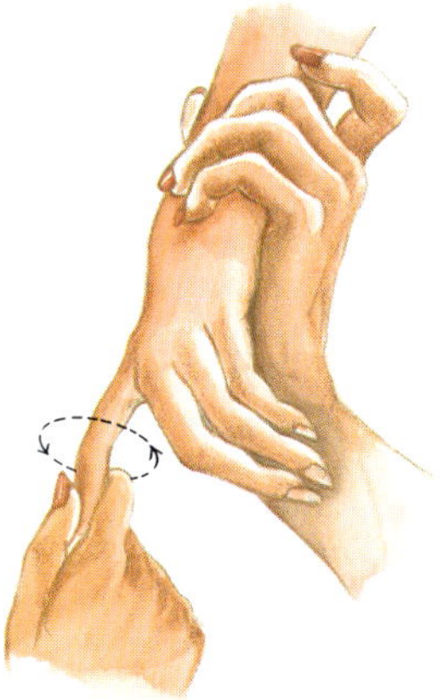

10.49 — Joint movement on fingers

3. **Circular movement in palm.** This is "effleurage" (**EF**-loo-rahzh)—light stroking that relaxes and soothes. Place client's elbow on the cushion and, with your thumbs in the client's palm, rotate in a circular movement in opposite directions. (Fig. 10.50)

4. **Circular movement on wrist.** Hold client's hand with both of your hands, placing your thumbs on top of client's hand, your fingers below the hand. Move your thumbs in a circular movement in opposite directions from the client's wrist to the knuckle on back of the client's hand. Move up and down, 3-5 times. The last time you rotate up, wring the client's wrist by bracing your hands around the wrist and gently twisting in opposite directions. This is a form of friction massage movement that is a deep rubbing action and very stimulating. (Fig. 10.51)

5. **Circular movement on back of hand and fingers.** Now rotate down the back of the client's hand using your thumbs. Rotate down the little finger and the client's thumb and gently

10.50 — Circular movement "Effleurage"

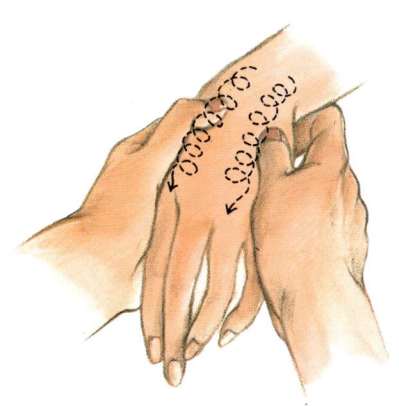

10.51 — Circular movement on wrist

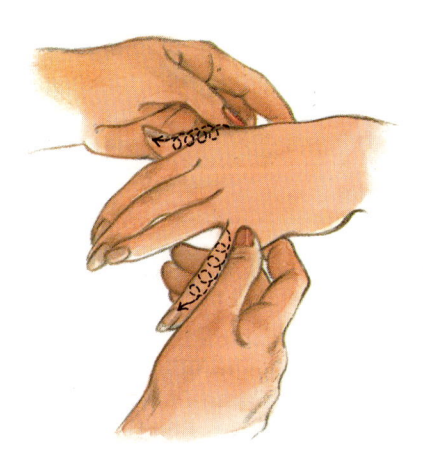

10.52 — Circular movement on back of hand and fingers

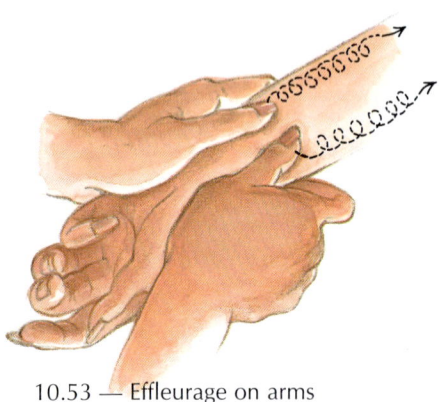

10.53 — Effleurage on arms

squeeze off at the tips of client's fingers. Go back and rotate down the ring finger and index finger, gently squeezing off. Now do the middle finger and squeeze off at tip. This restores blood flow to normal. (Fig. 10.52)

ARM MASSAGE TECHNIQUES

1. **Distribute cream or lotion.** Apply a small amount of cream to the client's arm and work it in. Work from the client's wrist toward the elbow, except on the last movement; work from the elbow to wrist, then squeeze off at fingertips, as you did at the end of hand massage. Apply more cream if necessary.

2. **Effleurage on arms.** Put client's arm down on the table, bracing the arm with your hands. Hold your client's hand palm up in your hand. Your fingers should be under the client's hand; your thumb side-by-side in your client's palm. Rotate your thumbs in opposite directions, starting at the client's wrist and working towards the elbow. When you reach the elbow, slide your hand down client's arm to the wrist and rotate back up to the elbow 3-5 times. Turn client's arm over and repeat 3-5 times on the top side of arm. (Fig. 10.53)

3. **Wringing movement on arm**—*friction massage movement.* A friction massage involves deep rubbing to the muscles. Bend client's elbow so the arm is horizontal in front of you, with the back of the hand facing up. Place your hands around the arm with your fingers facing the same direction as the arm, and gently twist in opposite directions as you would wring out a washcloth, from wrist to elbow. Do this up and down the forearm 3-5 times. (Fig. 10.54)

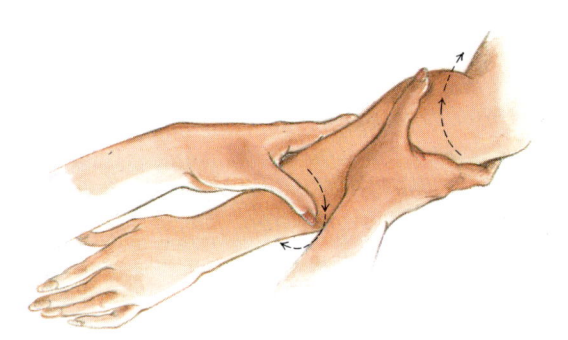

10.54 — Wringing movement on arm friction massage

4. **Kneading movement on arm.** This technique is called the petrissage (PE-tre-sahza) kneading movement. It is very stimulating and increases blood flow. Place your thumb on the top side of client's arm so they are horizontal. Move them in

opposite directions, from wrist to elbow and back down to wrist. This squeezing motion moves flesh over bone and stimulates the arm tissue. Do this 3-5 times. (Fig. 10.55)

5. **Rotation of elbow**—*friction massage movement.* Brace client's arm with your left hand and, with cotton-tipped orangewood stick, apply cream to elbow. Cup elbow with your right hand and rotate your hand over the client's elbow. Do this 3-5 times. To finish the elbow massage, move your left arm to the top of the client's forearm. Gently slide both hands down the forearm from the elbow to the fingertips as if climbing down a rope. Repeat this 3-5 times. (Fig. 10.56)

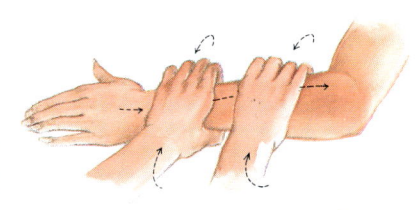

10.55 — Kneading movement on arm

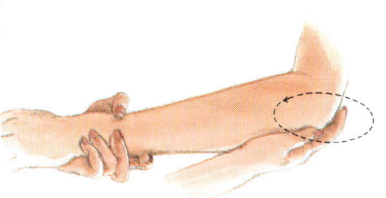

10.56 — Rotation of elbow

REVIEW QUESTIONS

1. When you give a manicure, you need equipment, implements, materials, and nail cosmetics. Give three examples of each of these manicuring supplies.
2. What are two reasons for having a manicuring table that is sanitary and properly equipped?
3. Describe the four basic nail shapes.
4. List the six steps in the water manicure pre-service.
5. Briefly describe the water manicure procedure.
6. Name the five types of polish applications.
7. List the five steps in the water manicure post-service.
8. List the four steps in the French manicure procedure.
9. What are the three benefits of the reconditioning hot oil manicure? How often should clients receive a reconditioning hot oil manicure?
10. What type of polish application is included in a man's manicure?
11. Name five hand massage techniques and five arm massage techniques.
12. What are two safety cautions for hand and arm massage?

Chapter 11
PEDICURING

LEARNING OBJECTIVES

After you have studied this chapter, you should be able to:

1. Identify the equipment and materials needed for a pedicure and explain what they are used for.
2. List the steps in the pedicure pre-service procedure.
3. Demonstrate the proper procedures and precautions for a pedicure.
4. Describe the proper technique to use in filing toenails.
5. Demonstrate your ability to perform foot massage properly.

CHAPTER 11   PEDICURING   ◆   **145**

INTRODUCTION

The information in this chapter will show you the pedicuring skills you need to care for clients' feet, toes, and toenails. A **pedicure** includes trimming, shaping, and polishing toenails as well as foot massage. Pedicures are a standard service performed by nail technicians. They are a basic part of good foot care for any client and they are particularly important for clients before summer beach visits. Proper foot care through pedicuring improves both personal appearance and basic foot comfort.

> **PROCEDURAL TIP**
>
> *When making an appointment for a pedicure, suggest that your client wear open-toe shoes or sandals so that polish will not smear. Also remind your client that hose will need to be removed before the pedicure can be performed.*

PEDICURE SUPPLIES

You will need to have the following supplies in addition to your standard manicure set-up to perform pedicures: (Figs. 11.1, 11.2)

Pedicuring station. A station includes a chair for the client, a footrest for the client, and a chair for the nail technician. Pedicure stations that combine all these items into one piece of furniture are available.

Pedicuring stool and footrest. A pedicuring stool is a low stool that will make it easier for you to work on your client's feet. Some pedicuring stools come with a footrest for the client, or a separate footrest can be used.

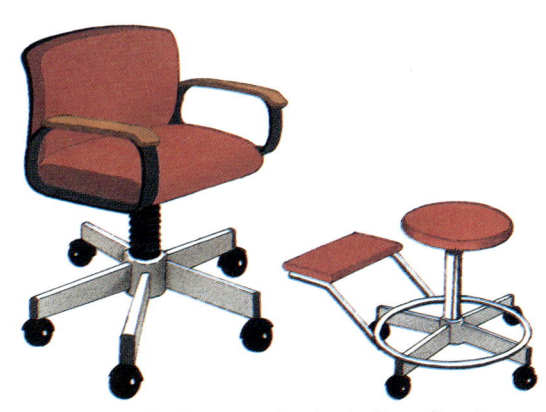

11.1 — Pedicure station including client's chair, footrest, and pedicuring stool

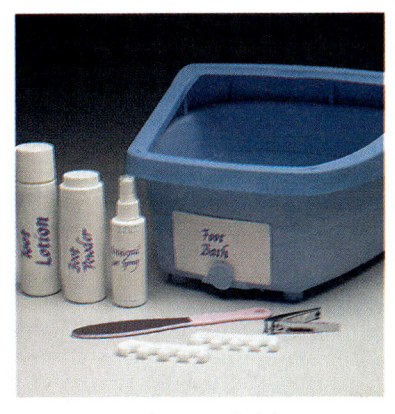

11.2 — Supplies needed for pedicure

Client's chair. The client's chair should be comfortable with arm rests.

Rinse and soap baths. These pedicure baths are filled with warm water and antibacterial soap in which to soak the client's feet. The bath must be large enough to immerse the client's feet. You will need two basins, one for warm water with soap or detergent and an antibacterial agent and the other for rinse water.

Toe separators. Foam rubber toe separators or cotton used to keep toes apart during the pedicure.

Foot file. Used to remove dry skin or **callus** growths.

Toenail clippers. Two types of toenail clippers are available; both are acceptable for a professional pedicure.

Antiseptic foot spray. Contains an **antifungal** (an-ti-**FUN**-gahl) agent as well as a mild antiseptic.

Antibacterial soap. Antibacterial (an-ti-bak-**TEER**-ee-ahl) soap for pedicuring contains a soap or detergent, an antifungal agent, and an antibacterial agent.

Foot lotion. Used during foot massage. Hand lotion can also be used.

Foot powder. Contains an antifungal agent for keeping feet dry after pedicure.

Pedicure slippers. These sanitized plastic or disposable paper slippers are optional.

PEDICURE

As with other procedures, a pedicure involves three parts: the Pre-Service, the Pedicure Procedure, and the Post-Service. In the Pre-Service you will sanitize your implements, greet your client, and do a client consultation. Next you will do the steps involved in the actual procedure. Then, in the Post-Service, you will schedule another appointment for your client, sell the retail products you discussed during the service, and sanitize.

PEDICURE PRE-SERVICE

Your pedicure area should be close to a sink so it is convenient when you fill the pedicure baths with water.

1. Complete your pre-service sanitation procedure. (This procedure is described on pages 32-33.)
2. Your station should be set up to include a pedicuring stool, client's chair, and a footrest for your client.
3. Spread one terry cloth towel on the floor in front of client's chair to put feet on during the pedicure. Put another towel over the stool to dry feet.

CHAPTER 11 PEDICURING ◆ 147

4. Set up your standard manicuring table in your pedicuring station. Add toe separators, foot file, toenail clippers, antiseptic antifungal foot spray, antibacterial soap, foot lotion, foot powder, and pedicure slippers to your table.

5. Fill both basins with warm water. Add a measured amount of antibacterial soap to the bath (follow manufacturer's directions). Add a few drops of antiseptic to the other bath for rinsing. Put baths in front of towel on the floor.

6. Greet client.

7. Complete client consultation. Use client record/health card to record responses and observations. Check for nail disorders and decide if it is safe and appropriate to perform a service on your client. If infection or inflammation is present, refer your client to his or her physician. If athlete's foot is present, you may not perform a pedicure.

Safety Caution

Be sure the floor around pedicure area is dry because wet floors are slippery and you or your clients can fall. When water is spilled, wipe it up immediately.

PEDICURE PROCEDURE

During the procedure, talk with your client about the products that are needed to maintain the service between salon visits. You might suggest polish, top coat, foot lotion, and foot powder.

1. **Remove shoes and socks.** Ask your client to remove shoes, socks, and hose and roll pant legs to the knees.

2. **Spray feet.** Spray feet with foot spray or wipe them with antiseptic. (Fig. 11.3)

3. **Soak feet.** Put client's feet in soap bath for 5-10 minutes to wash and sanitize the feet before you begin the pedicure. (Fig. 11.4)

4. **Rinse feet.** Remove both feet from soap bath and rinse in rinse bath.

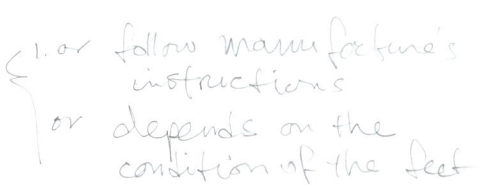

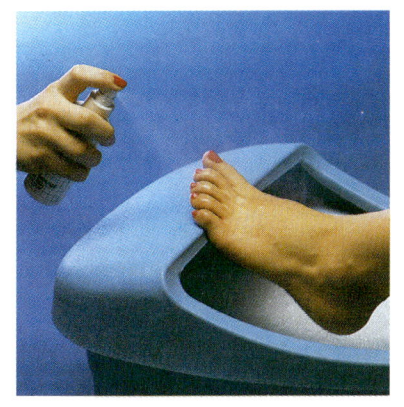

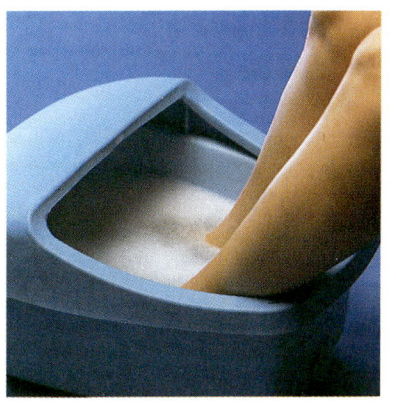

11.3 — Spray feet.

11.4 — Soak feet.

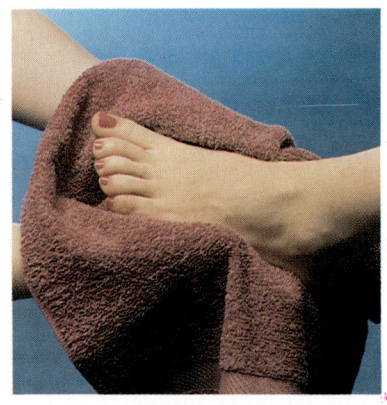

148 ◆ PART 3   BASIC PROCEDURES

5. **Dry feet.** Take one foot out of the rinse water and dry it off. Make sure you dry between the toes. Remove other foot from rinse bath and thoroughly dry. Ask client to place both feet on the towel you have placed on the floor. (Fig. 11.5)

6. **Remove polish.** Remove polish from little toe on left foot working towards big toe. Repeat with the right foot. (Fig. 11.6)

7. **Clip nails.** Clip the toenails of the left foot so that they are even with the end of the toe. (Fig. 11.7)

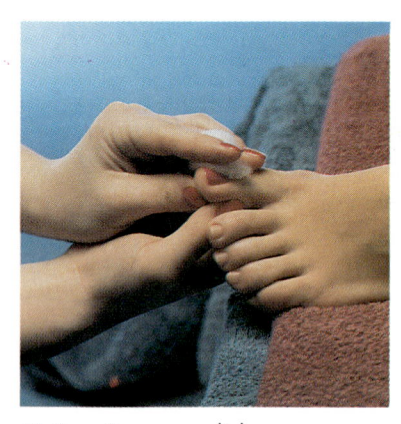

11.5 — Dry feet.

11.6 — Remove polish.

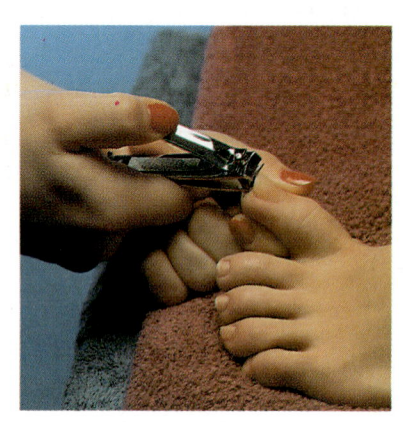

11.7 — Clip toenails.

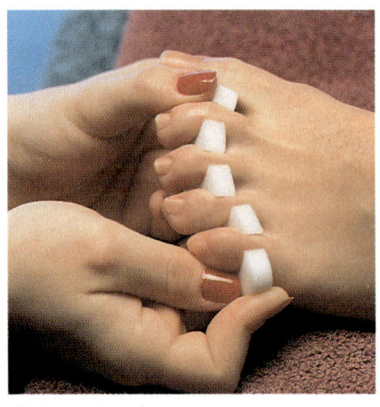

8. **Insert toe separators.** Use both hands to carefully insert toe separators or cotton between the toes of the left foot. (Fig. 11.8)

9. **File nails.** File the nails of the left foot with an emery board. File them straight across, rounding them slightly at the corners to conform to the shape of the toes. To avoid ingrown toenails, do not file into the corners of the nails. Smooth rough edges with the fine side of an emery board. (Fig. 11.9)

10. **Use foot file.** Use foot file on ball and heel of foot to remove dry skin and callus growths. Do not file too much because it can cause irritation and bleeding. (Fig. 11.10)

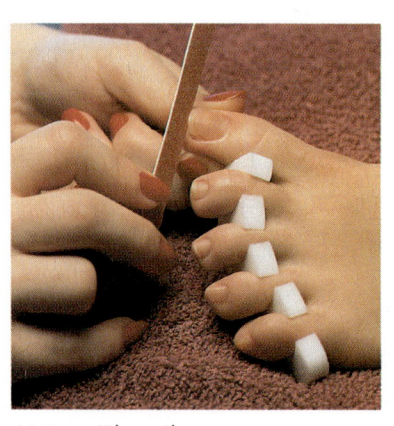

11.8 — Insert toe separators.

11.9 — File nails.

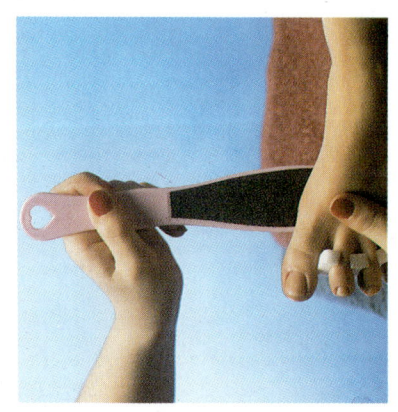

11.10 — Use foot file.

CHAPTER 11 PEDICURING ◆ **149**

> **STATE REGULATION ALERT**
>
> *A credo knife is a holder that supports a razor blade. Some states do not allow the use of the credo knife to remove callus growths because it can easily cut the client's foot. Be guided by your instructor about the use of a credo knife in your state.*

11. **Rinse foot.** Remove toe separators and place left foot in foot bath.

12. **Repeat steps 7-11 on right foot.** *[handwritten: Right foot begins, then R foot in foot basin again @ only 1st.]*

13. **Brush nails.** Remove left foot from foot bath and brush nails with nail brush. Rinse foot in rinse bath and dry thoroughly. Insert toe separators or cotton between toes. (Fig. 11.11)

14. **Apply cuticle solvent.** Use cotton-tipped orangewood stick to apply cuticle solvent to left foot. Begin with the little toe and work towards the big toe. You may apply solvent under free edge as well to soften excess skin beneath it. (Fig. 11.12)

15. **Push back cuticle.** On left foot, gently push cuticles with orangewood stick. If cuticle clipping is permitted in your state, clip only to remove a hangnail. (Fig. 11.13)

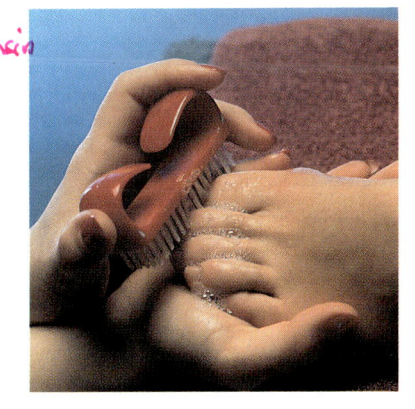

11.11 — Brush nails.

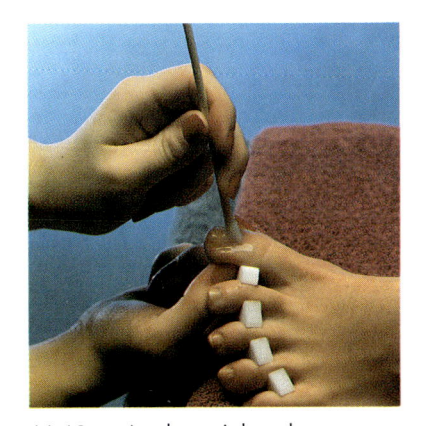

11.12 — Apply cuticle solvent.

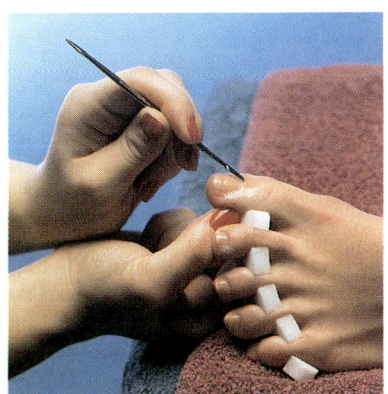

11.13 — Push back cuticle.

16. **Brush foot.** Remove toe separators. Ask your client to dip left foot into soap bath. With the left foot over the soap bath, brush with nail brush to remove bits of cuticle and solvent. Rinse foot in rinse bath and dry thoroughly. Place foot on towel.

17. **Apply lotion.** Apply lotion to foot for massage. Use a firm touch to avoid tickling your client's feet. (Fig. 11.14)

18. **Massage foot.** Perform foot massage on the left foot. Then place foot on a clean towel on the floor. (See massage techniques on pages 151-153.)

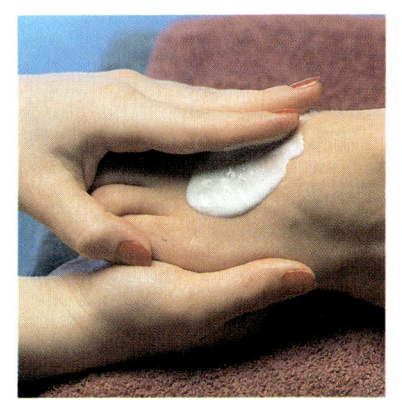

11.14 — Apply lotion.

Now for (R) foot

19. **Proceed with steps 13-19 on the right foot.**

20. **Remove traces of lotion.** Remove traces of lotion from toenails of both feet with a small piece of cotton that has been saturated with polish remover.

21. **Apply polish.** Reinsert the toe separators. Apply base coat, two coats of color, and top coat to toenails. Spray with instant nail dry. Place feet on a towel to dry.

22. **Powder feet.** When polish is dry, powder feet before the client puts shoes on.

Pushing Pedicures During Cold Weather

It's relatively easy to sell pedicures during the summer. The weather is warm and clients want their bare feet or sandal-clad feet to look in tip-top shape. But in the winter, feet are bundled up in layers of socks and leather footgear. For many clients it's out of sight, out of mind. To sell pedicures during cold weather, it helps to emphasize them as a pampering, luxury service. Feet that are confined uncomfortably in boots and often get wet from snow and sleet can suffer from dryness, cracking, fatigue and cramping. To soften and unkink feet, a pedicure is the ultimate time-out treatment that not only beautifies, but relaxes and coddles the entire client.

PEDICURE POST-SERVICE

Your pedicure is not complete. Follow the post-service procedure described below. (Fig. 11.15)

1. **Make another appointment.** Schedule another pedicure appointment for your client.

2. **Advise client.** Advise client about proper foot care. Remind client that wearing tight shoes and very high heels can cause ingrown toenails.

3. **Sell retail products.** Suggest that your client buy products you have discussed during the pedicure. Products such as polish, lotion, and top coat help to maintain the pedicure.

4. **Clean pedicure area.** Dump out basins and wipe them with a hospital-grade disinfectant to sanitize. Dry basins and put them away. Wipe table and footrest with a hospital-grade disinfectant.

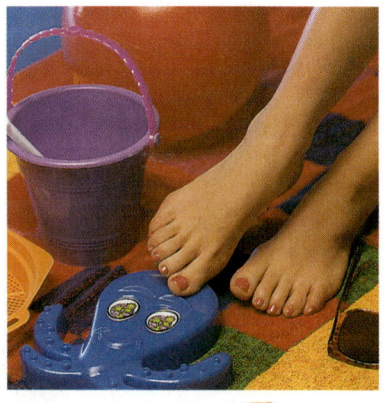

11.15 — Finished pedicure

5. **Discard used materials.** Place all used materials in the plastic bag at the side of the table. If the bag is full, discard it in a closed pail.

6. **Sanitize table and implements.** Perform the complete pre-service sanitation procedure. In most states this procedure calls for 20 minutes of proper sanitation before implements can be used on the next client. Return your table to its basic set-up.

FOOT MASSAGE

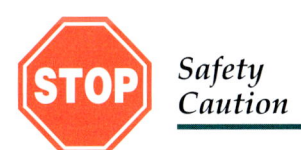

Foot massage during a pedicure stimulates blood flow and is relaxing to the client. These techniques and illustrations provide directions for massage of the left foot.

FOOT MASSAGE TECHNIQUES

1. **Relaxer movement to the joints of the foot.** Rest client's foot on footrest or stool. Grasp the leg just above the ankle with your left hand. This will brace the client's leg and foot. Use your right hand to hold left foot just beneath toes and rotate foot in a circular motion. (Fig. 11.16)

2. **Effleurage on top of foot.** Place both thumbs on top of foot at instep. Move your thumbs in circular movements in opposite directions down the center of the top of the foot. Continue this movement to the toes. Keep one hand in contact with foot or leg, slide one hand at a time back firmly to instep and rotate back down to toes. This is a relaxing movement. Repeat 3-5 times. (Fig. 11.17)

3. **Effleurage on heel (bottom of foot).** Use the same thumb movement that you did in the massage technique above. Start at the base of the toes and move from the ball of the foot to the heel, rotating your thumbs in opposite directions. Slide hands back to the top of the foot. This is a relaxing movement. Repeat 3-5 times. (Fig. 11.18)

STOP *Safety Caution*

DO NOT massage if client has high blood pressure, heart condition, or has had a stroke. Massage increases circulation and may be harmful to such a client. Have your client consult a physician before receiving a massage.

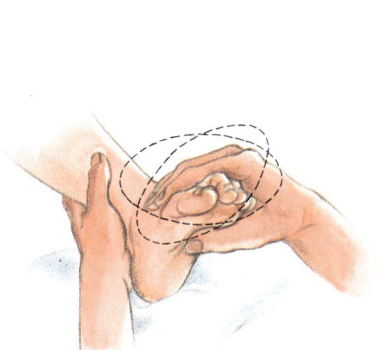

11.16 — Relaxer movement to the joints of the foot

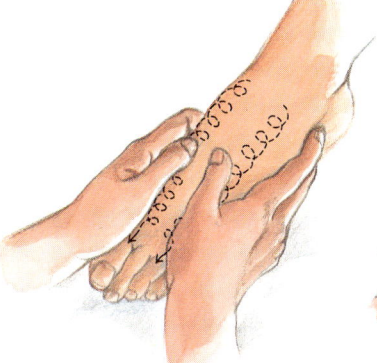

11.17 — Effleurage on top of foot

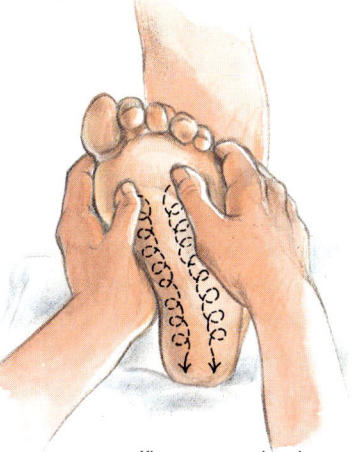

11.18 — Effleurage on heel

4. **Effleurage movement on toes.** Start with the little toe, using thumb on top and index finger on bottom of foot. Hold each toe and rotate with thumb. Start at base of toe and work towards the end of the toes. This is relaxing and soothing. Repeat 3-5 times. (Fig. 11.19)

5. **Joint movement for toes.** Start with the little toe and make a figure eight with each toe. Repeat 3-5 times. (Fig. 11.20)

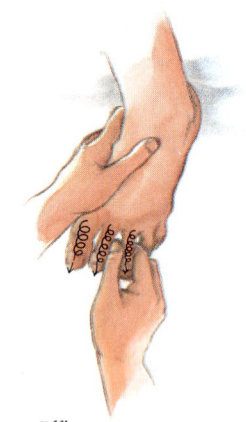

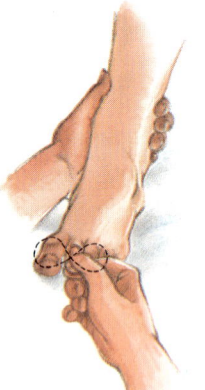

11.19 — Effleurage on toes

11.20 — Joint movement for toes

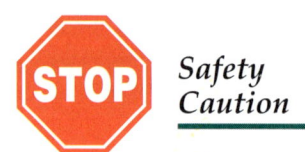

Safety Caution

If client has had a plantar's wart removed by a podiatrist either chemically or by excision, do not apply thumb compression to that area.

6. **Thumb compression**—*friction movement.* Make a fist with your fingers, keeping your thumb out. Apply firm pressure with your thumb and move your fist up the heel towards the ball of the foot. Work from the left side of foot and back down the right side towards the heel. As you massage over the bottom of the foot, check for any nodules or bumps. If you find one, be very gentle because the area may be tender. This movement stimulates the blood flow and increases circulation. (Fig. 11.21)

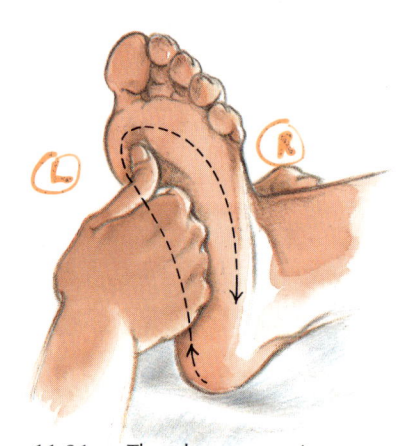

11.21 — Thumb compression "friction movement"

7. **Metatarsal scissors (a petrissage massage movement, kneading).** Place your fingers on top of foot along the metatarsal bones with your thumb underneath the foot. Knead up and down along each bone by raising your thumb and lower fingers to apply pressure. This promotes flexibility and stimulates blood flow. Repeat 3-5 times. (Fig. 11.22)

8. **Fist twist compression (a friction movement, deep rubbing).** Place left hand on top of foot and make a fist with your right hand. Your left hand will apply pressure while your right hand twists around the bottom of the foot. This helps stimulate blood flow. Repeat 3-5 times up and around foot. (Fig. 11.23)

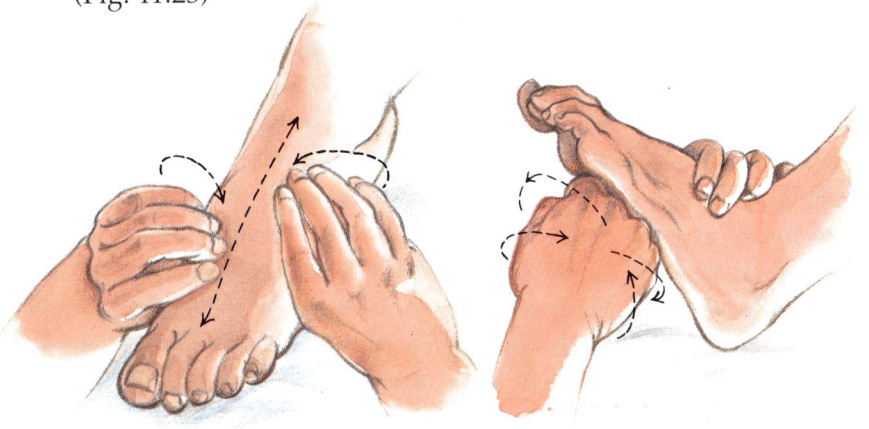

11.22 — Metatarsal scissors

11.23 — Fist twist compression

9. **Effleurage on instep.** Place fingers at ball of foot. Move fingers in circular movements in opposite directions. Massage to end of each toe, gently squeezing the tip of each toe. (Fig. 11.24)

10. **Percussion or tapotement movement.** Use fingertips to perform percussion or tapotement (tah-POT-mynt) movements to lightly tap over the entire foot to reduce blood circulation and complete massage.

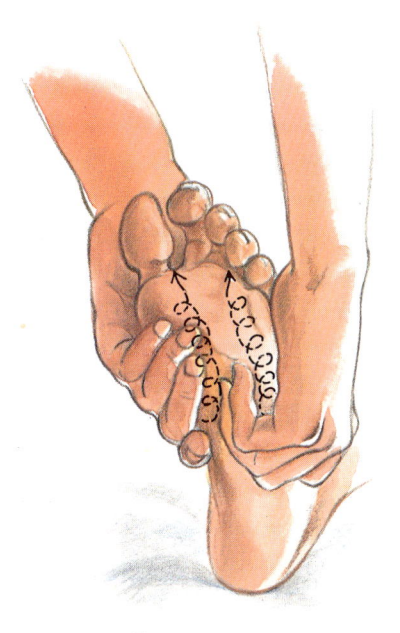

11.24 — Effleurage on instep

REVIEW QUESTIONS

1. Name five pedicure supplies.
2. List the seven steps in the pedicure pre-service.
3. Briefly describe the pedicure procedure.
4. Describe the proper technique to use in filing toenails.
5. List the six steps in the pedicure post-service.
6. Name six foot massage techniques.
7. What is a safety caution for pedicuring?

Part 4

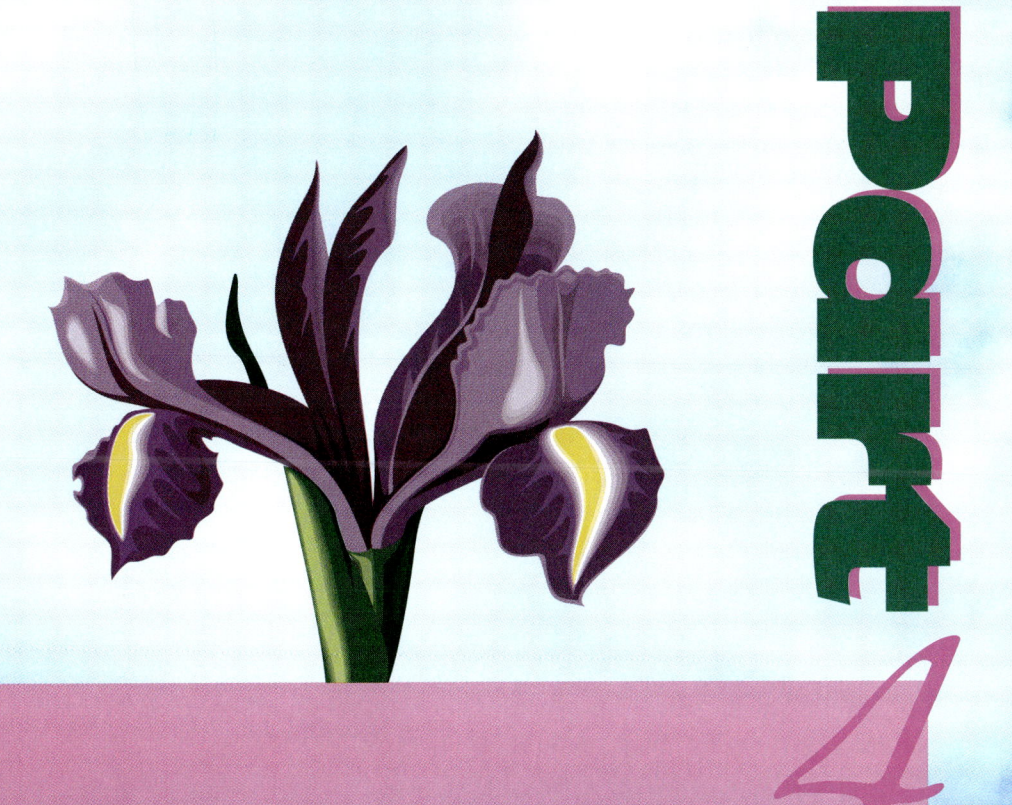

THE ART OF NAIL TECHNOLOGY

- ◆ *CHAPTER 12* - Nail Tips
- ◆ *CHAPTER 13* - Nail Wraps
- ◆ *CHAPTER 14* - Acrylic Nails
- ◆ *CHAPTER 15* - Gels
- ◆ *CHAPTER 16* - The Creative Touch

Chapter 12
NAIL TIPS

LEARNING OBJECTIVES

After you have studied this chapter, you should be able to:

1. Identify the supplies needed for nail tips and explain what they are used for.
2. Identify the two types of nail tips.
3. Demonstrate the proper procedure and precautions to use in applying nail tips.
4. Describe the proper maintenance of tips.
5. Demonstrate the proper removal of tips.

CHAPTER 12　　NAIL TIPS　　◆　　157

INTRODUCTION

A *nail tip* is an artificial nail made of plastic, nylon, or acetate. Tips are adhered to the natural nail to add extra length. Usually tips are combined with another artificial service, such as a fabric wrap or sculptured nail, since a tip worn with no overlay is very weak. If a client chooses to wear a tip with no overlay, the tip is considered a temporary service.

SUPPLIES FOR NAIL TIPS

In addition to the materials on your basic manicuring table, you will need the following supplies for nail tip application. (Fig. 12.1)

Abrasive. A rough surface that is used to shape or smooth the nail and remove the sine. It usually looks like a large emery board or disk, but it can be any shape or color.

Buffer block. Lightweight rectangular block that is abrasive and used to buff nails.

Nail adhesive. Glue or bonding agent used to secure the nail tip to the natural nail. It usually comes in a tube with a pointed applicator tip or one-drop applicator. Even the smallest amount of glue in the eyes can be very dangerous and can blind a person. A nail technician should always wear safety goggles when using and handling nail adhesives. Goggles should be offered to the client, as well.

Nail tips. All tips have a well that serves as the point of contact with the nail plate. The position stop is the point where the nail plate meets the tip before it is glued to the nail. Tips are designed with either a partial or full well. (Fig. 12.2) The tip should never cover more than 1/2 of the natural nail plate. Tips come in large boxes that have an assortment of sizes. Some nail technicians

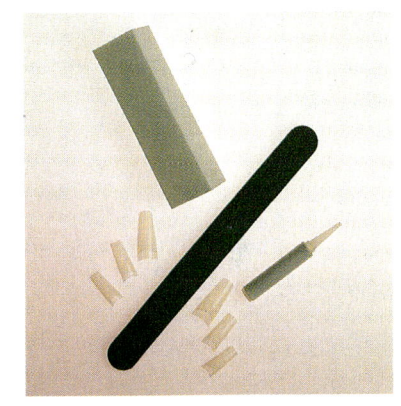

12.1 — Supplies needed for tip application

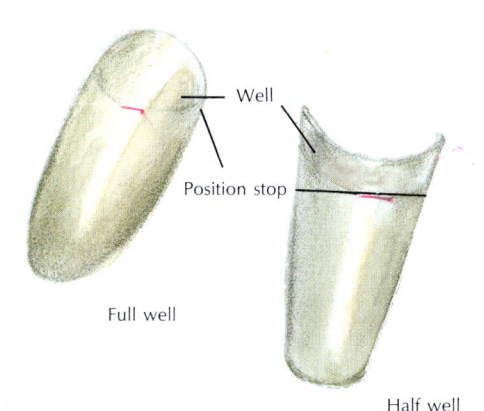

Well
Position stop
Full well
Half well

12.2 — Tip with half well and tip with full well

prefer to have tips from several different manufacturers, since they vary slightly in size and shape. With a wide assortment, it is easier to fit each client with precisely the right size and shape tip.

NAIL TIP APPLICATION

NAIL TIP APPLICATION PRE-SERVICE

1. Complete pre-service sanitation procedure. (This procedure is described on pages 32-33.)
2. Set up your standard manicuring table. Add abrasives, buffer blocks, nail adhesive, and nail tips to your table.
3. Greet client and ask her to wash hands with antibacterial soap. Thoroughly dry hands with a fresh towel.
4. Do client consultation, using client record/health card to record responses and observations. Check for nail disorders and decide if it is safe and appropriate to perform a service on this client. If the client should not receive service, explain your reasons and refer her to a doctor.
5. *Chemical card*

NAIL TIP APPLICATION PROCEDURE

During the procedure, discuss products such as polish, top coat, and lotion that will help your client maintain the service between salon visits.

1. **Remove old polish.** Begin with your client's left hand, little finger and work toward the thumb. Then repeat on the right hand.
    Remove the free edge (clip the nails)
2. **Push back cuticle.** Use a cotton-tipped orangewood stick to gently push back cuticle. Use a light touch because the cuticle is dry.
3. **Buff nail to remove shine.** Buff lightly over the nail plate with medium/fine abrasive to remove the natural oil. Do not use a coarse abrasive and be careful not to apply extreme pressure. (Fig. 12.3)
4. **Size tips.** Select the proper size tips. Make sure the tips you choose completely cover the nail plate from sidewall to sidewall but never cover more than half the length of the nail. (Fig. 12.4) Trim tips to the right size if the well covers too much of the nail. Nail tips should be pre-beveled along the edge closest to the cuticle to thin out the plastic. Tips that are pre-beveled require less filing on the natural nail after application. This cuts down the potential for damage to the natural nail. Put all sized tips on towel in order of finger size.

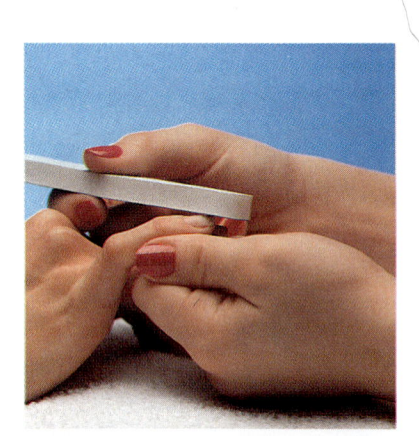

12.3 — Remove shine from nails.

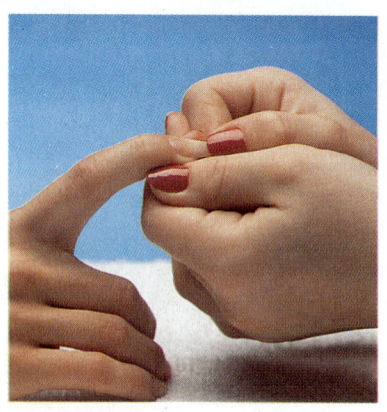

12.4 — Size tips.

CHAPTER 12   NAIL TIPS   ◆   **159**

5. **Apply nail antiseptic.** Use a cotton-tipped orangewood stick or spray to apply nail antiseptic to nails. Begin with the little finger on the left hand. The antiseptic will remove more of the remaining natural oil and dehydrate the nail for better adhesion. (Fig. 12.5)

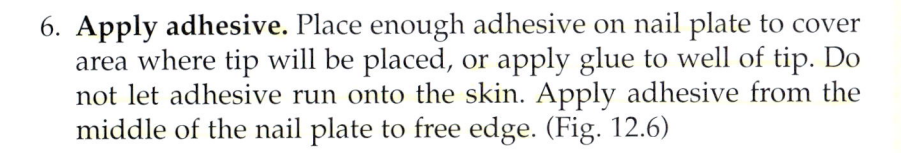

6. **Apply adhesive.** Place enough adhesive on nail plate to cover area where tip will be placed, or apply glue to well of tip. Do not let adhesive run onto the skin. Apply adhesive from the middle of the nail plate to free edge. (Fig. 12.6)

7. **Slide on tips.** Remember the stop, rock, and hold procedure. Stop—find stop against free edge at 45 degree angle. Rock—rock tip on slowly. Hold—hold in place 5 to 10 seconds until dry. (Fig. 12.7)

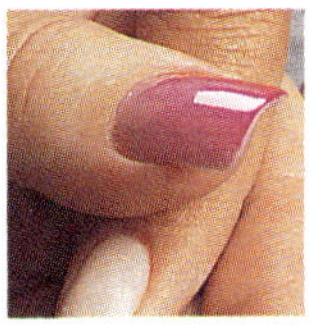

> *Sanitation Caution*
>
> If you accidently touch the nails after you apply antiseptic, you must clean them again and reapply antiseptic.

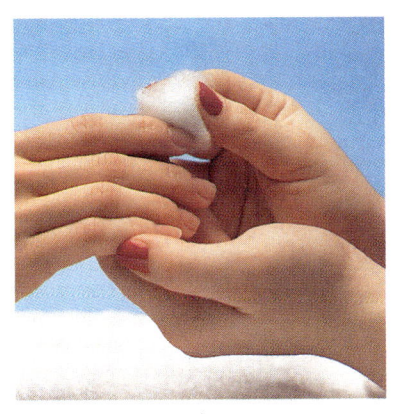

12.5 — Apply nail antiseptic.

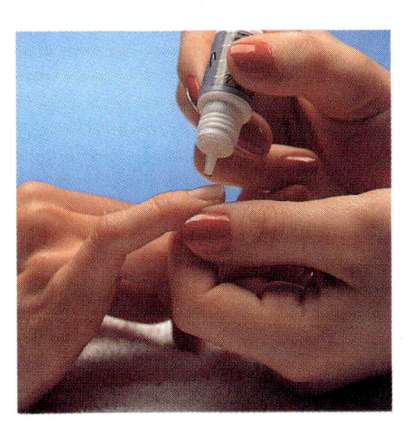

12.6 — Apply adhesive.

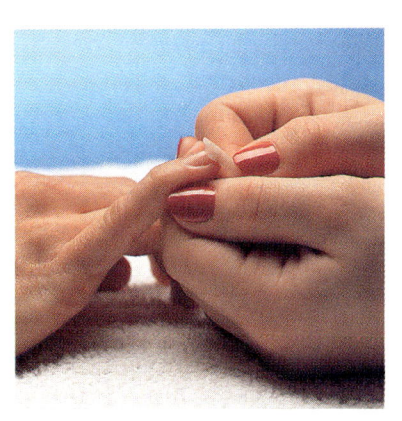

12.7 — Slide on tips.

PROCEDURAL TIP

An alternate method of applying adhesive is to apply to the well of the tip. This may ensure that fewer air bubbles are trapped in adhesive.

8. **Apply adhesive bead to seam.** Apply a bead of adhesive to seam between the natural nail plate and the tip to strengthen the stress point. (Fig. 12.8)

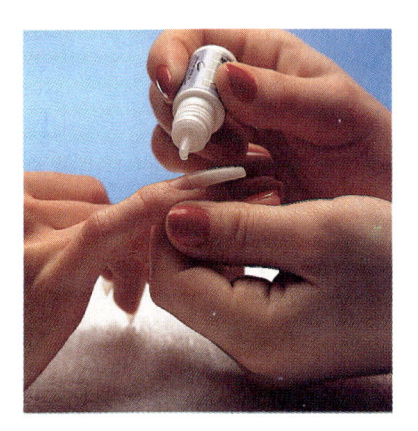

12.8 — Apply adhesive bead to seam.

9. **Trim nail tip.** Trim the nail tip to desired length using the large nail clippers. Cut from one side, the other. Cutting the tip straight across causes weakening of the plastic. (Fig. 12.9)

10. **Blend tip into natural nail.** Sand the shine off the tip with a semi-coarse abrasive. Make sure you keep the file flat on the nail at all times. Never hold file at an angle because filing at an angle can make a groove in the nail plate. (Fig. 12.10)

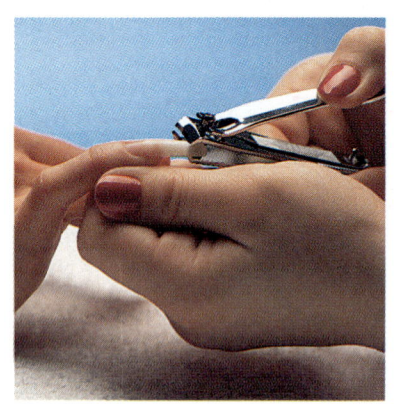

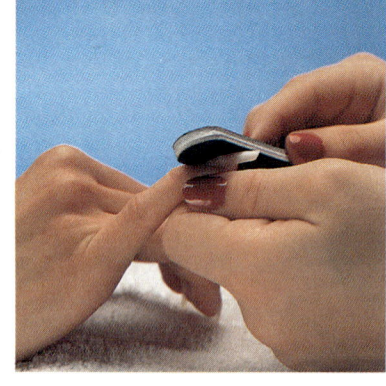

12.9 — Trim nail tip.

12.10 — Blend tip into natural nail.

11. **Buff tip for perfect blend.** Use the buffer block to gently buff down the area between the natural nail plate and the tip extension. The tip should blend with the natural nail so that there is no visible line or cloudiness between the two. (Fig. 12.11)

12. **Shape nail.** Use abrasive to shape new, longer nail. (Fig. 12.12)

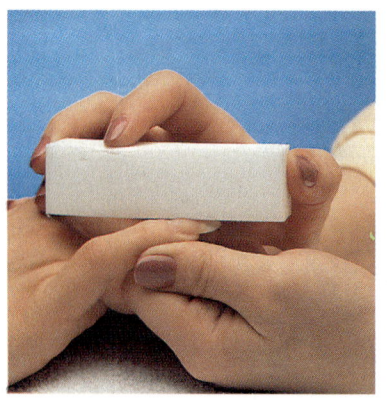

12.11 — Buff tip.

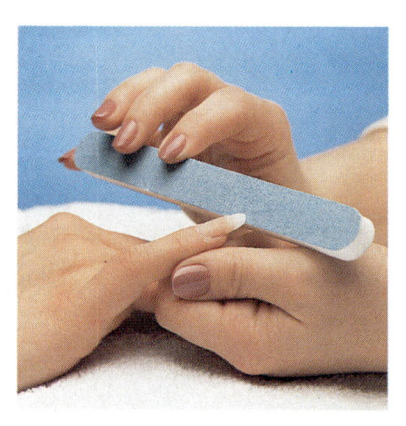

12.12 — Shape tip.

CHAPTER 12　NAIL TIPS ◆ **161**

13. **Proceed with desired service.** Your tip application is now complete. Although your client's tips blend perfectly with natural nails, tips are very seldom worn without an additional nail service such as wraps, acrylic nails, or gel nails. You are ready to proceed with the service that your client has chosen. (Fig. 12.13)

NAIL TIP POST-SERVICE

If your client is only wearing tips as a temporary service, add a drop of cuticle oil to each nail and buff.

1. **Make another appointment.** Schedule another appointment with your client to remove tips and condition nails and cuticles.
2. **Sell retail products.** Suggest that your client buy products necessary to maintain her nails throughout the week. Polish, lotion, top coat, etc. are valuable maintenance tools for her to have.
3. **Clean up around your table.** Take the time to restore the basic set-up of your table. Cap glue and clean applicator tips in acetone.
4. **Discard used materials.** Place all used materials in the plastic bag at the side of the table. If the bag is full or contains used materials from artificial nail services, discard it in a closed pail.
5. **Sanitize table and implements.** Perform the complete pre-service sanitation procedure. Implements need to be sanitized 20 minutes before they can be used on the next client.

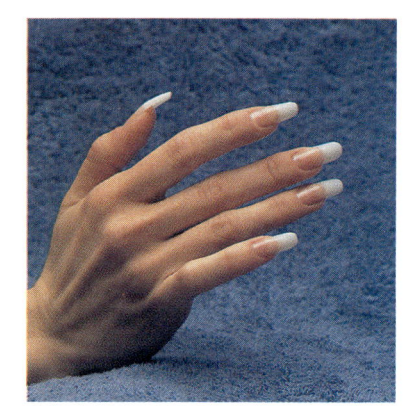

12.13 — Finished tip application

Profit with Temporary Tips

Consider selling tips as a temporary service. Tips have long been favored by individuals who desire length but can't seem to grow their nails, or by those who want longer nails without the wait. However, tips have a third following—women who want temporary length for a special occasion, such as a wedding or the prom. These people might work in jobs where long nails are a hindrance or they may find that longer lengths don't fit their lifestyle, but they still want the look for a day or two. For them, create a two-appointment service. During the first visit you apply and paint the tips. Schedule the second appointment to remove the extensions, then condition and manicure the client's own, natural nails.

MAINTENANCE AND REMOVAL OF TIPS

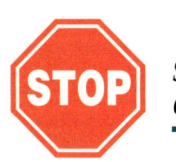

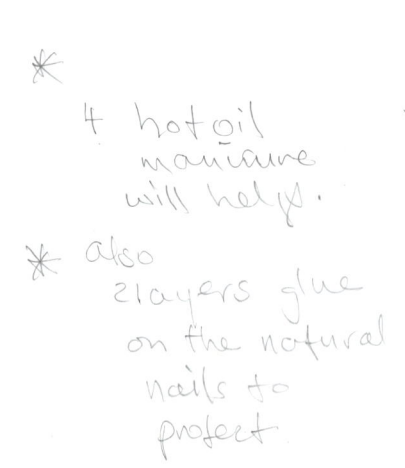

MAINTENANCE

Clients wearing tips will need weekly or biweekly manicures for regluing and rebuffing. Reglue at the seam between the natural nail and the tip. Most tips need non-acetone polish remover because acetone remover dissolves the tips.

Safety Caution

Never nip off nail tips because you might cause permanent damage to the nail bed.

TIP REMOVAL

Tips that have been glued to the nail plate can cause damage if removed improperly. Use a glue remover or acetone to remove tips.

1. **Complete nail tip application pre-service.** You will only need to add a buffer block to your manicuring table.

2. **Soak nails.** Place enough remover in a small glass bowl to cover nails. Soak nails for a few minutes.

3. **Slide off tip.** Use your orangewood stick to slide off softened tip. Be careful not to pry tip off because you can damage the nail bed and mantle. (Fig. 12.14)

4. **Buff nail.** Gently buff natural nail with fine block buffer to remove any glue residue. (Fig. 12.15)

5. **Condition cuticle and surrounding skin.** Condition cuticle and surrounding skin with cuticle oil and massage cream.

6. **Proceed to desired service.**

7. **Complete nail tip application post-service** if client is receiving no further service.

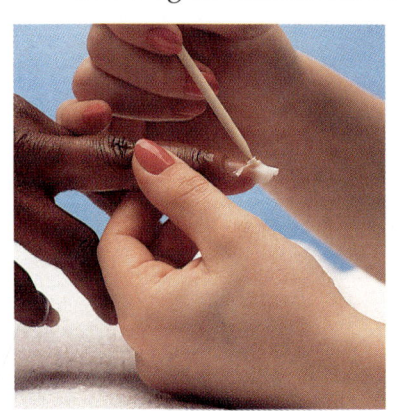

12.14 — Slide off tip; do not pry.

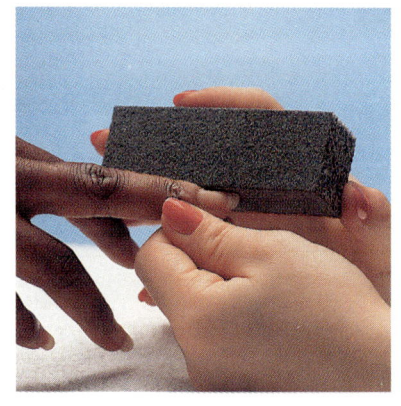

12.15 — Use fine buffer block to remove glue residue.

REVIEW QUESTIONS

1. List the four supplies, in addition to your basic manicuring table, that you need for nail tip application. *nail adhesive, nail tips, abrasive, buffer bk*
2. Name the two types of nail tips. *partial or full*
3. What portion of the natural nail plate should be covered by a nail tip? *< ½*
4. What type of tip application is considered a temporary service? Why? *a tip w/no overlay*
5. Briefly describe the procedure for nail tip application. *clean, sanitize, antiseptic, adhesive, file*
6. Describe the proper maintenance of nail tips. *remove polish, remove cut/push b/c buff, size tip*
7. Describe the procedure for the removal of tips.

Chapter 13
NAIL WRAPS

LEARNING OBJECTIVES

After you have studied this chapter, you should be able to:

1. List four kinds of nail wraps and what they are used for.
2. Explain benefits of using silk, linen, fiberglass, and paper wraps.
3. Demonstrate the proper procedures and precautions to use in fabric wrap application.
4. Describe the maintenance of fabric wrap. Include a description of the two-week and four-week follow-up.
5. Explain how fabric wrap is used for crack repair.
6. Demonstrate the proper procedure and precautions for fabric wrap removal.
7. List the supplies used in paper wrap.
8. Demonstrate proper procedures for paper wrap application.
9. Define liquid nail wrap and describe its purpose.

INTRODUCTION

Nail wraps, sometimes called *overlays,* are nail-size pieces of cloth or paper that are bonded to the front of the nail plate with nail adhesive. They are used to repair or strengthen natural nails or nail tips. Wraps can be cut from a swatch of cloth or piece of paper to fit a client's nail size and shape, or they can be purchased pre-cut. Pre-cut overlays have an adhesive back and are attached only to the front of the nail.

Fabric wraps are made from silk, linen, or fiberglass. **Silk** is a thin natural material with a tight weave that becomes transparent when adhesive is applied. A silk wrap is strong, lightweight, and smooth when applied to the nail. **Linen** is a closely woven, heavy material. It is much thicker than silk or fiberglass. Because it is opaque, even after adhesive is applied, a colored polish must be used to cover it completely. Linen is a strong wrap and lasts a long time. **Fiberglass** is a very thin synthetic mesh with a loose weave. The loose weave makes it easy for adhesive to penetrate. It is especially strong and durable.

Paper wraps are made of very thin paper and dissolve in both acetone and non-acetone remover. For this reason, paper wraps are temporary and must be reapplied when polish is removed. Paper wraps are glued both on top of the nail and under the free edge.

FABRIC WRAPS

SUPPLIES

In addition to the materials on your basic manicuring table, you will need the following items: (Fig. 13.1)

Fabric. Small swatches of linen, silk, or fiberglass material that can be cut to fit a client's nail size and shape. You may also find pre-cut wraps with an adhesive backing.

Nail adhesive. Glue or bonding agent used to secure the nail tip or fabric to the natural nail. It usually comes in a tube with a pointed applicator tip called an *extender tip.* When working with adhesives, be sure to protect your eyes with goggles; offer them to your client, as well.

Small scissors. Small and sharp for cutting fabric.
Nail block buffer.
Abrasive.
Adhesive dryer. Drop-on or spray that dries nail adhesive quickly.

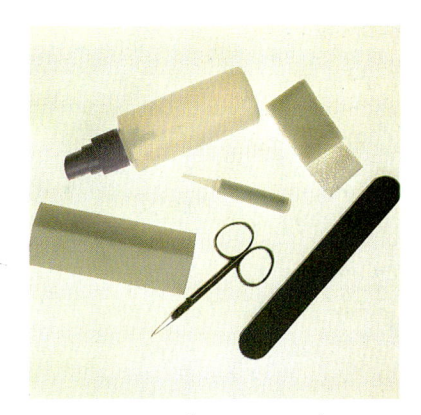

13.1 — Materials necessary for fabric wrap application

NAIL WRAP PRE-SERVICE

Use the following preparation for all nail wrap procedures.

1. Do the pre-service sanitation procedure. (This procedure is described on pages 32-33.)

2. Set up standard manicuring table. Add fabric, nail adhesive, small scissors, nail block buffer, abrasive, and adhesive dryer to your table.

3. Greet client and ask her to wash her hands in antibacterial soap. Dry hands and nails thoroughly with a fresh towel.

4. Do client consultation, using client record/health card to record the responses and your observations. Check for nail disorders. Decide if client's nails and hands are healthy enough for you to perform a service. If the client has a nail or skin disorder and should not receive a service, explain the reasons and refer the client to a doctor. If you proceed with the service, discuss you client's needs and wants.

NAIL WRAP PROCEDURE

During the procedure discuss with your client the products she will need to maintain the service between salon visits.

1. **Remove old polish.** Begin with the client's left hand, little finger. Saturate cotton with polish remover. If client is wearing artificial nails, use non-acetone remover to avoid damaging them. Hold saturated cotton on nail while you count to ten in your mind. Wipe the old polish off the nail with a stroking motion towards the free edge. If all polish is not removed, repeat this step until traces of polish are gone. It may be necessary to put cotton around the tip of an orangewood stick and use it to clean polish away from cuticle area. Repeat this procedure on each finger of both hands.

2. **Clean nails.** Dip nails in fingerbowls filled with warm water and antibacterial soap. Then use nail brush to clean nails over fingerbowl. Rinse nails briefly in clear water. DO NOT soak client's nails in water before you apply a nail wrap. When water is used to rinse the fingers, dip them very briefly in fingerbowl. Natural nails are porous and retain water. Water-soaked nails are a perfect breeding ground for mold and fungus under the nail wrap.

3. **Push back cuticle.** Use a cotton-tipped orangewood stick to gently push back cuticle. Use a light touch because the cuticle has not been soaked.

4. **Etch nail to remove shine.** Etch lightly over nail plate with medium/fine abrasive to remove the natural oil. Do not use a coarse file and be careful not to apply extreme pressure. Nail wraps can be done over natural nails or over a set of tips.

CHAPTER 13 NAIL WRAPS ◆ **167**

5. **Apply nail antiseptic.** Use a cotton-tipped orangewood stick, cotton, or spray to apply nail antiseptic to nails. Begin with the little finger on the left hand and work toward the thumb. The antiseptic will remove the remaining natural oil and dehydrate the nail for better adhesion.

6. **Apply adhesive.** Apply adhesive to the entire surface of all ten nails. This prepares them to receive wraps. Let adhesive dry. Use activator if needed to speed up process. (As if base coat)

7. **Cut fabric.** Cut fabric to approximate width and shape of nail plate. (Fig. 13.2)

8. **Apply fabric adhesive.** Apply a drop of adhesive to center of nail. Keep adhesive off the cuticle because it will cause the wrap to lift or separate from the nail plate. (Fig. 13.3)

9. **Apply fabric.** Gently fit fabric over nail, 1/16 inch away from cuticle. Press to smooth. (Fig. 13.4)

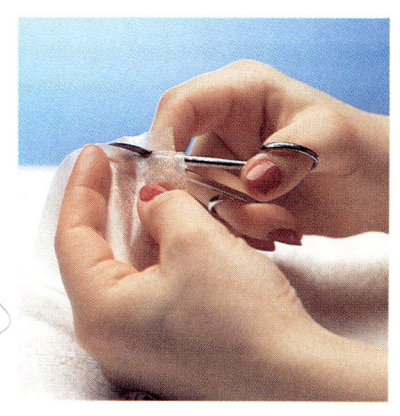

PROCEDURAL TIP

Using a thick plastic sheet to press fabric onto nail will prevent the transfer of bacteria from you to your client.

10. **Trim fabric.** Use small scissors to trim fabric 1/16 inch away from sidewalls and free edge. Trimming fabric slightly smaller than nail plate prevents fabric from **lifting** or separating from the nail plate. (Fig. 13.5)

11. **Apply fabric adhesive.** Draw a **thin** coat of adhesive down the center of the nail using the extender tip to apply. Do not touch the cuticle. The adhesive will penetrate the fabric and stick to the nail surface. (Fig. 13.6)

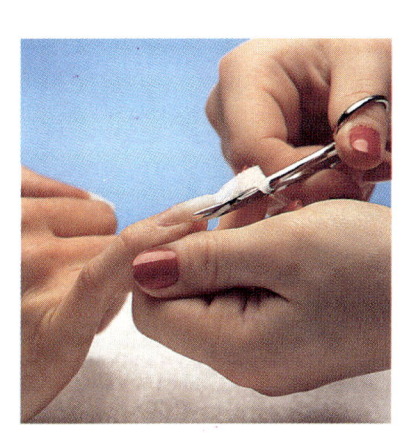

13.2 — Cut fabric.

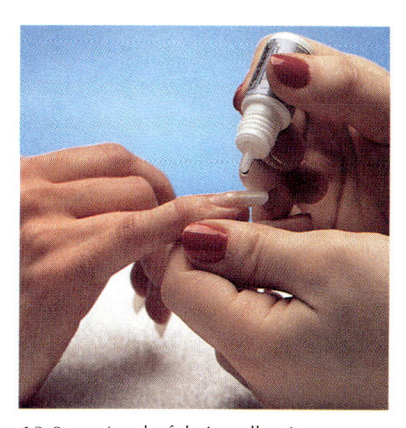

13.3 — Apply fabric adhesive.

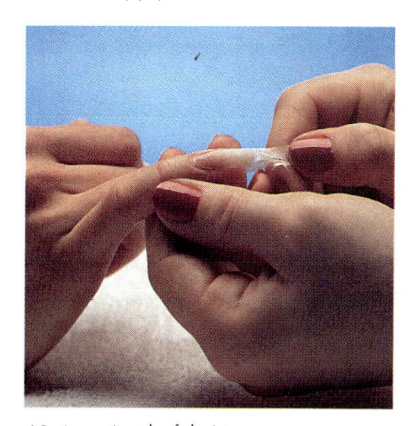

13.4 — Apply fabric.

13.5 — Trim fabric.

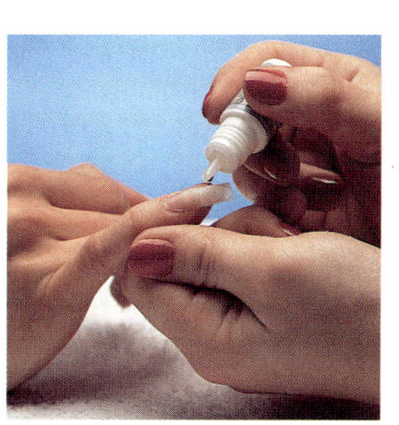

13.6 — Apply adhesive.

168 ◆ PART IV   THE ART OF NAIL TECHNOLOGY

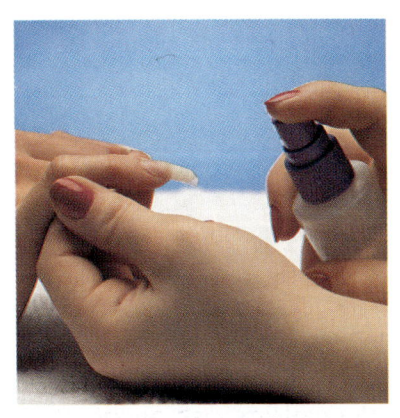

13.7 — Apply adhesive dryer.

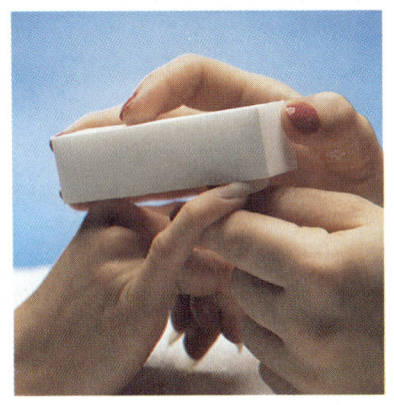

13.8 — Buff nails.

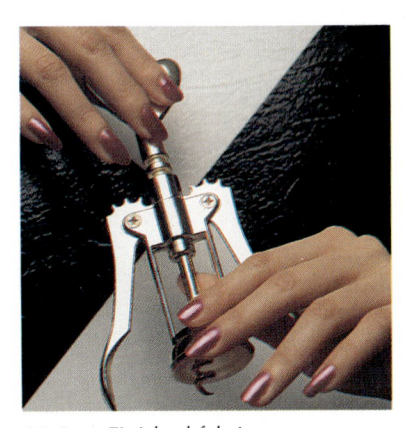

13.9 — Finished fabric wraps

12. **Apply adhesive dryer.** Spray or drop on adhesive dryer. Keep adhesive dryer off skin to prevent a heat sensation in your client's nail. (Fig. 13.7)
13. **Apply second coat of adhesive.** Apply and spread adhesive with extender tip. Seal free edge with adhesive by running the extender tip on the edge of the nail tip to prevent any lifting.
14. **Apply second coat of adhesive dryer.**
15. **Shape and refine nails.** Use medium/fine abrasive to shape and refine nails.
    * apply cuticle oil
16. **Buff nails.** Apply cuticle oil and buff to a high shine with block buffer. Brush block buffer over surface of nail to smooth out rough areas in fabric. Do not buff too much or too hard because you can wear through the wrap and weaken it. (Fig. 13.8)
17. **Remove traces of oil.** Use a small piece of cotton or a cotton-tipped orangewood stick to remove traces of oil from nail so alcohol or non-acetone polish will adhere. Send client to thoroughly wash at the sink with a nail brush and soap, not only to remove oil, but any dust or nail chemicals.
18. **Apply polish.** (Fig. 13.9)

NAIL WRAP POST-SERVICE

Follow this post-service for all your nail wrap services.

1. **Make another appointment.** Schedule another appointment with your client to maintain the nail wrap she has just received or for another service.
2. **Sell retail products.** Suggest that your client buy products necessary to maintain her nails throughout the week. Polish, lotion, top coat, etc. are valuable maintenance tools for her to have.
3. **Clean up around your table.** Take the time to restore the basic set-up of your table. Cap adhesive and adhesive dryer to prevent evaporation.
4. **Clean extender tips.** To clean clogged extender tips, place them in a covered glass jar with acetone. Poke a clean toothpick through hole.
5. **Store fabric.** Store fabric in a sealable plastic bag to protect from bacteria.
6. **Discard used materials.** Place all used materials in the plastic bag at the side of the table. If the bag is full or contains used materials from artificial nail services, discard it in a closed pail.
7. **Sanitize table and implements.** Perform the complete pre-service sanitation procedure. Implements need to be sanitized 20 minutes before they can be used on the next client.

Host Nail Fashion Nights

Whoever coined the phrase "seeing is believing" must have known that a person is more likely to purchase something she is familiar with. To acquaint customers firsthand with the latest manicure looks, try hosting a nail fashion night. For a $10.00–$15.00 admission fee, you showcase the latest nail looks by giving each attendee a manicure—using the season's most popular fashion colors and hottest new products, of course. To top off the evening, offer each client a nailcare fashion kit comprised of trial-sized products and a gift certificate for 15 percent off the next nailcare purchase or service. Spending an entire night focused on the products creates a buzz about them and shows clients how to use them. The sample size gets them hooked and the gift certificate gives them an incentive to return to you.

FABRIC WRAP MAINTENANCE, REMOVAL, AND REPAIRS

Fabric wraps need regular maintenance to keep them looking fresh. In this section you will learn how to maintain fabric wraps after two weeks and after four weeks. You will also learn how to remove fabric wraps and how to use fabric wraps for crack repair.

FABRIC WRAP MAINTENANCE

Fabric wraps are maintained with glue "fills" after two weeks and with glue and fabric "fills" after four weeks.

Two-Week Maintenance

After two weeks use the following procedure to maintain fabric wraps. You will need to add nail adhesive, a nail block buffer, and adhesive dryer to your standard table set-up.

1. **Complete nail wrap pre-service.**
2. **Remove old polish.** Use a non-acetone polish remover to avoid damaging wraps.
3. **Clean nails.**
4. **Push back cuticle.**
5. **File nail to remove shine.** Make sure the line between the new growth and the existing wrap is smooth.
6. **Apply nail antiseptic.**

7. **Apply adhesive to new nail growth area.** Apply a small drop of adhesive to new nail growth. Spread with extender tip, taking care not to touch skin.
8. **Apply adhesive dryer.**
9. **Apply adhesive to entire nail.** Apply a second coat of adhesive to entire nail to strengthen and reseal wrap.
10. **Apply adhesive dryer.**
11. **Shape and refine nail.** Use medium/fine abrasive over surface of nail to remove any peaks and imperfections.
12. **Buff nails.** Apply cuticle oil and buff to a high shine with block buffer.
13. **Apply hand lotion and massage hand and arm.**
14. **Remove traces of oil.** Use a small piece of cotton or a cotton-tipped orangewood stick to remove traces of oil from nail so polish will adhere.
15. **Apply polish.**
16. **Complete nail wrap post-service.**

Four-Week Maintenance

After four weeks use the following maintenance procedure to apply fabric and adhesive to new growth. You will need nail adhesive, a nail block buffer, fabric, small scissors, and adhesive dryer in addition to your standard table set-up.

1. **Complete nail wrap pre-service.**
2. **Remove old polish.** Use a non-acetone polish remover to avoid damaging wraps.
3. **Clean nails.** Use nail brush and antibacterial soap to gently clean nails.
4. **Push back cuticle.**
5. **Buff nail to remove shine.** Lightly buff over nail plates to remove natural oil and to remove any small pieces of fabric that may have lifted. Buff nail until smooth, without scratching natural nail plate. Totally refine nail until there is no line of demarcation between new growth and fabric wrap.
6. **Apply nail antiseptic.**
7. **Cut fabric.** Cut a piece of fabric large enough to cover the new growth area above the old wrap.
8. **Apply fabric.** Gently fit fabric over new growth area and smooth. (Fig. 13.10)
9. **Trim fabric.** Trim fabric 1/16 inch away from cuticle and sides of nail. Allow new fabric to slightly overlap existing fabric.

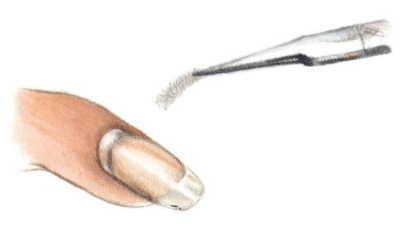

13.10 — Apply fabric to regrowth area.

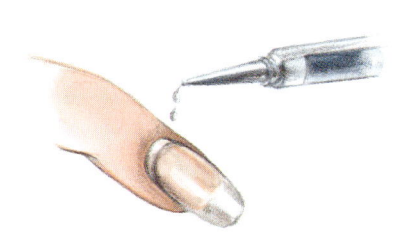

10. **Apply adhesive to regrowth area.** Apply a small drop of adhesive to fabric in new growth area. Spread throughout new growth area with the extender tip. Be careful to avoid cuticle or skin. (Fig. 13.11)
11. **Apply adhesive dryer.**
12. **Apply adhesive.** Apply a second coat of adhesive to regrowth area.
13. **Apply second coat of adhesive dryer.**
14. **Apply adhesive to entire nail.** Apply a thin coat of adhesive to entire nail to strengthen and seal wrap.
15. **Apply adhesive dryer.**
16. **Shape and refine nail.** Use medium/fine abrasive over surface of nail to remove any peaks and imperfections. Carefully stay away from cuticle so you do not cut and damage skin.
17. **Buff nails.** Apply cuticle oil and buff to a high shine with block buffer.
18. **Apply hand lotion and massage hand and arm.**
19. **Remove traces of oil.** Use a small piece of cotton or a cotton-tipped orangewood stick and acetone to remove traces of oil from nail so polish will adhere.
20. **Apply polish.**
21. **Complete nail wrap post-service.**

13.11 — Apply adhesive to regrowth area.

REPAIRS WITH FABRIC WRAPS

Small pieces of fabric can be used to strengthen a weak point in the nail or repair a break in the nail. A *stress strip* is a strip of fabric cut to 1/8 inch. The strip is applied to the weak point of the nail, using the four-week maintenance procedure. A *repair patch* is a piece of fabric that is cut so it completely covers the crack or break in the nail. Use the four-week fabric wrap maintenance procedure to apply your repair patch.

FABRIC WRAP REMOVAL

Be careful not to damage the nail plate when removing fabric wraps.

1. **Complete nail wrap pre-service.**
2. **Soak nails.** Put enough acetone in a small glass bowl to cover the nails. Immerse client's nails in bowl and soak for a few minutes.
3. **Slide off softened wraps.** Use an orangewood stick to slide softened wraps away from nail.

4. **Buff nails.** Gently buff natural nails with fine block buffer to remove the glue residue.

5. **Condition cuticles.** Condition cuticles and surrounding skin with cuticle oil and lotion.

PAPER WRAPS

Paper wraps are applied as a temporary method of strengthening the nail. Mending tissue, a thin paper, is applied over the nail plate to add strength to a nail just as a fabric does. Paper wraps are temporary because they are applied with mending liquid, which dissolves in polish remover. Therefore, the wrap is removed each time the polish is removed. Paper wraps provide added strength for a short period of time. These wraps are not recommended for extra long nails because they do not provide the strength that long nails require.

SUPPLIES

Mending tissue. A lightweight thin tissue paper.
Mending liquid. A heavy liquid adhesive that dissolves in polish remover. It is applied with a brush.
Ridge filler.

PAPER WRAP APPLICATION PROCEDURE

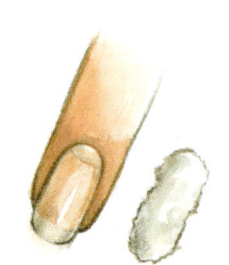

13.12 — Tear mending tissue.

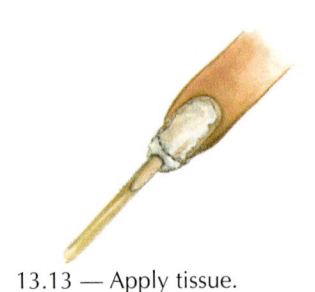

13.13 — Apply tissue.

1. **Complete nail wrap pre-service.** Add mending liquid, mending tissue, and ridge filler to your table.

2. **Remove old polish.**

3. **Clean nails.** Use nail brush and antibacterial soap to gently scrub nails.

4. **Push back cuticle.**

5. **Buff nails to remove shine.** Use medium/fine abrasive to remove shine from nails.

6. **Apply nail antiseptic.** Use cotton-tipped orangewood stick, cotton, or spray to apply nail antiseptic to all nails.

7. **Tear mending tissue.** Tear tissue to fit the shape of the nail, making sure it is feathered at the edges. The tissue should be long enough to tuck under the free edge. (Fig. 13.12)

8. **Apply mending liquid to tissue.** Saturate each piece of tissue with mending liquid.

9. **Apply tissue.** Place wrap over the nail using two fingers. (Fig. 13.13)

10. **Smooth the wrap.** Use a steel pusher or orangewood stick to push tissue toward the free edge and sidewalls. Dip pusher into polish remover repeatedly and pat tissue until it is smooth.

11. **Trim excess tissue.** Trim tissue 1/16 inch from the sidewalls. Leave enough tissue at the end to wrap under free edge. (Fig. 13.14)

12. **Apply mending liquid under free edge.** Turn the finger over and apply mending liquid under free edge.

13. **Smooth wrap.** Use pusher to smooth wrap under free edge. (Fig. 13.15)

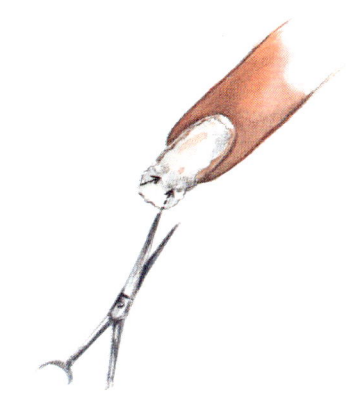

13.14 — Cut slits into tissue.

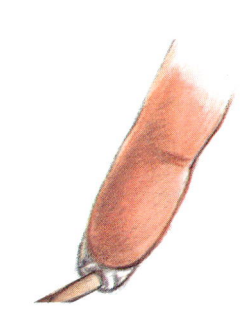

13.15 — Smooth wrap under free edge.

14. **Refine nail.** Gently smooth top of the wrap with the fine side of an emery board. This removes any minute particles that may cause bubbling.

15. **Apply mending liquid.** Apply two or three coats of mending liquid to the top and underside of the free edge of the nail.

16. **Apply ridge filler.** Apply a thin coat of ridge filler to top of nails to smooth surface. Allow filler to dry completely before applying polish.

17. **Apply polish.**

18. **Complete nail wrap post-service.** (Fig. 13.16)

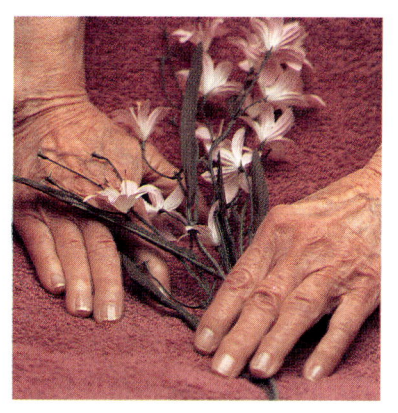

13.16 — Finished paper wrap

LIQUID NAIL WRAP

Liquid nail wrap is a polish made up of tiny fibers designed to strengthen and preserve the natural nail as it grows. It is brushed on the nail in several directions to create a network that, once hardened, protects the nail. It is similar to nail hardener, but thicker because it contains more fiber.

REVIEW QUESTIONS

1. List four kinds of nail wraps.
2. Explain the benefits of using silk, linen, fiberglass, and paper wraps.
3. Describe the procedure for fabric wrap application.
4. Explain how a fabric wrap is used as a crack repair.
5. Describe how to remove fabric wraps and what to avoid.
6. Describe the purpose of paper wraps and explain why they are not recommended for very long nails.
7. List the materials used for paper wraps.
8. Outline the procedures used in paper wraps.
9. Define liquid nail wrap and describe its purpose.

Chapter 14
ACRYLIC NAILS

LEARNING OBJECTIVES

After you have studied this chapter, you should be able to:

1. Identify the supplies needed for acrylic nail application.
2. Explain the chemistry of acrylic nails.
3. Demonstrate the proper procedure and precautions for the application of acrylic nails over forms.
4. Describe the safety precautions for applying primer.
5. Demonstrate the proper procedure and precautions for the application of acrylic nails over tips.
6. Demonstrate the proper procedure and precautions for the acrylic nails application over bitten nails.
7. Describe two basic types of maintenance for acrylic nails.
8. Describe the proper procedure for removing acrylics.
9. Explain how the application of odorless acrylics differs from the application of traditional acrylics.

INTRODUCTION

Acrylic (a-**KRYL**-yk), nails (also known as sculptured or build-on nails) are made by combining a liquid acrylic product with a powdered acrylic product. The two products form a soft ball that can easily be molded into a nail shape. After it is applied, the soft acrylic hardens into a strong artificial nail. Acrylic nails can be applied to natural nails, nail tips, or nail forms to strengthen or extend the nail. They can also be used to repair weak, bitten, or torn nails. The nail technician builds the nail to conform to the shape of the client's fingers and hands for natural-looking, durable nails.

The basic chemistry of acrylic nails is simple. There are three basic ingredients in the acrylic nail process. A *monomer* (**MON**-oh-mehr) is something made up of many small molecules that are not attached to one another. Liquid acrylic is a type of monomer. A *polymer* (**POL**-i-mehr) is made up of molecules that are attached in long chains and usually form something hard. Finished acrylic nails are polymers. A *catalyst* (**CAT**-a-lyst) is an ingredient that speeds up the hardening process. The hardening process is also referred to as **curing**. The powdered acrylic used is a combination of ground-up polymer and a catalyst. The process of forming the nail is called **polymerization** (pol-i-mehr-i-**ZAY**-shun).

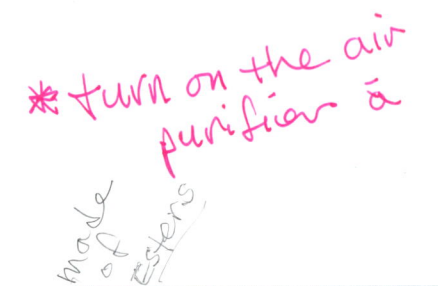

ACRYLIC NAILS OVER FORMS

There are two acrylic nail methods—one-color and two-color. The one-color method uses a single color of acrylic powder (clear, natural, or pink) for the entire nail and produces a nail that is usually worn with polish. The two-color method uses white acrylic powder for the free edge and clear, natural, or pink powder for the nail plate. It produces a nail that looks as if it has a French manicure and needs no polish.

SUPPLIES FOR ACRYLIC NAILS

In addition to the supplies in your basic manicuring set-up, you will need the following items: (Fig. 14.1)

Acrylic liquid. Combined with the acrylic powder to form the sculptured nail. Also referred to as a monomer.

Acrylic powder. White, clear, natural, and pink powder is available. The color(s) you chose will depend on the acrylic nail method you are using.

Primer. Applied to the nail so that the acrylic product will adhere to the natural nail. Primer can be non-etching or etching.

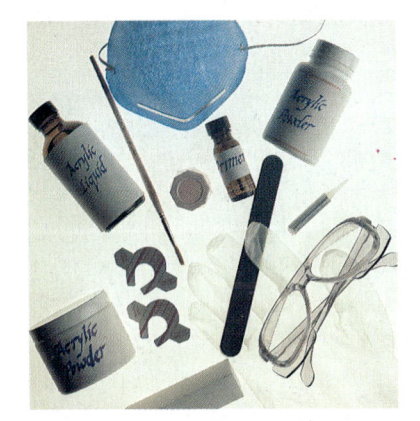

14.1 — Materials needed for application of acrylic nails

Non-etching primer is easier to use safely but may not be as effective as etching primer. *Etching primers* chemically dissolve nooks and crannies into the natural nail to help the acrylic to hold on to the nail plate. Primers are very effective but can cause serious, sometimes irreversible, damage to skin and eyes. Never use primer without plastic gloves and safety glasses.

Abrasive.

Small containers for liquid and powdered acrylic.

Nail forms. Can be disposable or reusable. Disposable forms have an adhesive backing that holds the form in place. Reusable forms are made of aluminum, Teflon, or plastic and have no adhesive backing.

Sable brush. Used to apply and shape the soft balls of acrylic on the nail.

Safety glasses.

Plastic gloves.

Safety mask. (optional)

ACRYLIC NAIL PRE-SERVICE

1. Complete Pre-Service Sanitation Procedure. (This procedure is described on pages 32-33.)

2. Set up your standard manicuring table. Add the acrylic materials to your table.

3. Greet client and ask her to wash hands with antibacterial soap. Be sure to dry hands thoroughly with a fresh towel.

4. Do client consultation, using client health/record card to record responses and observations. Check for nail disorders and decide if it is safe and appropriate to perform a service on this client. If the client should not receive a service, explain your reasons and refer her to a doctor.

14.2 — Clean nails.

ACRYLIC NAIL PROCEDURE

1. **Remove** polish. Begin with your client's left hand, little finger, and work toward the thumb. Then repeat on the right hand.

2. **Push back cuticle.** Use a cotton-tipped orangewood stick to gently push back cuticle.

3. **Buff nail to remove shine.** Buff lightly over nail plate with medium/fine abrasive to remove the natural oil. Brush off filings. (Fig. 14.3)

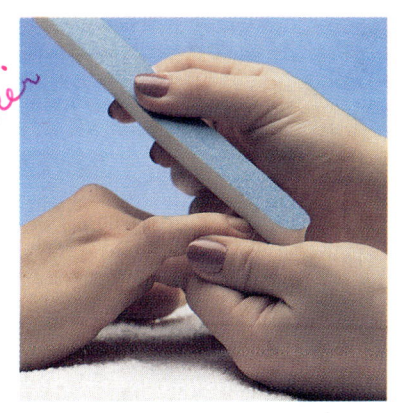

14.3 — Buff nail to remove shine.

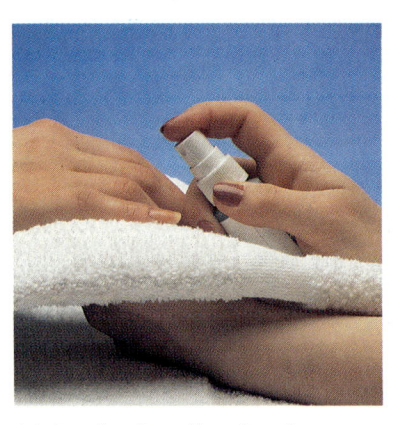

178 ◆ PART IV   THE ART OF NAIL TECHNOLOGY

— Kills bacteria dehydrate the nail

4. **Apply nail antiseptic.** Apply nail antiseptic to nails with cotton-tipped orangewood stick, cotton, or spray. Begin with the little finger on the left hand and work toward the thumb. (Fig. 14.4)

5. **Position nail form.** Position nail form on nail. If you are using disposable forms, peel a nail form from its paper backing and, using the thumb and index finger of each of your hands, bend the form into an arch to fit the client's natural nail shape. Slide the form onto your client's finger and press adhesive backing to sides of the finger. Check to see that the form is snug under the free edge and level with the natural nail.

   If you are using reusable forms, slide the form onto the client's finger, making sure the free edge is over the form and that it fits snugly. Be careful not to cut into the part of the skin under the free edge. Tighten the form around the finger by squeezing lightly. (Fig. 14.5)

6. **Apply primer.** Put on plastic gloves and a pair of safety glasses. Offer a pair of safety glasses to your client. Apply a dot of primer on nail with cotton-tipped orangewood stick. The primer prepares the nail surface for bonding with the acrylic material. Primer should be applied very sparingly. Allow primer to dry on nail to a chalky white. (Fig. 14.6, 14.7)

   * Spray of baking soda - helps neutralizer

7. **Prepare acrylic liquid and powder.** Pour acrylic liquid and acrylic powder into separate small containers. If you are using the two-color method, you will need three small containers—one for the white tip powder, one for the clear, natural, or pink powder, and one for the acrylic liquid. (Throughout this chapter, pink and white acrylic powders are used for the two-color method. Your client may select the one-color method or she may pick clear or natural powder instead of pink.)

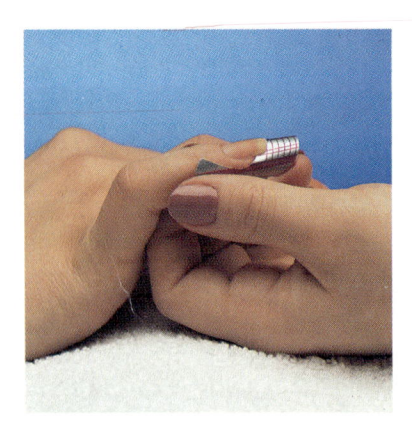

14.4 — Apply nail antiseptic.

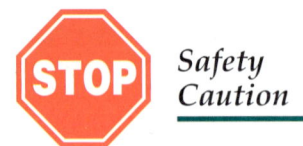

STOP — **Safety Caution**

Be very careful not to allow primer to touch your client's skin or your own. If you accidently spill primer on your clothing, remove the soiled garment immediately.

14.5 — Position nail form.

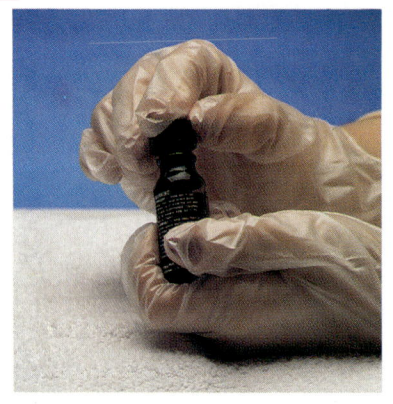

14.6 — Always use plastic gloves when applying primer.

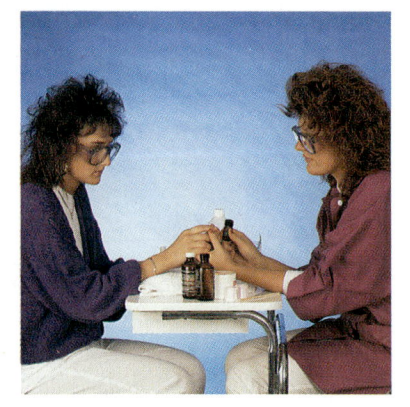

14.7 — Always wear safety glasses when applying primer.

CHAPTER 14 ACRYLIC NAILS ◆ 179

8. **Dip brush into acrylic liquid.** Dip brush fully into the liquid and wipe on the edge of the container to remove the excess. (Fig. 14.8)

9. **Form acrylic ball.** Dip the tip of the same brush into the white acrylic powder and rotate slightly. You will pick up a ball of acrylic product of medium-dry consistency that is large enough for shaping the entire free edge extension. (Fig. 14.9)

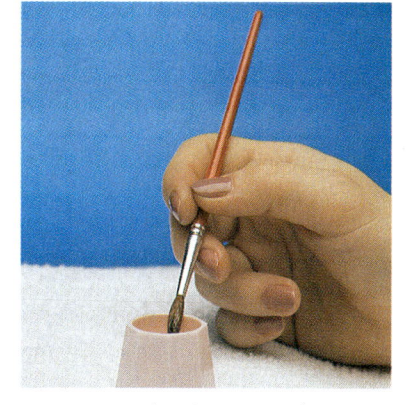

14.8 — Dip brush into acrylic liquid.

PROCEDURAL TIP

Do not touch primed area of the nail with wet brush until you apply acrylic on the area. The acrylic will lift if the area has been touched with the wet brush.

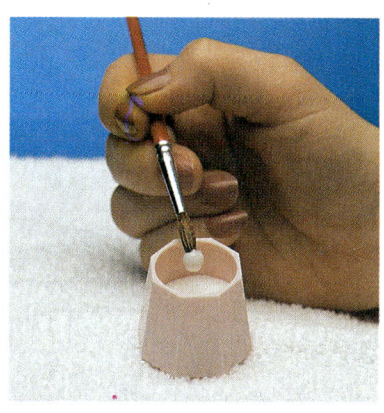

10. **Place ball of acrylic.** Place acrylic ball on the nail form at the point where the free edge joins the nail form. (Fig. 14.10, 14.11)

14.9 — Form ball of acrylic.

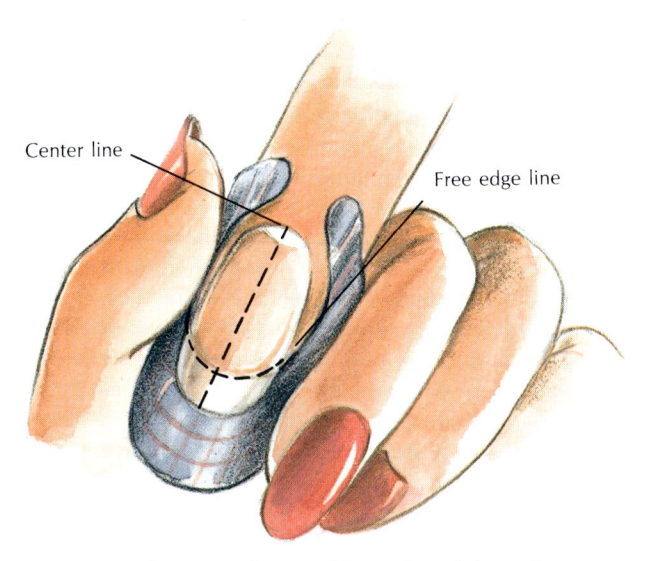

14.10 — The center line and free edge of the nail

11. **Shape free edge.** Use the middle portion of your sable brush to dab and press the acrylic to shape an extension. Do not "paint" the acrylic onto the nail. Dabbing and pressing the acrylic is more accurate than "painting" and produces a more natural-looking nail. Keep sidewall lines parallel and shape acrylic continuously along free edge line. If you are using the

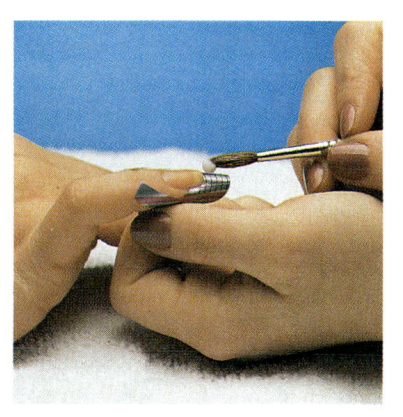

14.11 — Place ball of acrylic on nail form.

two-color acrylic method, make sure you follow the natural free edge line with the white powder to produce the French manicure look. (Fig. 14.12, 14.13)

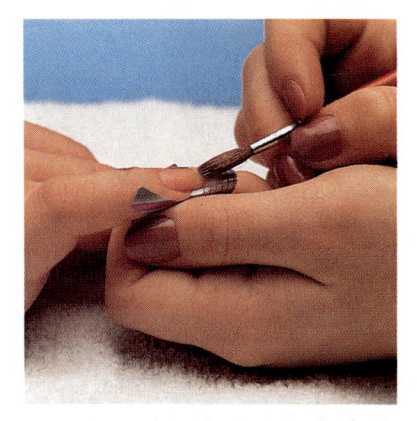

14.12 — Dab and press acrylic with the middle portion of brush.

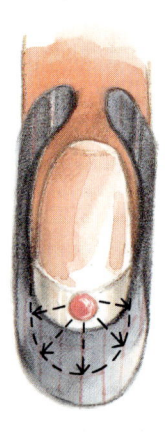

14.13 — Shape free edge.

12. **Place second ball of acrylic.** Pick up a second ball of acrylic of medium consistency and place it on natural nail next to the free edge line in center of nail. (Fig. 14.14)

13. **Shape second ball of acrylic.** Dab and press product to sidewalls, making sure the product is very thin around all edges. If you are using a two-color acrylic product, use the pink powder in this step. (Fig. 14.15)

14. **Apply acrylic beads.** Pick up small wet beads of pink acrylic powder on your brush and place at cuticle area. Use the moisture in the brush to smooth these beads over entire nail plate. Glide brush over nail to smooth out imperfections. Acrylic application near cuticle, sidewall, and free edge should be extremely thin for a natural-looking nail. (Fig. 14.16)

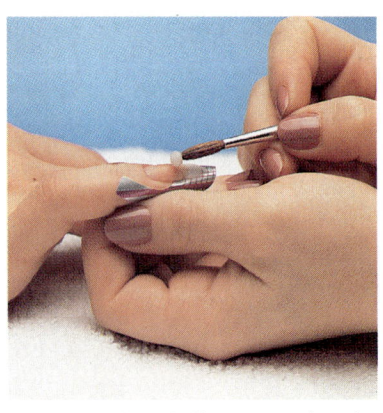

14.14 — Place ball on natural nail.

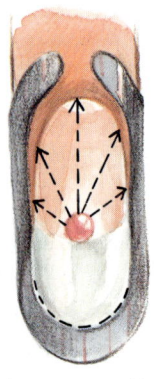

14.15 — Shape second ball of acrylic.

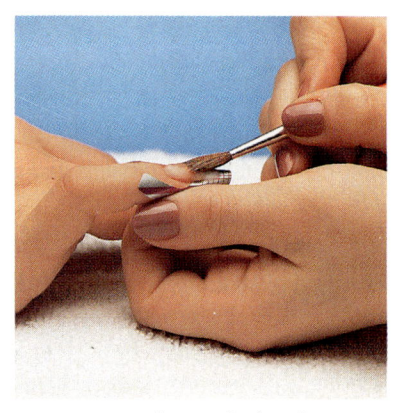

14.16 — Apply acrylic beads.

CHAPTER 14　ACRYLIC NAILS　◆　**181**

PROCEDURAL TIP

Acrylic applied too thickly near cuticle can cause acrylic nail to lift.

15. **Apply acrylic to remaining nails.** Repeat steps 5-14 on remaining nails.

16. **Remove forms.** When nails are thoroughly dry, loosen forms and slide them off. Nails are dry when they make a clicking sound when lightly tapped. (Fig. 14.17)

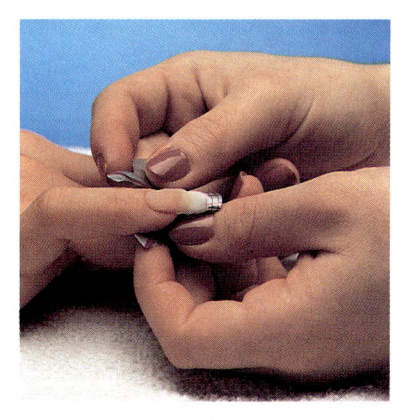

14.17 — Remove forms.

17. **Shape nails.** Use coarse/medium abrasive to shape free edge and to remove imperfections. Glide abrasive over each nail with long sweeping strokes to further shape and perfect nail surface. Make nails thinner toward cuticles, free edge, and sidewalls.

18. **Buff nails.** Buff nails with block buffer until entire surface is smooth.

19. **Apply cuticle oil.** Use a cotton-tipped orangewood stick to apply cuticle oil to cuticles, surrounding skin, and nails. (Fig. 14.18)

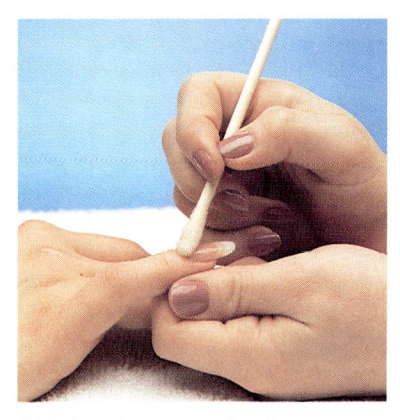

14.18 — Apply cuticle oil.

20. **Apply hand cream and massage hand and arm.**

21. **Clean nails.** Ask client to dip nails in fingerbowl filled with antibacterial soap. Then use nail brush to clean nails over fingerbowl. Rinse with water. Dry thoroughly. If your client selected the two-color method, her acrylic nails are finished. (Fig. 14.19)

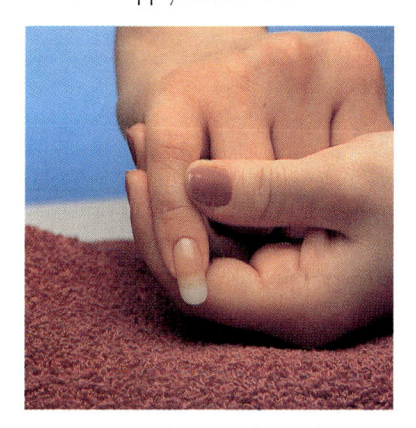

22. **Apply polish.** If your client selected one-color acrylic nails, apply the polish she has chosen.

14.19 — Finished acrylic nail

ACRYLIC NAIL POST-SERVICE

1. **Make another appointment.** Schedule another appointment with your client for maintaining her acrylic nails. A fill-in will be necessary in two or three weeks, depending on how quickly the nails grow. Encourage your client to return for a water manicure between acrylic maintenance appointments if her acrylic nails are polished.

2. **Sell retail products.** Suggest that your client buy products necessary to maintain her acrylic nails between appointments. Polish, lotion, and top coat may be helpful.
3. **Clean up around your table.** Take the time to restore the basic set-up of your table. Be sure that all your acrylic product bottles are closed tightly.
4. **Clean brush.** Clean brush in acetone or in manufacturer's cleaner. Never pull out bristles of brush because you will loosen the remaining bristles. Clip one stray hair if necessary but never trim bristles because you will ruin the accuracy of the brush.
5. **Store acrylic products.** Store acrylic powders in covered containers. Store all primers and acrylic liquids in a cool, dark area. Do not store products near heat.
6. **Discard used materials.** Never save used primer or liquid that has been removed from original bottle. Use on one client only. In order to dispose of leftover liquid or primer, pour it into a very absorbent paper towel or cloth and then place the towel or cloth in a plastic bag. Never pour the liquid directly into the plastic bag! Place all used materials in the plastic bag at the side of the table. After all used materials have been placed in the bag, seal it, and discard it in a closed pail. Since acrylic products can produce harmful vapors, it is important to remove items soiled with acrylic product from your manicuring station after each client.
7. **Sanitize table and implements.** Perform the complete pre-service sanitation procedure. Implements must be sanitized for 20 minutes before they can be used on another client. Reusable forms must be sanitized for at least 20 minutes in an approved disinfectant since they will be used again.

ACRYLIC NAILS OVER TIPS OR NATURAL NAILS

PROCEDURE

1. **Complete acrylic nail pre-service.** This procedure is described on page 177.
2. **Remove polish.** Begin with your client's left hand, little finger, and work toward the thumb. Then repeat on the right hand.
3. **Clean nails.** Ask client to dip nails in fingerbowl filled with antibacterial soap. Then use nail brush to clean nails over fingerbowl. Rinse nails briefly in clear water.
4. **Push back cuticle.** Use an orangewood stick to gently push back cuticle.
5. **Buff nail to remove shine.** Buff lightly over nail plate with medium/fine abrasive to remove the natural oil. Brush off filings.

6. **Apply nail antiseptic.** Apply nail antiseptic to nails with cotton-tipped orangewood stick, cotton, or spray. Begin with the little finger on the left hand and work toward the thumb.

7. **Apply tips.** Apply tips if your client desires them, using the technique described in Chapter 12.

8. **Apply primer.** Put on plastic gloves and a pair of safety glasses. Offer a pair of safety glasses to your client. Apply a dot of primer on nail and nail tip (if instructed by tip manufacturer) with a cotton-tipped orangewood stick. Allow primer to dry to chalky white color before applying acrylic.

9. **Prepare acrylic liquid and powder.** Pour acrylic liquid and acrylic powder into separate small containers. If you are using the two-color system, you will need three small containers—one for the white tip powder, one for the pink powder, and one for the acrylic liquid.

10. **Dip brush into liquid.** Dip brush fully into the liquid and wipe on the edge of the container to remove the excess.

11. **Form acrylic ball.** Dip the tip of the same brush into the white acrylic powder and rotate slightly. You will pick up a medium/dry ball of acrylic product that is large enough to shape the entire free edge.

12. **Place ball of acrylic on free edge.** Place acrylic ball on the free edge of tip or natural nail. (Fig. 14.20)

13. **Shape free edge.** Use the middle portion of your sable brush to dab and press the acrylic to shape the free edge. Keep sidewall lines parallel. Do not "paint" acrylic onto nail. If you are using the two-color acrylic method, make sure you follow the natural free edge line with the white powder to produce a French manicure look.

14. **Place second ball of acrylic.** Pick up a second ball of acrylic of medium consistency and place it on the nail bed next to the free edge line in center of nail. (Fig. 14.21)

15. **Shape second ball of acrylic.** Dab and press product to sidewalls and cuticle, making sure the product is very thin around all edges. If you are using a two-color acrylic product, use the pink powder in this step.

16. **Apply acrylic beads.** Pick up small wet beads of acrylic powder on your brush and place at cuticle area. Use the moisture in the brush to smooth these beads over entire nail. Glide brush over nail to smooth out imperfections. Keep acrylic application near cuticle, sidewall, and free edge extremely thin for the most natural-looking nail. For the two-color method use pink powder to form acrylic beads. (Fig. 14.22)

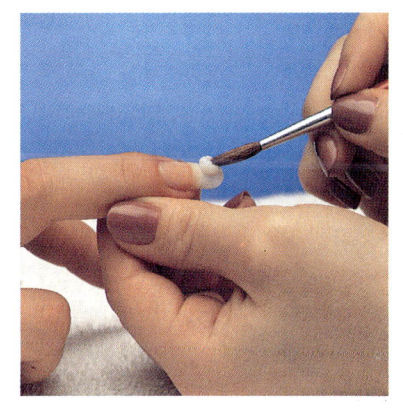

14.20 — Place ball of acrylic on free edge.

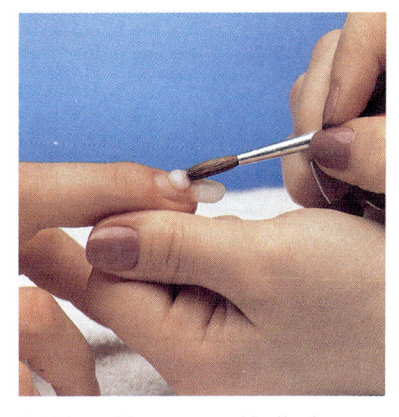

14.21 — Place second ball of acrylic on nail bed.

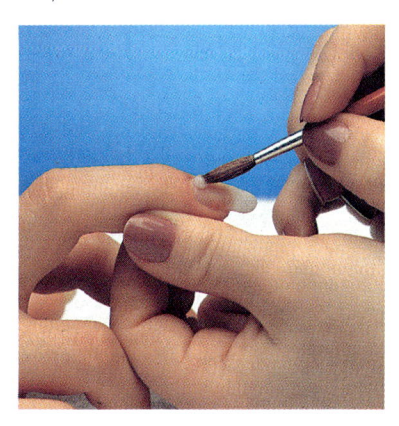

14.22 — Apply acrylic beads.

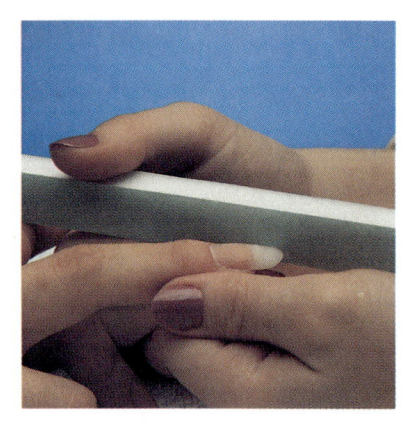

14.23 — Shape and refine nail.

17. **Shape and refine nail.** Use coarse abrasive to shape free edge and to remove imperfections. Then refine with medium/fine abrasive. (Fig. 14.23)
18. **Buff nails.** Buff nail with block buffer until entire surface is smooth. (Fig. 14.24)
19. **Apply cuticle oil.** Rub cuticle oil into cuticles surrounding skin and nails surface.
20. **Apply hand cream and massage hand and arm.**
21. **Clean nails.** Ask client to dip nails in fingerbowl filled with antibacterial soap. Then use nail brush to clean nails over fingerbowl. Rinse with water. Dry thoroughly. If your client selected the two-color method, her acrylic nails are finished. (Fig. 14.25)
22. **Apply polish.** Polish one-color acrylic nails.
23. **Complete acrylic post-service procedure.**

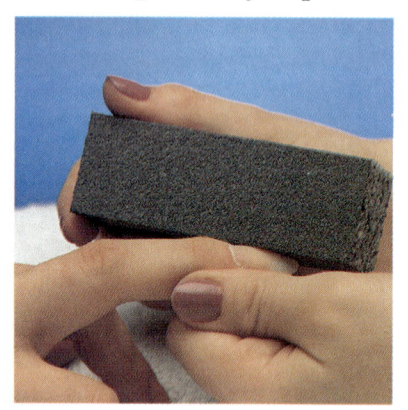

14.24 — Buff nails until smooth.

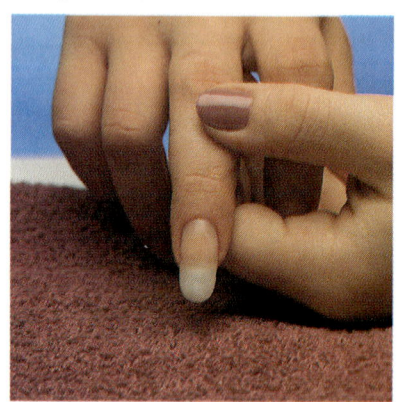

14.25 — Finished acrylic nail over tip

ACRYLIC NAIL APPLICATION OVER BITTEN NAILS

PROCEDURE

The procedure for applying acrylic nails over bitten nails is similar to the application of acrylic nails over forms. However, you must create a portion of the nail plate before applying the nail form.

1. **Complete acrylic application pre-service.**
2. **Remove polish.** Begin with your client's left hand, little finger, and work toward the thumb. Then repeat on the right hand.
3. **Clean nails.** Ask client to dip nails in fingerbowl filled with antibacterial soap. Then use nail brush to clean nails over fingerbowl. Rinse nails briefly in clear water.
4. **Push back cuticle.** Use a cotton-tipped orangewood stick to gently push back cuticle.

5. **Buff nail to remove shine.** Buff lightly over nail plate with medium/fine abrasive to remove the natural oil. Brush off filings.
6. **Apply nail antiseptic.** Apply nail antiseptic to nails with cotton-tipped orangewood stick, cotton, or spray. Begin with the little finger on the left hand and work toward the thumb.
7. **Apply primer.** Put on plastic gloves and a pair of safety glasses. Offer a pair of safety glasses to your client. Apply a dot of primer on nail with cotton-tipped orangewood stick. Primer is meant for the nail plate only. People with bitten nails often have rough cuticles and damaged surrounding skin. Be very careful to avoid touching any of the client's skin with primer.
8. **Prepare acrylic** liquid and powder. Pour acrylic liquid and acrylic powder into separate small containers.
9. **Form acrylic ball.** Pick up a small ball of acrylic product of medium-dry consistency. Use white for the two-color method.
10. **Place ball of acrylic on skin.** Apply a small ball of acrylic product on the skin near bitten nail. (Fig. 14.26)
11. **Create nail plate.** Use the middle of your brush to dab and press to shape a nail plate or a base for the form on which the acrylic nail will be built. Do not place acrylic product beyond the sidewall line. (Fig. 14.27)
12. **Pull skin away.** Allow the acrylic to dry completely. You should be able to hear a click when you tap it with a brush. Then gently pull the client's skin away at the free edge line. You will now have a free edge that is large enough to support a nail form. (Fig. 14.28)

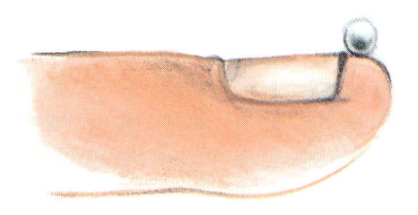

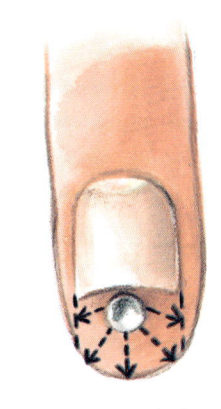

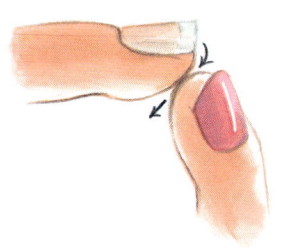

14.26 — Place ball of acrylic on skin.

14.27 — Create nail plate.

14.28 — Pull skin away.

13. **Position nail form.** Position nail form under newly created free edge.
14. **Place ball of acrylic.** Pick up ball of acrylic of medium consistency and place it on the nail form where the nail meets the nail form.
15. **Shape free edge.** Use the middle of your brush to dab and press the acrylic to shape an extension. Make free edge extend only slightly beyond fingertip because people with bitten nails are not used to having long nails.

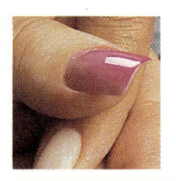

Sanitation Caution

Check primer for clarity on a regular basis to make sure it is not contaminated with bacteria. If bacteria are present, the primer will appear grainy and cloudy.

16. **Place second ball of acrylic.** Pick up a second ball of acrylic of medium consistency and place it next to the free edge line in center of nail. If you are using the two-color method, use pink powder.
17. **Shape second ball of acrylic.** Dab and press product to sidewalls and cuticle area, making sure the product is very thin around all edges.
18. **Apply acrylic beads.** Pick up small wet beads of acrylic powder and place at cuticle area. Use the moisture in the brush to smooth these beads over cuticle and entire nail plate. If you are using a two-color product use pink powder.
19. **Remove forms.** When nails are thoroughly dry, loosen forms and slide them off. Nails are dry when they make a clicking sound when lightly tapped.
20. **Shape nails.** Use coarse/medium abrasive to shape free edge and to remove imperfections.
21. **Buff nails.** Buff nails with block buffer until entire surface is smooth.
22. **Apply cuticle** oil. Rub cuticle oil into surrounding skin and nails surface.
23. **Apply hand cream and massage hand and arm.**
24. **Clean nails.** Ask client to dip nails in fingerbowl filled with antibacterial soap. Then use nail brush to clean nails over fingerbowl. Rinse with water. Dry thoroughly. Your two-color acrylic nails are finished.
25. **Apply polish.** Polish one-color acrylic nails.
26. **Complete acrylic application post-service.**

ACRYLIC NAIL MAINTENANCE AND REMOVAL

Regular maintenance helps prevent acrylic nails from lifting or cracking. When acrylic nails lift, crack, or grow out with no maintenance, moisture and dirt can become trapped under the acrylic nail and fungus can begin to grow.

ACRYLIC MAINTENANCE

There are two basic types of maintenance for acrylic nails—rebalancing and crack repair.

Rebalancing

Rebalancing is the addition of acrylic to the new growth area of the nails. Acrylic nails should be filled in every two to three weeks, depending on how fast the nail grows. Without a rebalancing, the nail will begin to look unnatural and uneven as it grows longer. The new growth area near the cuticle will be noticeably lower than the rest of the nail.

Use the following procedure for rebalancing.

1. **Complete acrylic application pre-service.**

2. **Remove old polish.**

3. **Smooth ledge between new growth and acrylic nail.** Use a medium/fine abrasive to smooth the ledge of acrylic in the new growth area so that it blends into nail plate. (Fig. 14.29)

4. **Refine entire nail.** Hold abrasive flat and glide it over entire nail to reshape and refine nail and thin out free edge.

5. **Buff nail.** Use buffer block to buff acrylic and blend it into new growth area.

6. **Blend acrylic that has lifted.** Use a file to smooth out any acrylic that might have lifted.

7. **Clean nail.** Use fingerbowl filled with warm water and antibacterial soap and a nail brush to gently wash nails. Do not soak nails.

8. **Push back cuticle.** Use a cotton-tipped orangewood stick to gently push back cuticle.

9. **Buff nail to remove shine.** Buff lightly over nail plate with medium/fine abrasive to remove the natural oil. Brush off filings.

10. **Apply nail antiseptic.** Apply nail antiseptic to nails with cotton-tipped orangewood stick, cotton, or spray.

11. **Apply primer.** Put on plastic gloves and a pair of safety glasses. Offer a pair of safety glasses to your client. Apply a dot of primer to the newly grown natural nail.

12. **Prepare acrylic liquid and powder.** Pour acrylic liquid and acrylic powder into separate small containers.

13. **Place balls of acrylic.** Pick up one or more small balls of acrylic and place them on the new growth area. Be sure to use pink acrylic if you are using a two-color method.

14. **Shape balls of acrylic.** Use middle of brush to dab and press the acrylic until it blends into the existing sculptured nail.

15. **Place balls of acrylic.** Pick up one or more small wet balls of acrylic and place them at the base of the nail bed towards the cuticle.

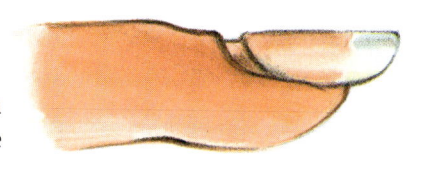

14.29 — New growth area that needs fill-in acrylic maintenance

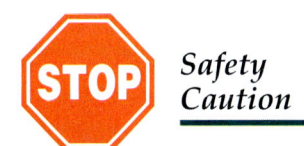

Safety Caution

Do not use a nipper to clip away loose acrylic. Nipping may perpetuate the lifting problem and can damage the nail plate. If lifting is excessive, soak off acrylic and start fresh with a new nail application.

16. **Shape beads of acrylic.** Use the moisture in the brush to smooth these beads over entire nail plate. Glide brush over nail to smooth out imperfections. Acrylic application near cuticle, sidewall, and free edge should be extremely thin for a natural-looking nail. If you are using a two-color acrylic product, use the pink powder in this step.

17. **Shape nails.** Allow nails to dry thoroughly. Nails are dry when they make a clicking sound when lightly tapped. Use a coarse/medium grit abrasive to shape free edge and remove any imperfections. Use medium/fine abrasive to glide over nail with long sweeping strokes to further shape and perfect nail surface. Taper nail shape towards cuticle, nail tip, and sidewalls, making it thin at all edges. (After four or five weeks of growth and two rebalancings, the white acrylic free edge created with the two-color method grows beyond the natural free edge. At this time, your client may want to start wearing polish, and she may want you to file back the white free edge to create a one-color nail.)

18. **Buff nail.** Smooth entire surface of nail using block buffer until it is smooth.

19. **Apply cuticle oil.** Rub cuticle oil into surrounding skin, cuticle, and nail surface using a cotton-tipped orangewood stick.

20. **Apply hand cream and massage hand and arm.**

21. **Clean nails.**

22. **Apply polish.**

23. **Complete acrylic application post-service.**

Crack Repair

Acrylic crack repair is the addition of extra acrylic to fill the crack in an acrylic nail and reinforce the rest of the nail.

1. **Complete acrylic application pre-service.**
2. **Remove old polish.**
3. **File cracked acrylic.** File a "V" shape into the crack or file flush to remove crack.
4. **Clean nails.** Ask client to dip nails in fingerbowl filled with warm water and antibacterial soap. Then use nail brush to clean nails over fingerbowl. Rinse nails briefly in clear water. Dry nails thoroughly.
5. **Apply nail antiseptic.** Apply nail antiseptic to nails using cotton-tipped orangewood stick, cotton, or spray.
6. **Apply primer.** If natural nail plate is exposed, put on plastic gloves and a pair of safety glasses and apply a dot of primer to the area.

7. **Apply nail form.** If the crack is large, apply a nail form for added support.

8. **Prepare acrylic** liquid and powder. Pour acrylic liquid and acrylic powder into separate small containers.

9. **Place balls of acrylic.** Pick up one or more small beads of acrylic and apply them to the cracked area. If you are using the two-color system, be sure to use the correct color acrylic.

10. **Shape balls of acrylic.** Dab and press the acrylic to fill crack. Be careful not to let acrylic seep under form or under existing nail.

11. **Place additional balls of acrylic.** Apply additional acrylic, if needed, to fill in crack or reinforce the rest of the nail. Shape acrylic and allow it to dry thoroughly.

12. **Remove form (if used).**

13. **Reshape nail.**

14. **Buff until smooth.**

15. **Clean nails.**

16. **Apply cuticle oil.**

17. **Apply hand cream and massage hand and arm.**

18. **Clean nails.**

19. **Apply polish.**

20. **Complete acrylic application post-service.**

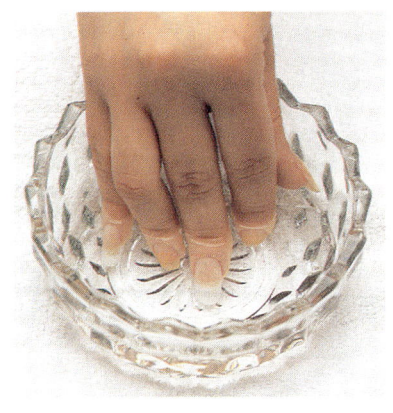

14.30 — Soak fingertips in acetone.

ACRYLIC REMOVAL

1. **Fill bowl with acetone.** Fill glass bowl with enough acetone to cover client's fingertips.

2. **Soak fingertips.** Soak client's fingertips for 15 minutes or as long as needed to remove acrylic product. Refer to your manufacturer's directions for acrylic removal. (Fig. 14.30)

3. **Remove acrylic with orangewood stick.** Use orangewood stick and gently push off softened acrylic nail. Repeat until all acrylic has been removed. Do not pry off acrylic with nippers, as this will damage natural nail plate. (Fig. 14.31)

4. **Buff nails.** Gently buff natural nail with fine block buffer to remove the acrylic residue.

5. **Condition cuticle.** Condition cuticle and surrounding skin with cuticle oil and hand lotion.

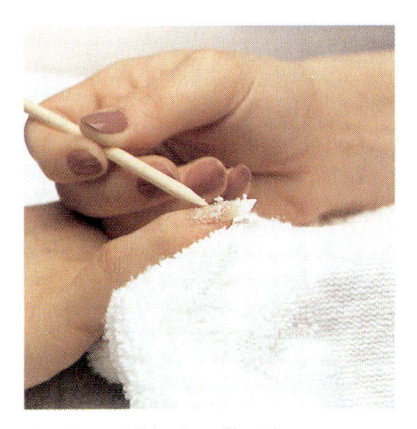

14.31 — Slide tip off with orangewood stick.

ODORLESS ACRYLICS

Odorless acrylics are acrylic products that do not smell as strongly as traditional acrylic products. They are useful if you or your clients are bothered by the odor of acrylic liquid. Although they are not completely odorless, they have less odor and are drier than the traditional acrylic product.

Most odorless acrylics are self-leveling. As the product sets, it automatically levels off, so there is less shaping required. The shaping that is required can be done at a more leisurely pace, because the product has a longer drying time.

When the nails are dry, the surface has a tacky, gummy residue. As you refine the nails, this residue rolls off. The refining process is finished when the product stops rolling off.

You cannot mix traditional acrylics and odorless products because they are not chemically compatible.

Celebrate The Holidays

Taking advantage of gift-giving holidays like Christmas, Chanukah, St. Valentine's Day, Secretary's Day and Mother's Day bring you a 20 to 50 percent temporary surge in retail sales. To make money during the holidays, you must do two things: Decorate festively to encourage clients to consider shopping for presents, and offer a wide range of gifts that customers can conveniently buy while they're at their appointments. Try creating two or three festive packages with different product combinations and sizes, priced from $5.00 to $15.00. People buy these for stocking stuffers or to give as office or church/synagogue gifts. Also, don't forget to offer gift certificates in any denominations.

REVIEW QUESTIONS

1. List the supplies needed for acrylic nail application.
2. Briefly describe the chemistry of acrylic nails.
3. Describe the procedure for the application of acrylic nails over forms.
4. Describe the safety precautions for applying primer.
5. Describe the procedure for applying acrylic nails over tips.
6. How does the procedure for acrylic nail application over bitten nails differ from other acrylic nail procedures?
7. Describe the two basic types of maintenance for acrylic nails.
8. Describe the proper procedure for acrylic removal.
9. Explain how the application of odorless acrylics differs from the application of traditional acrylics.

Chapter 15

GELS

LEARNING OBJECTIVES

After you have studied this chapter, you should be able to:

1. Describe the two basic types of gels.
2. List the supplies needed for light-gel application.
3. Demonstrate the proper procedure and precautions for light-cured gel application.
4. Demonstrate the proper procedure and precautions for light-gel cured application over forms.
5. Demonstrate the proper rocedure and precautions for no-light gel applications.

INTRODUCTION

The following pages introduce the services you can perform with gels. *Gels* are strong, durable artificial nails that are brushed on the nail plate like polish. They have a chemical consistency very similar to the consistency of acrylic nails, but they require a separate catalyst to harden. There are two types of gels. *Light-cured gels* harden when they are exposed to a special light source—either an ultraviolet light or a halogen light. *No-light gels* harden when a gel activator is sprayed or brushed on, or when they are soaked in water.

Gels are available in colors that need no polish. These nails look as if they have already been polished and stay the same color until the gel itself is removed. Polish may be worn over colored gels. When polish is removed, the gel color will remain the same. Colored gels are a great base for nail art.

LIGHT-CURED GEL ON TIPS OR NATURAL NAILS

SUPPLIES

In addition to the materials in your basic manicuring set-up, you will need the following items:

Light-cured gel.

Curing light. A box that has an *ultraviolet* or *halogen* bulb to cure or harden the gel nail. The type of light and the shape of the box varies from manufacturer to manufacturer.

Brush. Some nail technicians prefer to use a synthetic brush with small, flat, square bristles to hold and spread the gel.

Nail forms.

Primer (if recommended by gel manufacturer).

Block buffer.

Nail tips.

Adhesive.

GEL APPLICATION PRE-SERVICE

1. Do your Pre-Service Sanitation procedure. (This procedure is described on pages 32-33.)

2. Set up your standard manicuring table. Place light-cured gel materials on your table.

3. Greet client and ask her to wash her hands with antibacterial soap. Dry hands thoroughly with a fresh towel.

4. Do client consultation, using health/record card to record responses and observations. Check for nail disorders and decide if it is safe and appropriate to perform a service on this client. If the client should not receive a service, explain your reasons and refer him or her to a doctor.

LIGHT-CURED GEL PROCEDURE

1. **Remove polish.** Begin with your client's left hand, little finger, and work toward the thumb. Then repeat on the right hand.

2. **Clean nails.** Ask client to dip nails in fingerbowl filled with antibacterial soap. Then use nail brush to clean nails over fingerbowl. Rinse nails briefly in clear water. Dry hands thoroughly with a fresh towel.

3. **Push back cuticles.** Use a cotton-tipped orangewood stick to gently push back cuticles.

4. **Buff nails to remove shine.** Buff lightly over nail plate with a medium/fine abrasive to remove the natural oil. Brush off filings.

5. **Apply nail antiseptic.** Apply nail antiseptic to nails. Begin with the little finger on the left hand and work toward the thumb.

6. **Apply tips if desired.** If your client wants tips, apply them according to the procedure described in Chapter 12.

7. **Apply primer if recommended by gel manufacturer.** If primer is recommended by the manufacturer of the gel you are using, put on plastic gloves and a pair of safety glasses. Offer a pair of safety glasses to your client. Apply a dot of the primer recommended by the manufacturer on nail plate with a cotton-tipped orangewood stick. Allow primer to dry to a chalky white.

PROCEDURAL TIP

The procedure recommended for applying and curing gel varies from one manufacturer to another. Some systems recommend applying gel to four nails on one hand and curing, and then repeating this procedure on the other hand before applying and curing gel on the thumbnails. Other manufacturers provide light sources that cure only one finger at a time. Be sure to follow the instructions recommended by the manufacturer of the system you are using.

CHAPTER 15   GELS   ◆   **195**

8. **Apply gel.** Brush gel onto entire nail. Cover with a thin, even layer as you would nail polish. Do not brush on cuticle because gel will lift. (Fig. 15.1)

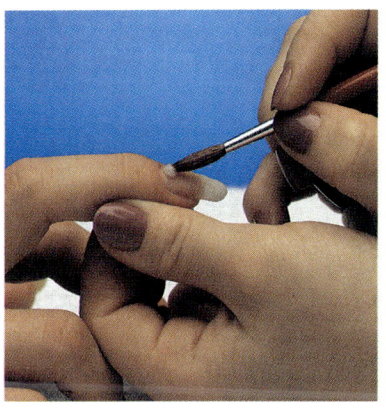

9. **Cure gel.** Place nails under light source and set timer for time recommended by manufacturer. (Figs. 15.2, 15.3)

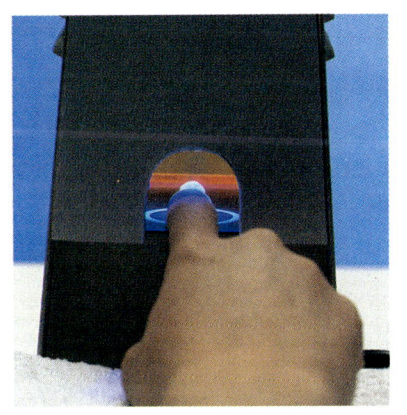

15.1 — Apply gel to entire nail.

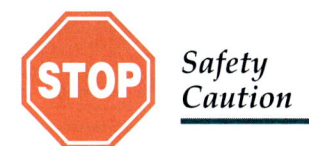

15.2 — Cure gel.

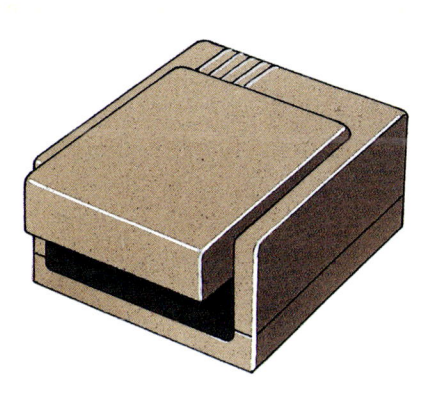

15.3 — Ultraviolet light source

Safety Caution

Inadequately shielded ultraviolet lamps can damage eyes and skin.

PROCEDURAL TIP

During the procedure keep brush and gel away from light to prevent hardening of gel.

10. **Repeat steps 8 and 9 on the other hand.**

11. **Apply second coat of gel to the first hand.** Apply gel in a thin and even coat that looks like a glossy top coat. Do not leave any imperfections in application because the finished nail will not be smooth.

12. **Cure gel.**

13. **Repeat steps 11 and 12 on the other hand.**

14. **Repeat steps 11-13.**

15. **Clean nails.** Wipe nails with alcohol or manufacturer's suggested cleanser to remove residue and tackiness on cured acrylic nails. Cured nails have a shiny gloss that needs no buffing if applied smoothly.

16. **Apply cuticle oil.** Rub cuticle oil into surrounding skin and nail surface.

17. **Apply hand lotion and massage hand and arm.**

18. **Clean nails.** Ask client to dip nails in fingerbowl filled with antibacterial soap. Then use nail brush to clean nails over fingerbowl. Rinse with water and dry thoroughly.

19. **Apply polish.**

GEL APPLICATION POST-SERVICE

Your light-cured gel service is complete. Follow the post-service procedure described below.

1. **Make another appointment.** Schedule another appointment with your client to maintain the service she has just received or to perform another service.

2. **Suggest retail products.** Suggest that your client buy products necessary to maintain her nails throughout the week. Polish, lotion, top coat, etc. are valuable maintenance tools for her to have.

3. **Clean up around your table.** Take the time to restore the basic set-up of your table.

4. **Discard used materials.** Place all used materials in the plastic bag at the side of the table. Empty the bag frequently when you are doing gel nails.

5. **Sanitize table and implements.** Perform the complete pre-service sanitation procedure. In most states, this procedure calls for 20 minutes of proper sanitation before implements can be used on the next client.

LIGHT-CURED GEL OVER FORMS

Clients who want to strengthen and lengthen their natural nails with a light-weight artificial nail may choose gel nails over forms.

1. **Complete gel application pre-service.** Place light-cured gel supplies on your manicuring table.

2. **Apply nail forms.** Fit forms onto all ten fingers just as you would for acrylic nails over forms.

3. **Apply gel to natural nail.** Apply gel first to the natural nail only, not the nail form. (Fig. 15.4)

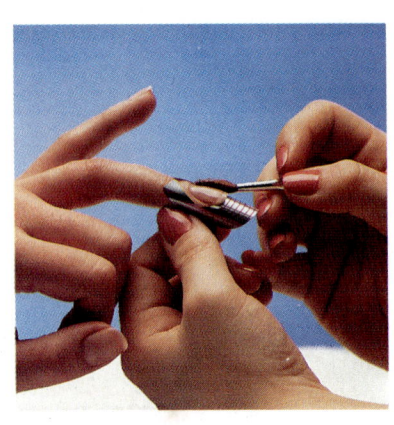

15.4 — Apply gel to natural nail.

4. **Cure gel.** (Fig. 15.5)

5. **Create free edge.** Apply gel to the nail form to create a free edge. (Fig. 15.6)

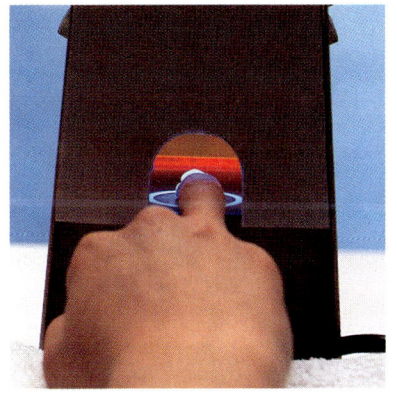

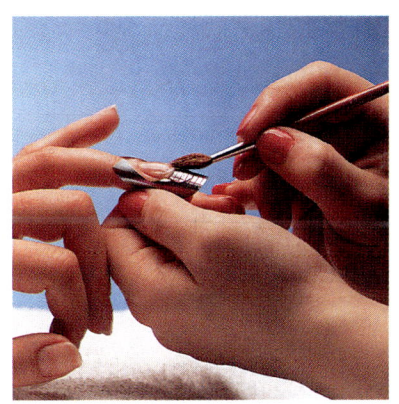

15.5 — Cure gel.

15.6 — Create free edge.

6. **Cure gel.**

7. **Apply gel to entire nail.** Apply gel to entire nail-both the natural nail and the free edge.

8. **Cure gel.**

9. **Remove forms.**

10. **Shape free edge.**

11. **Apply gel to entire nail without form.**

12. **Cure gel.**

13. **Remove residue.** Wipe nails with alcohol or manufacturer's suggested cleanser to remove residue and tackiness on cured acrylic nails. Cured nails have a shiny gloss that needs no buffing if applied smoothly.

14. **Apply cuticle oil.** Rub cuticle oil into surrounding skin and nail surface.

15. **Apply hand cream and massage hand and arm.**

16. **Clean nails.** Ask client to dip nails in fingerbowl filled with antibacterial soap. Then use nail brush to clean nails over fingerbowl. Rinse with water and dry thoroughly.

17. **Apply polish.**

18. **Complete gel application post-service.**

NO-LIGHT GEL APPLICATION

No-light gels come in many varieties with different curing agents. Some are soaked in water and some are sprayed with an activator. The following is a generic procedure designed to show you how no-light gels are applied. For actual application you will need to follow your manufacturer's instructions carefully.

1. **Complete gel application pre-service.**
2. **Remove polish.** Begin with your client's left hand, little finger, and work toward the thumb. Then repeat on the right hand.
3. **Clean nails.** Ask client to dip nails in fingerbowl filled with antibacterial soap. Then use nail brush to clean nails over fingerbowl. Rinse nails briefly in clear water.
4. **Push back cuticles.** Use a cotton-tipped orangewood stick to gently push back cuticles.
5. **Buff nails to remove shine.** Buff lightly over nail plate with a medium/fine abrasive to remove the natural oil. Brush off filings.
6. **Apply nail antiseptic.** Apply nail antiseptic to nails. Begin with the little finger on the left hand and work toward the thumb.
7. **Apply tips if desired.** If your client wants tips, apply them according to the procedure described in Chapter 12.
8. **Apply gel.** Use brush to paint on gel or use bottle to spread a thin coat of gel onto entire nail. Apply gel to the five nails of one hand. Do not brush on cuticle because gel will lift.

PROCEDURAL TIP

Some gels run and must be applied and cured one finger at a time. Be guided by manufacturer's instructions.

9. **Cure gel with activator or water.** *Activator-Cured:* Spray or brush gel activator (also called adhesive dryer) onto nail plate. If you use a spray, hold it at least 8 inches away from the client's nails to reduce the chance of having your client experience a heat reaction from the activator. *Water-Cured:* Immerse nails in lukewarm water for 2-5 minutes, depending on manufacturer's directions.
10. **Repeat steps 8 and 9 on the other hand.**
11. **Apply second coat of gel and cure if necessary.** With no-light gels, a second application of gel may not be necessary. Follow your manufacturer's directions for correct application.

12. **Shape and refine nails.** Shape and refine the entire surface of the nail with a medium/fine abrasive. Use a light touch to remove any imperfections.

13. **Buff nail. Buff nail with block buffer to shine.**

14. **Apply cuticle oil.** Rub cuticle oil into surrounding skin and nail surface.

15. **Apply hand cream and massage hand and arm.**

16. **Clean nails.** Ask client to dip nails in fingerbowl filled with antibacterial soap. Then use nail brush to clean nails over fingerbowl. Rinse with water and dry thoroughly.

17. **Apply polish.**

18. **Complete gel application post-service.**

GEL MAINTENANCE AND REMOVAL

GEL MAINTENANCE

Both light-cured and non–light-cured gels should be maintained every two to three weeks, depending on how fast the client's nails grow. Use a medium abrasive file and buff entire nail to remove shine. Eliminate regrowth ledge by gliding file over ledge area. Hold file flat at ledge, not at an angle, because this can make a groove and damage the natural nail plate. Shape nail and blend it into the natural nail. Continue buffing until there is no line between hardened gel and natural nail plate. Be careful not to damage the natural nail plate by buffing too roughly. When the nail is smooth, follow the procedure for the application of gel on natural nails.

GEL REMOVAL

Soak client's nails for a few minutes in small glass bowl containing enough acetone (or gel remover recommended by gel manufacturer) to cover nails. Use orangewood stick to slide off softened tip. Gently buff natural nail with fine block buffer to remove the glue residue. Condition cuticle and surrounding skin with cuticle oil and lotion.

Teen Time

Take advantage of teenagers' interest in good grooming by introducing them to professional nail care. Ideal lures include a 20 percent discount on all prom and graduation nail services. Contact local schools to see when these events take place; then spread the word by advertising the promotion in high school newspapers six to eight weeks ahead of time. Another option is to hold a "back to school night." Decorate the salon in fun colors, provide refreshments, and invite teens to pay a $10.00 registration fee for a night of nail education and fashion manicures, plus a take-home bag of trial-sized products. Many technicians report success with discounted nail extensions offered to the cheerleading squad, sports manicures to the volleyball team, or even a "good grade" discount for any teen earning a 3.0 or higher grade point average.

REVIEW QUESTIONS

1. Describe the two basic types of gels.
2. List the supplies needed for light-gel application.
3. Describe the proper procedure and precautions for light-cured gel application.
4. Describe the proper procedure and precautions for light-gel application over forms.
5. Describe no-light gel application.

Chapter 16
THE CREATIVE TOUCH

LEARNING OBJECTIVES
After you have studied this chapter, you should be able to:

1. Describe three different nail art supplies.
2. Describe techniques for using these supplies
3. Demonstrate one nail art application.
4. Describe airbrush equipment.
5. Demonstrate proper airbrush techniques.
6. Describe the two-color fade.

INTRODUCTION

Nail art offers endless opportunities for you to express your creativity and your client's unique personality. For example, you can create a nail extension with red gel, polish half of it with blue polish, and paint it with stars, stripes, cats eyes, or tiger lilies highlighted with a rhinestone dew drop. With a creative touch, your imagination and your client's desires are your only limits. (Fig. 16.1)

CREATING NAIL ART

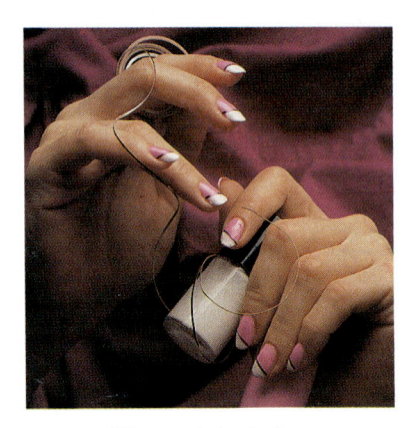

16.1 — Wear artistic designs on your own nails.

Nail art is an exciting and creative part of a nail technician's job. It turns nails into small canvases on which you can paint pictures, create designs, and make collages with tiny gems, foils, tapes, or whatever your client will wear.

This section will provide you with a brief introduction to creating artistic nails with gems, foils, tape, and air brushing. You will also learn the procedures for creating holly berries, a design called "the sweep," and marbled gold.

If you are interested in providing nail art services for your clients, you might want to wear artistic designs on your own nails. This will give your clients a chance to see examples of the type of work you can do.

You may not have to schedule extra time to do nail art because often only one finger is done. Creating nail art on one finger takes only 2 or 3 minutes; but all ten fingers or a very complex design will take longer.

Every nail technician is an artist. This is your chance to be creative. The colors and designs in the world around you will give you ideas for new art. Even mistakes you make could be the beginning of a new creation. Make mistakes into some abstract design. Don't forget there is always nail polish remover to wipe the nail canvases clean so you can start again.

GEMS

Tiny rhinestones are popular nail art materials. They come in different shapes, colors, and sizes. **Gems** give sparkle to a design and add texture.

Use a wet orangewood stick to pick up small gems on the shiny side of the stone. Put them on while the top coat of the polish is still tacky so gems will adhere. Allow nail to dry and apply another top coat over gems. Reapply top coat every three or four days to seal gem to nail and revitalize the shine.

You can use either tweezers or an orangewood stick to pick up large gems. If you use the orangewood stick, dip it in top coat and touch the shiny surface of the gem with the sticky tip of the orangewood stick.

Use acetone to remove gems from your clients' nails. These gems can be reused if the silver backing stays in place. If the silver backing comes off a gem, it must be thrown away because it will no longer reflect color.

STRIPING TAPE

Striping tape comes in rolls of different colors, although silver, gold, and black are the most popular. Tape has a tacky backing and is stuck to a dry, polished nail. Lift the edge of the tape when it is on the nail and, using nippers, cut it 1/16 inch away from cuticle and free edge. This will prevent the tape from peeling and rolling off the nail. Seal tape on nail with top coat and reapply top every three to four days.

FOIL

Foil is very fragile leafing that is available in gold, silver, and copper. It comes in sheets that are packaged approximately ten to a bag. Sheets should be stored in the bag to protect them from cracking. Use tweezers to remove the piece you need. Put the leaf on your table, and rip off little pieces with tweezers or an orangewood stick. Put these small pieces of foil on the tacky top coat.

Foil leaf is used to accentuate parts of a nail. As an example, if you paint half a nail red and the other half black, you can use gold foil to highlight the black portion of each nail or the line between the two colors. Seal the foil with a top coat and reapply the top coat every three to four days.

NAIL TAPE APPLICATION

Polish nails in regular manner. Apply top coat and let dry completely. (Fig. 16.2) If applying nail tape over another design, the design must be dry.

You can have a pattern in mind when you start or use your imagination to create an original design every time.

1. Hold the end of tape in one hand and hold the roll of tape, sticky side down, in the other.

2. Place tape on the nail in desired spot and cut the tape off at end of roll. (Leave the ends long until pattern is complete.)

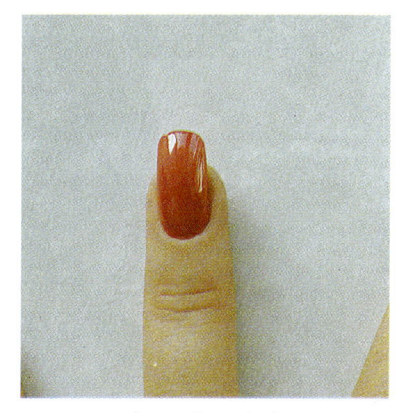

16.2 — A dry nail ready for tape

204 ◆ PART 4 THE ART OF NAIL TECHNOLOGY

3. Use orangewood stick to firmly press tape into place. Be sure there are no air bubbles under tape and that ends are well pressed down.
4. Continue applying tape to complete design, leaving the ends hanging over the free edge and cuticles. (Fig. 16.3)
5. Trim all tape ends with nippers or scissors. Trimming all the ends at the same time assures the tape will meet evenly. (Fig. 16.4)
6. Check to see that all tape ends are pressed down and stuck to nail. If ends won't stay down, you can apply a small amount of clear polish under the, let it dry a little, then press ends down with an orangewood stick. (Fig. 16.5)

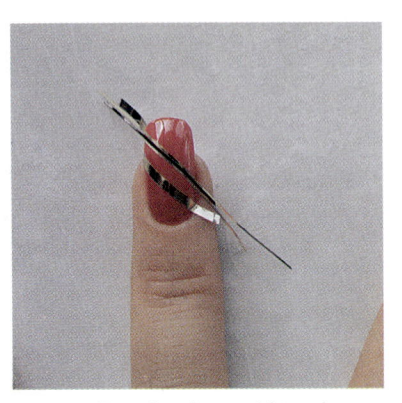

16.3 — Tape in place with ends extending beyond nail.

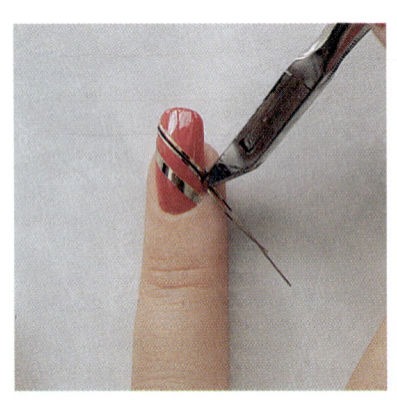

16.4 — Trimming the tape ends with nippers.

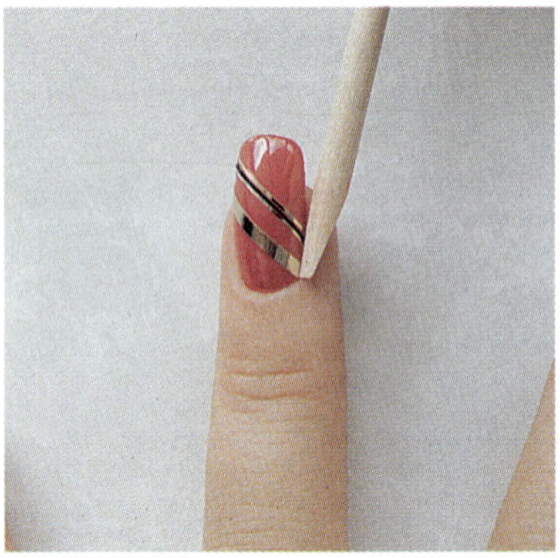

16.5 — Press tape ends down with orangewood stick.

7. Apply clear polish over nail, covering tape and edges of nail completely. (Fig. 16.6)
8. Let dry and check tape ends to be sure they are secure. If they are not, gently press with an orangewood stick until they stay down. Apply another layer of clear polish to secure tape ends. (Fig. 16.7)

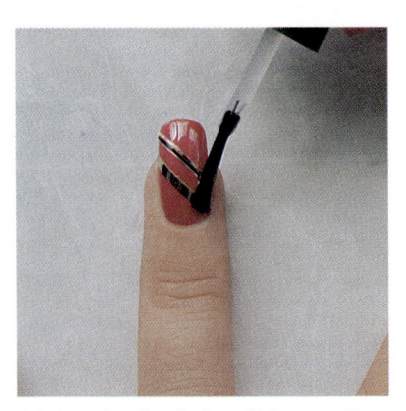

16.6 — Apply clear polish on nail and tape.

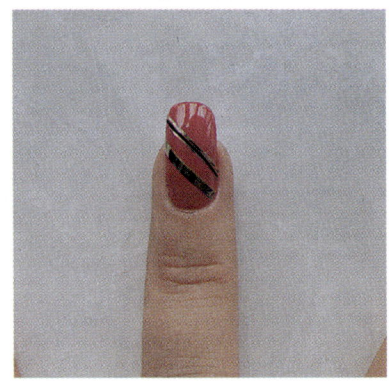

16.7 — Finished tape design

GOLD LEAF APPLICATION

Complete design or polish desired. Cover with clear polish and let dry.

1. Apply clear nail polish on area you want covered with gold. (Fig. 16.8)

2. Using tweezers and orangewood stick, place bits of gold on nail and gently press into wet polish. (Fig. 16.9) Continue doing this until design is complete. (Fig. 16.10)

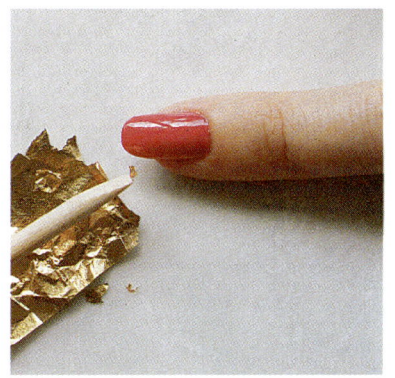

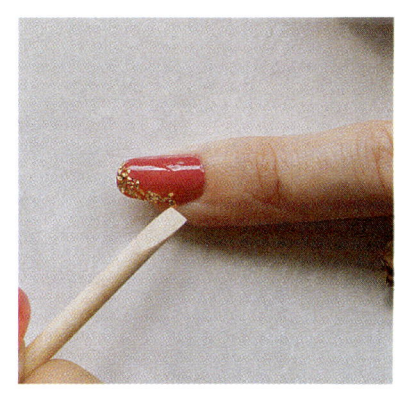

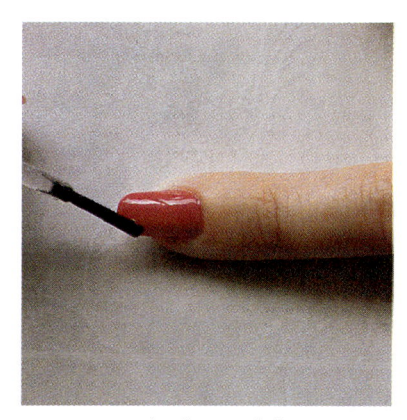

16.8 — Apply clear polish to area of nail on which you want gold leaf to adhere.

16.9 — Apply gold leaf to wet polish.

16.10 — Complete the design.

3. Use orangewood stick to press gold leaf flat on nail. (Fig. 16.11)

4. Apply clear polish over gold leaf to seal. Let dry. (Fig. 16.12) If you are going to add striping tape or a gemstone, do it before applying the final coat of clear polish. (Fig. 16.13)

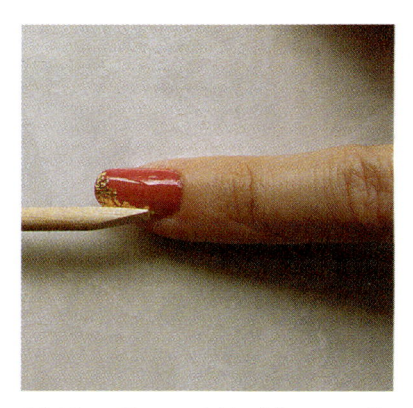

16.11 — Press gold leaf flat on nail.

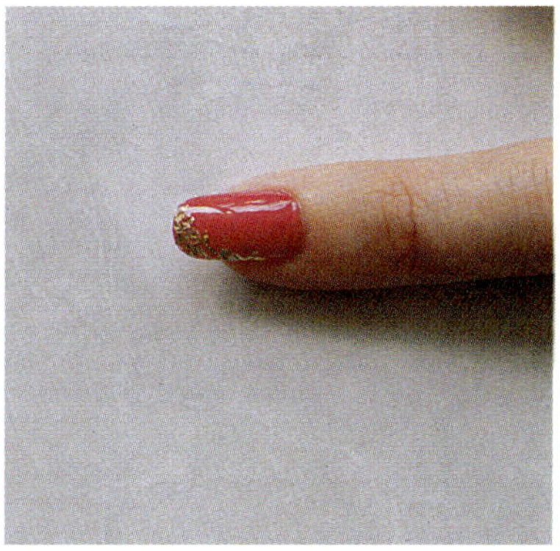

16.12 — Apply clear polish over gold leaf to seal design.

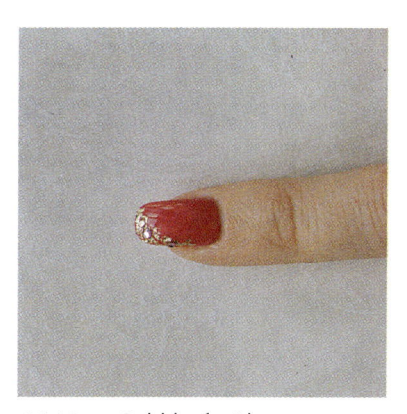

16.13 — Gold leaf with gems

5. A second or third coat of clear polish may be applied if needed to cover nail design. Let each layer dry slightly before applying the next.

206 ◆ PART 4 THE ART OF NAIL TECHNOLOGY

FREEHAND PAINTING

Polish nails in regular manner. Apply top coat and let dry.

1. Using an orangewood stick place a small amount of color on palette.

2. Dip a small brush into water to moisten the bristles.

3. Dip brush in paint.

4. Make a circle of small dots on nail, then put one dot in the middle. To make several flowers use the same process but make some smaller and some larger.

5. Use a striping brush to make the stems.

6. Let the paint dry completely before applying the clear polish. When applying the clear polish, be sure the brush is wet enough to cover the nail. If there is not enough polish on the brush it can damage your painting by smearing the paint instead of covering it.

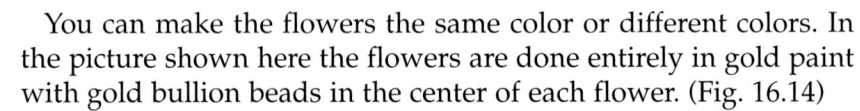

You can make the flowers the same color or different colors. In the picture shown here the flowers are done entirely in gold paint with gold bullion beads in the center of each flower. (Fig. 16.14)

You can make the same design with less flowers. Paint them in any color and add green stems. Use your imagination to create your own flower design.

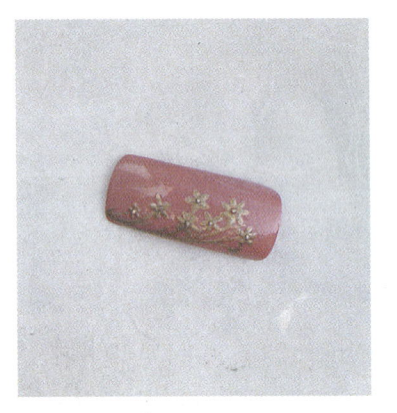

16.14 — Gold flowers with bullion beads

USING AN AIRBRUSH FOR NAIL COLOR AND NAIL ART

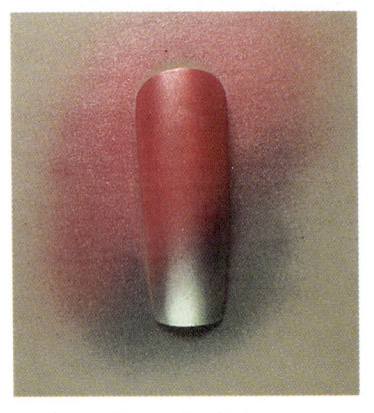

Airbrushing nails has become a popular salon service. Many nail technicians are offering their clients an alternative to traditional nail color by airbrushing the nail color for their clients. Subtle color combinations may be achieved by airbrushing two or more colors on the nails at the same time. This technique is called a color fade or color blend. (Fig. 16.15) By airbrushing the nail color the nail technician may charge an additional price for the special nail color technique.

16.15 — Two color fade

CHAPTER 16   THE CREATIVE TOUCH   ◆   **207**

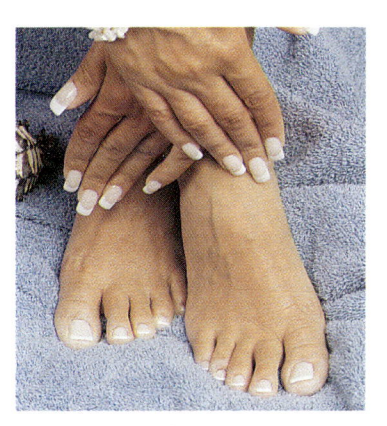

16.16 — French manicure

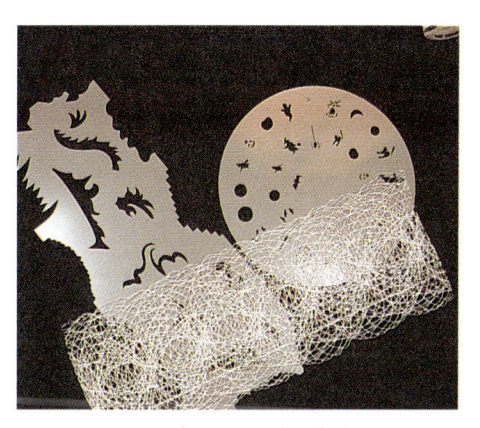

16.17 — Stencils are made of plastic, paper, or fabric

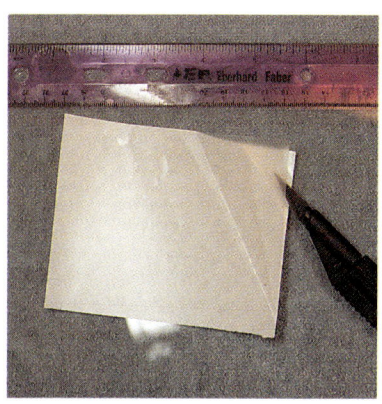

16.18 — Customized mask stencil with mask paper and mask knife

The most popular technique used in airbrushing is the **French manicure.** (Fig. 16.16) The airbrushed French manicure has no bumps or unevenness at the white tip. The application is very smooth and the white tip has a perfect shape every time. The airbrushed French manicure is accomplished as quickly as hand polishing, yet you may charge more for the airbrushed service.

The nail is a hard surface and has no ability to absorb like a fabric—such as a T-shirt does. It is impossible to draw with an airbrush on the nail—the paint will bead up and drip off the nail. You must use a **design tool**, like a **stencil** or **mask paper.** (Fig. 16.17) There are pre-cut stencils and mask paper on the market that have designs already in them. You may custom-cut your own designs by using a mask knife on uncut stencil or mask paper. (Fig. 16.18) Place the material to be cut on a glass plate and carefully cut your design out with the **mask knife.** Use the full edge of the knife, not just the point of the blade.

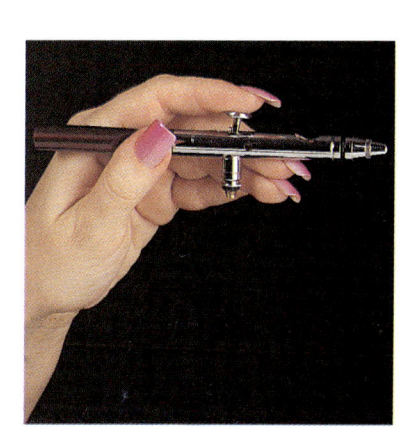

16.19 — Double action airbrush with self centering nozzle

AIRBRUSH EQUIPMENT AND OPERATION

An airbrush looks like a small spray gun. It uses compressed air to force paint out of its tip creating a fine mist of paint. There are many types of airbrushes available that are suitable for airbrushing fingernails. Some airbrushes are made with metal parts. Other airbrushes made of solvent-resistant resin are now available. (Fig. 16.19)

All airbrushes work on the same principle. They combine air and paint to form an atomized spray for painting. Airbrushes differ in the (1) type of trigger action, (2) location of air and paint mixing, (3) ease of use and maintenance. Each airbrush has a small cone shaped **fluid nozzle,** also called a **tip,** (Fig. 16.20) that a tapered

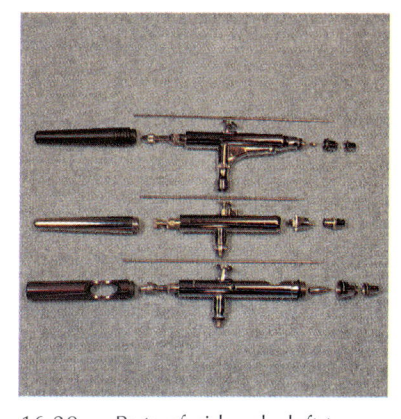

16.20 — Parts of airbrush, left to right, handle, shell/body, nozzle/tip, cap and needle

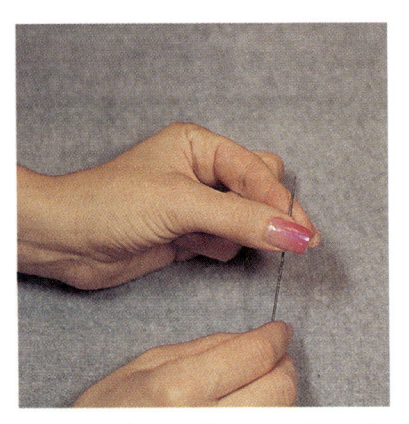

16.21 — The needle passes through a seal (O-ring) in the airbrush body, and keeps liquids out of the back of the airbrush.

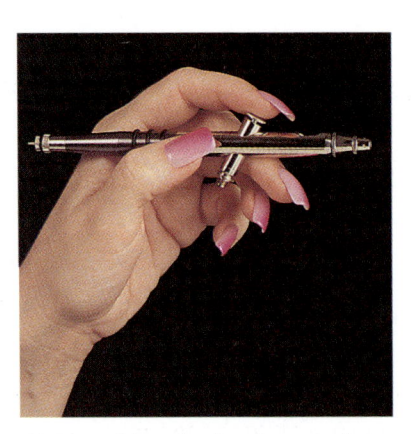

16.22 — No paint is released when the trigger is depressed.

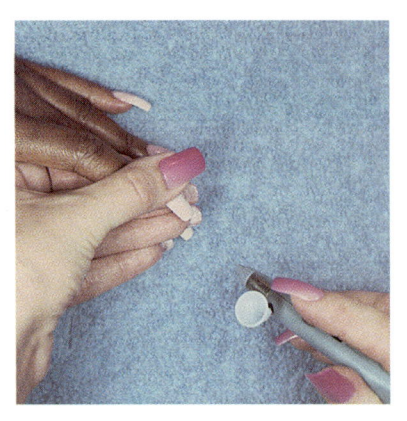

16.23 — The airbrush begins to release paint.

needle fits into. (Fig. 16.21) When the needle fits snugly in the fluid nozzle, no paint is released when the trigger is depressed. (Fig. 16.22) When the needle is drawn back, the airbrush begins to release paint. (Fig. 16.23) The further the needle is drawn back, the more paint is released. Control of the amount of paint released varies with different types of airbrushes.

There are many different makes of airbrushes available on the market today. You want to avoid airbrushes that are designed for volume paint application; they are not economical or practical choices for airbrushing nails. Airbrushes that have a large siphon bottle attached below the body of the airbrush take too long to change colors and do not offer the features you will want as a nail airbrush artist.

You want to choose an airbrush that is **designed for small quantities of paint,** is **gravity-fed** (gravity pulls the paint into the airbrush) and **mixes the paint with air inside the airbrush** (**internal mix**). This type of airbrush usually has a **well** or **small color cup** for the paint to be placed in the airbrush. A well (also called a **reservoir**) is a hole in the top of the airbrush, where drops of paint may be placed. If the airbrush has a color cup, it may be located on top of the airbrush or it may be attached to the side of the airbrush for the paint.

Even though we have narrowed the scope of airbrushes to choose from, there are still many differences in airbrushes available. When you purchase an airbrush, retain the manufacturer's airbrush diagram that comes with it for future reference. This diagram outlines the correct assembly of your airbrush as well as the order numbers for parts in case you lose or break something.

The **air hose** connects the airbrush to the **air source.** Each airbrush has a unique size fitting; be sure that the size fitting on your hose will fit your airbrush. It is best if you buy them at the same time. The end of the hose that attaches to your air source is usually a 1/4" thread, although there are a few air sources that have a different size fitting. If you find that you have a hose that does not attach to one or both pieces of equipment, adapters are available.

The most common choice for an air source for airbrushing nails is a small compressor. (Fig. 16.24) The compressor takes air from the room you are working in and compresses it. You may require an air pressure regulator attached to the compressor in order to control the air pressure being released into your air hose. (Fig. 16.25) Most airbrush nail technicians work at a pressure between 25 pounds per square inch (psi) to 35 psi. You will require a moisture trap or moisture separator for your airbrush system since you are using air from the environment that you are working in. There is moisture or water in the air. When the compressed air from the compressor reaches the air hose, the moisture begins to accumulate in the air hose. The moisture will form water droplets which will eventually spit out from the airbrush. A moisture separator will prevent this from happening.

You will need airbrush paint, airbrush cleaner and appropriate nail polishes to protect the airbrush paint on the nail. Check that the literature and product labeling clearly state that the products you are using are recommended for use on nails. Use the airbrush products per manufacturer's directions to ensure that you have the manufacturer's liability. If you are unsure about whether the airbrush product is recommended for use on nails, check with the manufacturer prior to use. Ask for a written document for your files if the labeling is not clear.

Consult your professional beauty or nail distributor to see the different types of equipment and airbrush products available. Many manufacturers offer complete systems for airbrushing nails, which include everything you need to get started. Your school may have different types or brands of equipment available for you to experiment with. Look for seminars that may permit you to rent the equipment before committing to a purchase.

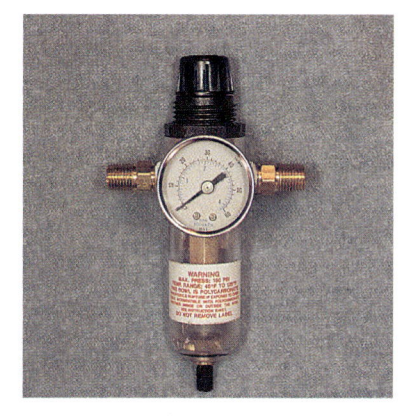

16.24 — Diaphragm compressor is portable and the most economical compressor available.

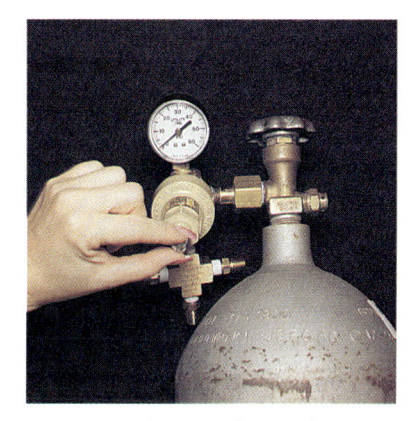

16.25 — Adjust regulator valve to release desired air pressure into the air hose.

GETTING STARTED AND FINISHED

SET-UP AND PRACTICE

When you begin practicing, you will need a table, good lighting, a comfortable chair, your airbrush equipment and supplies. Prepare a number of nail tips to be airbrushed by mounting them to a surface and base coating them. Assemble your airbrush, hose and compressor per the manufacturer's directions. Place your airbrush paints and airbrush polishes in an accessible tray, roll cart, drawer or polish rack. Have your design and cleaning tools in a tray, drawer or rollcart ready for use. Put your airbrush cleaner in a squirt bottle.

Set up a cleaning area for the airbrush off to the side of the work area. Either side is fine as long as it is comfortable for you. The best set-up is to have a separate roll-cart for all of your airbrush nail equipment and supplies storage. You could also use one of the drawers that is at a comfortable height when you sit at your work table. Pull out the drawer and line it with terry or paper toweling. Inside the drawer, place your cleaning station, plastic tray or jar that you will spray your airbrush into when cleaning it. If you are using an open tray, bowl or jar, place absorbent material at the bottom to prevent your overspray from bouncing off the bottom surface of your container and spreading all over. Place your cleaning brushes, airbrush cleaner bottle and other cleaning items in the open drawer. Avoid spraying into your wastebasket—it looks unsanitary and unprofessional.

Begin practicing on absorbent paper. When you start airbrushing, place a few drops of cleaner into your airbrush and spray it out into your cleaning station. This wets the airbrush inside and your airbrush nail paints will move through the airbrush better. To become familiar with how your airbrush operates, start spraying onto the paper approximately two to three inches from the surface of the paper. The first thing most people notice, if you are spraying properly, is that you will not see the airbrush paint leave your airbrush. It will seem to appear magically on the paper in front of you.

To airbrush properly, you need to move your whole arm up and down, diagonally, or side to side in order to move the airbrush spray around on your surface. Do not move from the wrist! Your wrist must remain straight and relaxed. If you move from the wrist, you will find the airbrush color will be inconsistent in coverage and intensity. This will occur because the airbrush starts out far from the surface, moves closer as your wrist straightens out and then further away as your wrist completes the movement. If you find you are moving your wrist, grasp your wrist with your other hand while practicing and consciously move your whole arm. After awhile, your movements will correct themselves and you will be fine.

Practice spraying a consistent row of dots. When the dot appears where you expect it to, you have learned how to properly aim your airbrush. The next practice step is to draw lines. To draw crisp lines, you must have the airbrush nozzle very close to the paper. The further you pull the airbrush away from the paper the wider and softer the line will become. After experimenting with dots and lines, draw a grid on your paper by drawing horizontal and vertical lines overlapping each other. This will create rows of boxes. Place a dot in each of the boxes. You are now ready to practice the technique used for airbrushing nails.

When airbrushing nails, the distance from the nail will vary according to the type of airbrush you are using. Most people will use the airbrush two to three inches from the nail surface. On your paper, spray a smooth even box of color by moving your arm back and forth slowly. Develop even color with no lines by moving back and forth over the same area a few times. If you are seeing streaks or lines on the paper and not a smooth even box of color, the airbrush is either too close to the paper or you are releasing too much paint at a time. Practice this technique until you can achieve an even coating of color on the paper with no streaks! (Fig. 16.26)

Now you are ready to practice on nail tips. Place your nail tips about two to three inches apart on your practice surface. Lightly coat the nail with your airbrush color. Repeated passes over the nail will build up the airbrush nail color. When first learning, most people are impatient and want to see the color right away. If you are too close to the nail tip or release too much paint at one time on the nail surface, the airbrush paint will puddle and begin to run off the nail. (In Fig. 16.27, the first nail is sprayed too quickly or too closely. The second nail tip has the correct, dry appearance.) When correctly applying airbrush nail color, the airbrush paint on the nail should appear dull, with a powdery look to it. If the airbrush paint is shiny or appears as droplets, wipe the nail tip off and try again. The best way to apply airbrush nail color is to work on five nail tips at a time, as if you were working on a client's hand. Apply one dry layer of color to each nail tip. Usually three passes of the airbrush up and down over the nail tip will cover it with color lightly. Move to the next nail tip and repeat the procedure until you have airbrushed each nail tip once. Start with the first nail tip and repeat the procedure on each nail tip until you have reached your desired airbrushed nail color. When you have successfully completed applying the airbrushed nail color to the five nail tips, you are ready to move on to practicing a color fade or French manicure.

REAL PEOPLE

One of the benefits of adding airbrushing to your services, is that you do not require live models to practice your skills. You should become proficient at airbrushing your nail tips prior to working on live models. When you are skilled at airbrushing on nail tips, you are ready to practice on a few close friends or relatives to become

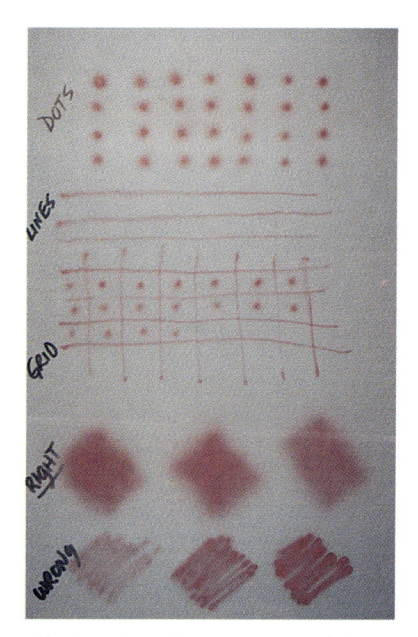

16.26 — Practice on paper achieving an even coating of color.

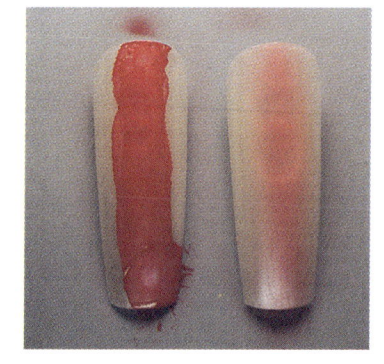

16.27 — The nail tip at left shows what happens if you spray too close to the nail tip or release too much paint onto the surface. The paint will puddle and run off the nail. The nail on the right has the correct appearance, achieved by light passes of the airbrush to build up color.

212 ◆ PART 4 THE ART OF NAIL TECHNOLOGY

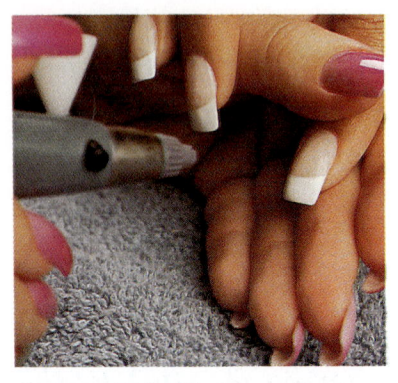

16.28 — By holding your client's hand, you can catch the overspray and lessen the amount of clean-up time on her hand.

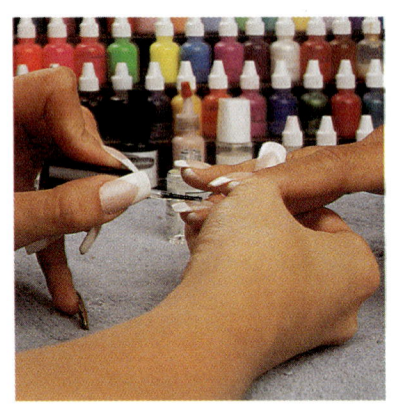

16.29 — Keep polish brush parallel to the nail guiding liquid down the nail.

comfortable holding the client's hand and cleaning up the overspray when done.

1. Complete your nail service and have the client pay the bill prior to the airbrush nail color service. Have them put on a coat and dig in the pockets or purses for necessary items prior to clean-up.

2. Have the client use a nail brush and cleanse the hands and nails of any dust or oils from the nail service. Dry the nail and cuticle area thoroughly, checking for droplets of water or missed oils and dust that would interfere with the airbrush nail color application.

3. Apply your base coat(s) to the nails. Be sure to bumper the sides and free edge of the nails.

4. Airbrush your client's nails just as you practiced on the nail tips. Hold the client's hand in yours. Your hand should encircle each of your client's finger as you spray it. Your hand catches the overspray as you work so it doesn't fall onto the other nails on your client's hand. Place your thumb on the finger just above the cuticle area. Most of the overspray lands on your thumb and little on the client's finger. This reduces cleanup on your client. (Fig. 16.28) Use a similar procedure when airbrushing toenails. The paint washes off your hands with airbrush paint hand cleaner, when you sanitize prior to your next client.

5. Apply paint bonder or thin top coat to the dry airbrush nail paint. Keep your polish brush parallel to the nail, guiding the liquid down the nail. (Fig. 16.29) Do not use the bristles of the brush since this may scratch or drag the paint. Be sure to have enough bonder on the polish brush; a dry polish brush or bristle may also damage your paint. Apply paint bonder to all ten nails. Be sure to saturate all the paint and to bumper the sides and free edge of the nails.

6. Any airbrush paint that is not sealed to the nail may be washed away later. Allow paint bonder to dry two to three minutes. Clean your airbrush and put it away at this time.

7. Apply one or two coats of protective airbrush nail glaze. Be sure to bumper the sides and free edge of the nails. While applying the protective glaze, instruct your client on proper home maintenance of airbrushed nail color or nail art. Allow client's nails to dry for ten minutes.

8. Cleanse the fingers or toes per manufacturer's directions. This may be accomplished at the nail table, pedicure station, or, with some airbrush skin cleaner products, at a sink. Have the client pat hands or feet on a towel to dry the skin, but avoid pressure on nails for another ten minutes. Use an orangewood stick or cotton-wrapped implement saturated with polish remover to remove any paint sealed to skin by paint boner or protective nail glaze. (Fig. 16.30)

9. You may apply a quick-dry product if desired. Use spray-on products instead of brush-on products for proper sanitation and less-risk of injury to the airbrushed nail service. Airbrushed nail color is usually surface dry in ten minutes and completely dry within a half hour since only clear nail polish is applied.

10. Airbrushed nail color will last as well or better than traditional nail polish. Since it is a thinner coating, it tends to be a longer-lasting coating. If you don't get these results, evaluate your airbrush nail paint and airbrush nail polishes. You may need to experiment with different brands or combinations of products for maximum durability. Follow manufacturer's directions.

11. Airbrushed nail color is generally removed with regular nail polish remover (acetone will work quickest) unless manufacturer of your paint stipulates otherwise.

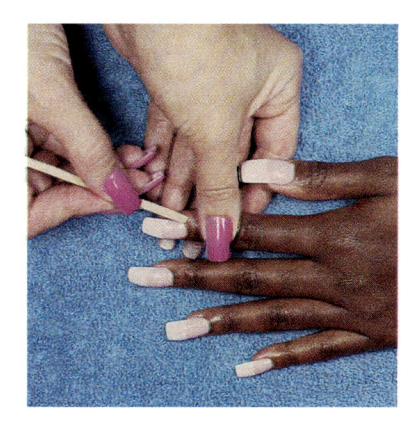

16.30 — Remove paint sealed to skin.

Airbrush nail color artists vary in their client skin cleaning procedures. Some nail technicians cleanse the airbrush paint on the skin after the paint bonder is applied and allowed to dry. Others send their clients home with a small container of airbrush paint skin cleanser for use at home after the color has dried. Experiment with different procedures to find which one works best for you.

In order to offer airbrushed nail color successfully to every client you service, it is necessary to have your airbrush equipment and supplies ready to use at all times. Many people have airbrush systems that are in a box collecting dust. When an opportunity arises for them to use their airbrush equipment, they are not prepared and usually do not have the time in their schedule to set up their airbrush system. Having your airbrush system in a roll-cart by your side or set up at a nail table/pedicure station, provides you with the ability to airbrush at a moment's notice, simply by plugging in or turning on your compressor.

TWO-COLOR FADE

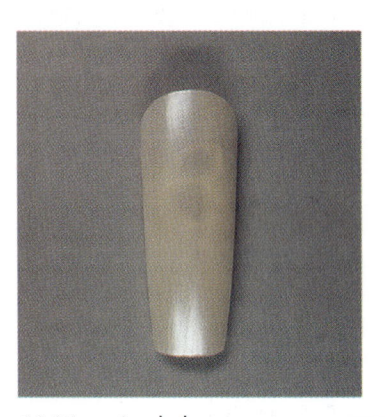

The nail color fade, or color blend, is one of the most used airbrushed nail color services. It will appeal to every client that you service; the airbrush paint colors selected are key to the success of this design for each individual. A conservative client might prefer subtle, soft hues of similar colors while an outgoing client might choose bold colors that strongly contrast. This multi-color airbrush nail service justifies an additional charge for the nail color application. This technique may be used as the background for an airbrushed nail design or on its own as an airbrushed nail color service.

1. Apply your base coat to the nail. If the nail to be covered is a dark tone that may influence your nail color or if you are using a transparent airbrush nail paint, apply a crystalline, special effect or white base coat. (Fig. 16.31)

2. Place a couple drops of airbrush cleaner into your airbrush and completely spray out the airbrush cleaner into your cleaning station or cleaning receptacle. Place your airbrush paint color into your airbrush. Always start feeding your paint into your airbrush by spraying onto the surface next to your nails. When the airbrush paint is loaded into your airbrush and it is spraying correctly, you are ready to begin application on the nail. *When using pearlescent paints, you will find the airbrush may clog more easily. (You should use pearlescent airbrush paints only after you have mastered opaque and transparent airbrush paints!)* Apply a dry, even coat going back and forth diagonally over the top two-thirds of the nail, moving your whole arm. If you are working on more than one nail, apply this light, dry coat diagonally to all the nails. *With the pearlescent paint, you may have to pull your hand further away from the nail and release slightly more paint to get an even spray. Practice will make the adjustment smoother.* Apply more coats of the airbrush paint at the cuticle area, with fewer coats toward the center of the nail to create a soft edge for the second color to overlap. (Fig. 16.32)

3. Continue applying light, dry coats of airbrush paint diagonally until you have reached the desired color or opacity in the nail cuticle area fading towards the center. (Fig. 16.33)

4. Clean your airbrush of the first color paint. Choose a color that is appropriate for your client—one that contrasts and creates a transition color. When airbrushing the second color, start at the bottom of the nail tip and move up two-thirds of the nail.

16.31 — Apply base coat.

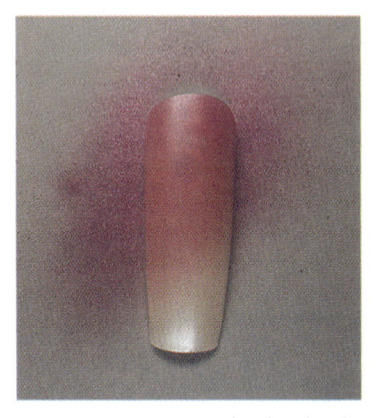

16.32 — Create a soft edge for the second color to overlap.

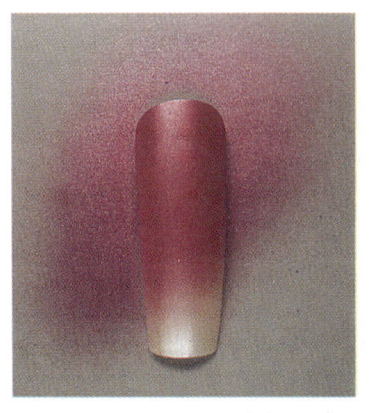

16.33 — Continue applying paint until your desired color is released.

Apply more coats or passes of the airbrush over the free edge or nail tip, with fewer passes or coats of paint through the center of the nail. If the colors chosen mix when overlapped, you will begin to see a transition color start to develop. (Fig. 16.34)

5. Continue to apply a dry, even coat going back and forth diagonally over the bottom two-thirds of the nail, until you have achieved the desired color at the free edge of the nail. If a transition color does develop, you control how much of the color is on the nail by the amount the two paint colors overlap. (Fig. 16.35) Remember when working on your client, the airbrushed color fade on the right hand should be a mirror image of the color fade on the left hand. Many nail technicians prefer to have the colors travel from the outer corner of the nail (towards the pinkie finger) the inner corner of the cuticle (towards the thumb) but each airbrush artist has his or her own style.

6. After you have completed all nails, apply your nail paint bonder and let it dry for three minutes. If you are not going to continue airbrushing, clean your airbrush at this time. Apply the airbrush paint protective glaze for durability. Instruct your client on home maintenance of the airbrushed nail color.

The color fade is one of the most popular airbrushed nail color service. It demonstrates a technique one can accomplish only with an airbrush: the subtle color change from one to another with no bump, line, or demarcation in the nail color coating. The photo (Fig. 16.36) shows a few possible variations of this design. The nail tip on the left is a subtle blend for the conservative client. It is a cognac nail color with a transparent gold shimmer splashed at the free edge. The center nail is a bit more daring; pearl red in the cuticle fading into a true pink nail tip. The nail tip on the right is the nail tip completed in the step-by-step directions above. This nail color selection is for a bold client who wants people to notice her nails!

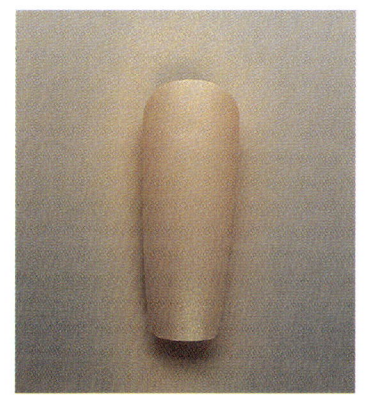

16.34 — When airbrushing the second color, start at the bottom of the nail tip and move up two thirds of the nail.

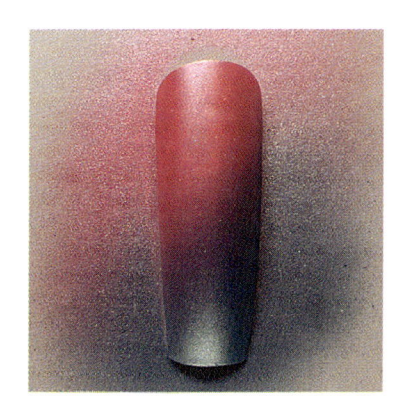

16.35 — Continue to apply a dry, even coat going back and forth diagonally over the bottom two-thirds of the nail.

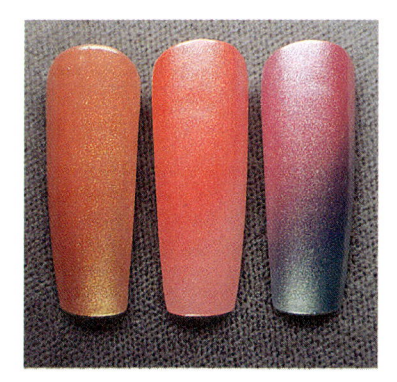

16.36 — Three variations of the design

TRADITIONAL FRENCH MANICURE (WITH OPTIONAL LUNULA)

The French manicure is the reason why most nail technicians look into airbrushed nail color. The hand-polished French manicure cannot compare to the airbrushed version! The airbrushed French is easier, quicker, and more attractive than the hand-polished version. The airbrushed French manicure has a clean, sophisticated look yet retains a neutral color application that matches all clothing. Each airbrush nail technician has a favorite method of achieving the traditional French manicure, which is a skin toned nail bed with a curved French white tip. There are three popular methods for achieving the curved nail tip, demonstrated for you in the following steps. All three methods may add the white lunula or moon to the cuticle area if desired (for a slight additional charge.)

1. **Apply a clear base coat to the nail**(s). (You may use a French manicure polish to achieve the nail bed color if desired. Allow plenty of time for the nail polish to dry. If you choose not to airbrush the nail bed color, skip to step 4.) You can use a crystalline base coat to neutralize the color of the nail tip. (Fig. 16.37)

2. **Choose your French manicure airbrush paint**. Mist the French manicure color over the nail lightly. If you desire the color to be opaque, continue the passes of your airbrush over the nail until the desired color or opacity is achieved. If you client desires a transparent French manicure color, you may mist the opaque color lightly. Most airbrush paint colors may be made slightly transparent by adding a couple drops of distilled water.

3. **Optional:** Add a shimmer to your French manicure paint by misting a gold highlight or shimmer evenly over the French beige. (Fig. 16.38)

4. French tip application with a stencil: You will use a curved edge to cover the nail bed color and expose the nail tip to be sprayed white. This is an excellent method for a soft-edged French nail tip.

   • You may cut a curved piece of paper, but there are many ready-made stencils on the market.

   • Hold the stencil as close to the nail as possible, exposing the nail tip to be sprayed. Keep the stencil parallel to the nail to avoid scratching the paint on the nail.

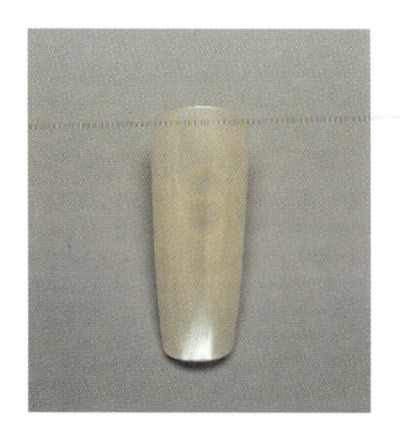

16.37 — Apply a base coat.

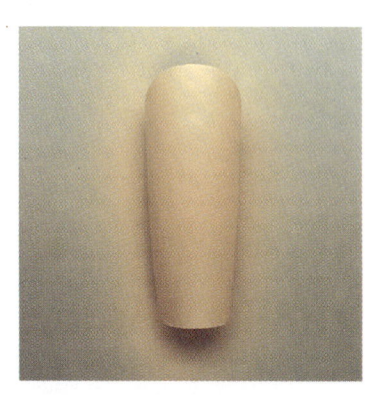

16.38 — Add a shimmer to your French manicure by misting a gold highlight.

CHAPTER 16 THE CREATIVE TOUCH ◆ **217**

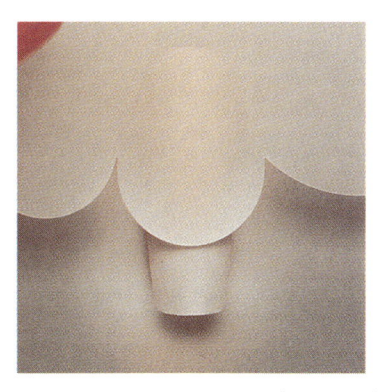

16.39 — Mist paint over the stencil.

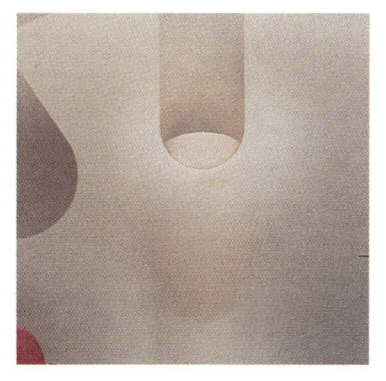

16.40 — Add a lunula or moon with a stencil.

- When you have the stencil lined up, mist the nail tip white. Build the color slowly, to avoid getting the paint wet and runny. (Watch the edge of your stencil if it is plastic. The paint easily accumulates and may run down onto the nail. Dry the stencil with air from your airbrush without moving it, as it is difficult to line up the stencil in precisely the same position.)

- When working with stencils, mist paint then blow air to dry the nail tip and stencil. Repeat the process until the nail tip is the desired color. (Fig. 16.39)

5. If the nails you are working on are very curved, you may have to touch up the stenciled nails. Using the stencil, roll the finger sideways and carefully line up the stencil with the white tip already sprayed. Mist the sides of the nail to match and complete the white tip.

6. **Optional:** Adding a lunula or moon with a stencil creates the "real" look. Mist the lunula slightly lighter than nail tip color. (Fig. 16.40)

7. After you have completed all nails, apply your nail paint bonder and let it dry for three minutes. Apply the airbrush paint protective glaze for durability.

8. This procedure is easily accomplished on toes. Use your preferred method to apply the French manicure to the toes. (Fig. 16.41)

9. Cleanse the toes with airbrush paint cleanser after they have been bonded and glazed. (Fig. 16.42)

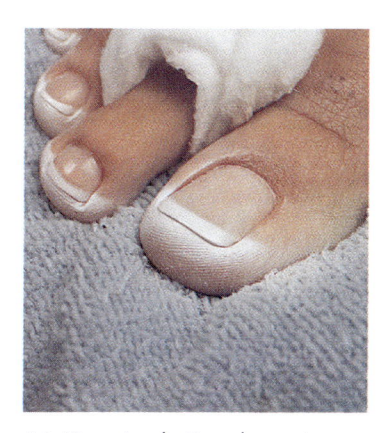

16.41 — Apply French manicure to the toes.

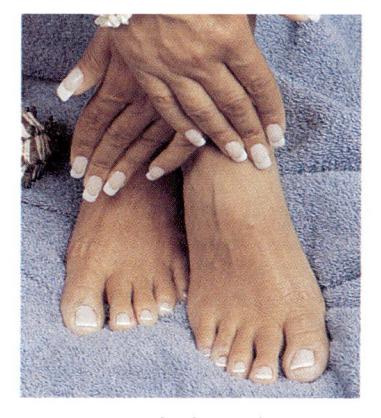

16.42 — Finished French manicure on toes

The Artistic Touch

If you're like most nail techs, you have a specific number of customers who are enthusiastic nail art fans. But that shouldn't stop you from selling the service to other segments of your clientele. The secret behind selling nail art is introducing the right design to the right client at the right time. An understated geometric design, or two similarly-toned blocks of neutral color may be just right for the more conservative client who normally wouldn't even consider nail art. Others who might not be interested in this service could find it difficult to resist a jack-o-lantern sitting on the pinkie near Halloween or a cupid on the index finger to celebrate Valentine's Day.

REVIEW QUESTIONS

1. Why should you develop nail art skills?
2. What is the technique called for airbrushing two or more colors on the nail at the same time?
3. How does the finished airbrushed French manicure differ from the traditional application?
4. Describe the parts of the airbrush and how they work together to release the paint.
5. Describe the best airbrush to use for nails.
6. What is the most common choice for an air source for airbrushing nails?
7. What is the most common air pressure used by nail technicians when airbrushing?
8. Describe the procedure for an airbrushed version of a French manicure.

Part 5

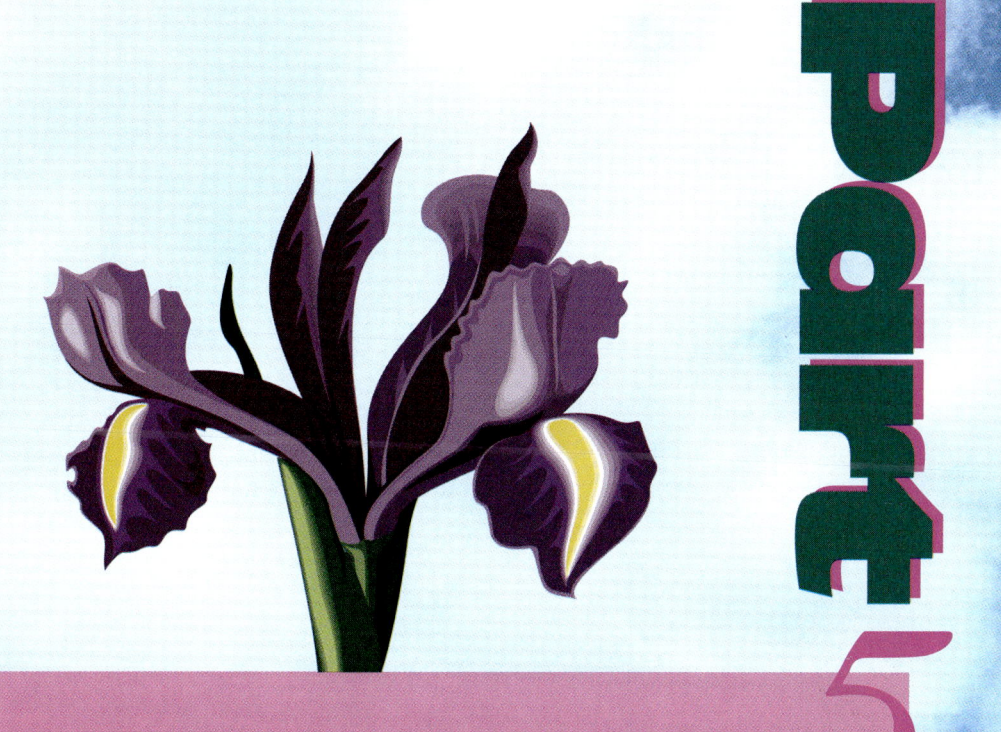

THE BUSINESS OF NAIL TECHNOLOGY

◆ *CHAPTER 17* - Salon Business

◆ *CHAPTER 18* - Selling Nail Products and Services

chapter 17
SALON BUSINESS

LEARNING OBJECTIVES

After you have studied this chapter, you should be able to:

1. Discuss the advantages and disadvantages of working in a full-service salon.
2. Discuss the advantages and disadvantages of working in a nails-only salon. Identify the two types of nail tips.
3. List ten questions you will need to ask before deciding what salon is right for you.
4. List eight questions that will help you determine if a salon has safe working conditions.
5. Explain the difference between income and expenses and give two examples of each.
6. List the practical uses for business records that are required by local, state, and federal laws.
7. List the types of information that a salon can gather by keeping accurate business records.
8. Discuss the advantages of keeping proper service, inventory, and personal appointment records.
9. List the guidelines that should be followed in booking appointments.

INTRODUCTION

You are training to become part of a $2 billion nail care industry. If you want to be financially successful in this business, you must know more than how to give clients manicures, pedicures, or artificial nail services. You should also be a good business person. From the moment you receive a job offer, you have to negotiate how much money you are paid. When you develop a clientele, you will handle tips and, possibly, a commission.

If you someday decide to open your own salon, you will be responsible for the complicated business of renting or buying a shop, and paying expenses such as electricity, telephone, advertising, safety systems, employee salaries, and taxes. You may be an expert nail technician, but if you can't handle the business part of nail care, you will not make as much money as nail technicians who can.

YOUR WORKING ENVIRONMENT

Good business sense begins with the decisions you make when you look for your first job. Should you work for a full-service or a nails-only salon? There are advantages and disadvantages to each choice.

THE FULL-SERVICE SALON

Unless they are large and very successful, *full-service salons* often employ only one nail technician. The arrangement is a convenient one for both the nail technician and the salon. You automatically get all of the nail-care business in the salon, and your services make it convenient for clients to have their nails done when they are there for hair-care or skin-care services. You might make arrangements with the salon to attract clients by offering them special rates for nail care when they have other services performed.

On the other hand, at a full-service salon, there won't be other nail technicians with whom to share ideas and experience. There also won't be someone to fill in for you when you are sick or on vacation. If the salon is a traditional one, you may be limited in the variety of artificial nail services that you are allowed to perform. (Fig. 17.1)

17.1 — Full-service salon

THE NAILS-ONLY SALON

In a *nails-only salon* you will work with several other nail technicians. In addition to having the opportunity to share ideas and experiences, you could increase your business by serving their clients when they are sick, on vacation, or retire. (Fig. 17.2)

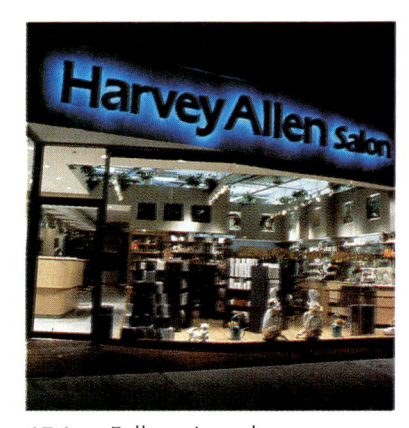

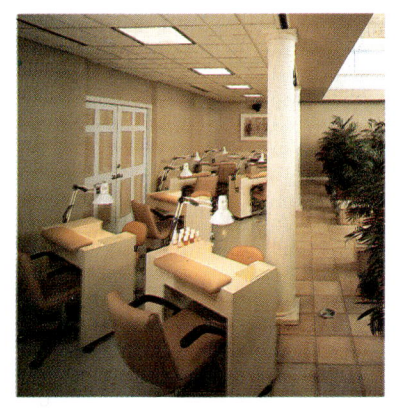

17.2 — Nails-only salon

The client who patronizes a nails-only salon may take nail care more seriously than clients who have their nails done in full-service salons. Your clients may have special nail problems, or want more creative artificial nail services. If this is the case, you will gain valuable experience. A nails-only salon is a good place for a nail technician to establish a serious clientele. On the other hand, there could be competition for clients in a nails-only salon where there are many nail technicians.

MAKE YOUR DECISION

Before you make a decision about what salon is right for you, visit several full-service and several nails-only salons. Observe the working environment and decide which feels comfortable to you.

You will want to consider the following factors in deciding on the salon that is right for you:

1. Will the salon provide additional training for you or encourage you to attend training outside the salon?
2. Will the salon help you build a clientele? Will they spend money on advertising low-price specials? Will they refer customers to you?
3. Will you be considered an employee, or will you be an independent contractor who rents a booth? If you are an independent contractor, what are the terms of the booth rental?
4. If you are an employee, how will the salon pay you? Will you receive a weekly salary or salary plus commission? Will you receive a commission on retail products sold? Is there a regular salary review?
5. Will the salon provide nail-care products or will you have to bring your own?
6. Does the salon offer benefits such as medical, liability, life insurance, or paid sick days?
7. Are there fixed or flexible working hours?
8. What is the dress code?
9. Does the salon close for a regular vacation period, or does each employee take a separate vacation?
10. What is the salon's reputation? There is an advantage to working in a successful "upscale" salon where you can make good contacts and learn valuable tricks of the trade from your employer and coworkers.
11. Does the salon have safe working conditions?
    a) Does it have proper ventilation, like an exhaust system to the outside?
    b) Does it provide separate refrigerators for food and nail product storage?

CHAPTER 17   SALON BUSINESS   ◆   **223**

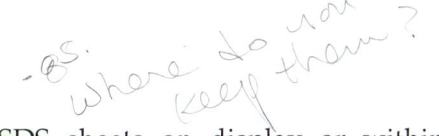

c) Are MSDS sheets on display or within easy access to employees?
d) Are work stations well-equipped and clean, with plastic disposal bags that can be closed?
e) Are nail technicians required to wear dust masks?
f) Are nail technicians required to wear safety glasses?
g) Are aerosol cans used or are safe application methods used, such as pumps or drop-on products?
h) Are salon workers ready for emergencies? Are the telephone numbers for poison control, the hospital, paramedics, the fire station, or the police posted in a visible place?

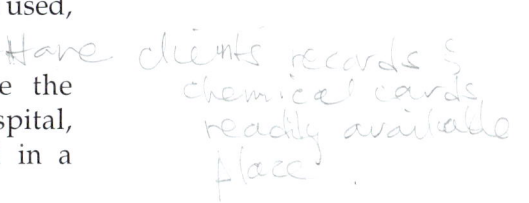

KEEPING GOOD PERSONAL RECORDS

Although you may not be required to keep business records for your salon, you will want to develop a simple and efficient system for keeping track of your own income and expenses. you will also want to save all of your check stubs, cancelled checks, receipts, and invoices. Basically, *income* is the money you make and *expenses* are what you spend. Another valuable personal record is your appointment calendar.

INCOME

To keep a correct, concise, and complete record of your income, you should create a form with room to list each source of income. It might include salary, commission from services, commission from retail products sold, and tips.

EXPENSES

Your expenses working in the salon could include equipment, supplies, magazines or books that explain techniques, comfortable shoes, uniforms (if required), and tuition for special courses on nail techniques.

APPOINTMENTS

Use a personal appointment calendar to help you arrange your work time. If you keep this calendar with you, you can plan each day's schedule before you arrive at the salon. You will know who your clients are, when each one will arrive, and the services you will perform. With this information, you can prepare all your supplies ahead of time, so you are more efficient.

UNDERSTANDING SALON BUSINESS RECORDS

Most salons use the services of an accountant to help them keep accurate records that meet the requirements of local, state, and federal laws. These records are used to:

1. Determine income, expenses, and profit or loss.
2. Prove the value of your clientele or the worth of the salon to prospective buyers.
3. Get a bank loan.
4. Compute income tax, social security, unemployment, and disability insurance, among others.

Businesses hold daily sales slips, the appointment book, and the petty cash book for at least one year. The payroll book, canceled checks, monthly and yearly records, and service and inventory records are usually held for at least seven years for tax purposes. (Fig. 17.3)

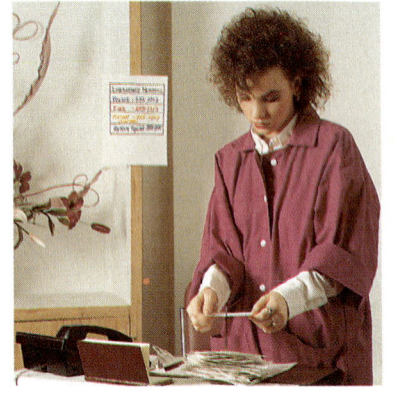

17.3 — Keep accurate and neat business records.

USING BUSINESS RECORDS

Accurate records will help you and your employer gather the following valuable information.

1. **Profit and loss comparisons with other weeks, months, or years.** As an example, over a period of time, you can see which are the slow months and which are the busiest in your business. This will allow you to cut expenses by not being overstocked during slow months, and being fully stocked during busy periods. You can also schedule vacations or renovations during the slow months and have a full staff and full service during the busy months.

2. **Changes in demands for services.** If the demand for a service is growing, your salon may choose to hire more nail technicians to service this growing demand.

3. **Inventory.** If you keep accurate records of inventory, you can cut costs by keeping the appropriate stock levels. This means that you are neither overstocked nor running short of supplies needed for services. Daily inventory records also help you quickly detect any loss of stock from theft.

4. **Net income.** Net income refers to all the income you make less all the expenses. Accurate net income records can help you establish the net worth of the business at the end of the year.

5. **Materials and supply levels.** Records will help you compare the use of materials and supplies with the services rendered to make sure that neither too much nor too little is being used.

KEEPING CLIENT RECORDS

A *client service record* lists services rendered and merchandise sold to each client. All service records should contain the name and address of the client, date, amount charged, product used, results obtained, and client's preferences and tastes. Most salons use a card file system or a memorandum book to keep service records. With the service record for each client should be any release statements that he or she has signed. Service records are especially valuable if another nail technician has to fill in for a client's usual nail technician. If the client's usual service is explained in detail on the card, it can be done accurately and efficiently.

The client health/record card lists clients' personal information, such as what types of jobs they have, what hobbies they have and what sports they enjoy. It is a good idea to start your day by reading the records of clients scheduled for services during the day. Your clients will be happy to know you remembered the things that are important to them. See Chapter 9 for a complete discussion of client records.

KEEPING INVENTORY RECORDS

Keep a running inventory of all supplies. Classify them by use and retail value. Those used in the business are *consumption supplies.* Those that are sold to the customer are *retail supplies.*

BOOKING APPOINTMENTS

The system used in your salon will determine whether you book appointments with clients or they are booked by a receptionist. Keeping a proper record of appointments will cut down on the confusion, annoyance, and stress of overbooking and help prevent clients from arriving at the wrong time and having no wait.

Regardless of who books the appointments, the following guidelines should be followed: (Fig. 17.4)

1. Always have a supply of appointment books, pencils, erasers, pens, a calendar, and a message pad.

2. Be prompt. Whether you are answering the phone or acknowledging your client's presence at the counter, try not to keep them waiting.

3. Identify both yourself and the salon by name when you answer the telephone.

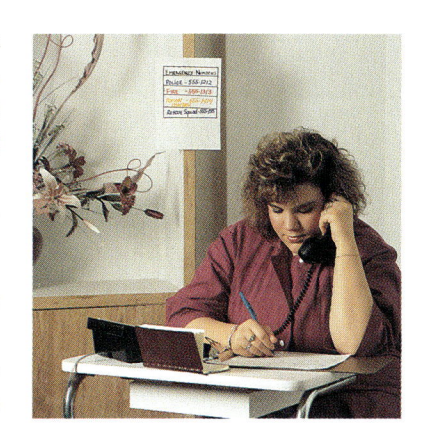

17.4 — Keep an accurate record of appointments.

4. **Be pleasant.** Let clients know you are pleased to talk with them.

5. Make sure to take the following information when a client calls to make an appointment: client's name and phone number, type of service to be performed, date, and time of appointment. Repeat the information to the client to be sure you are correct, then block out the amount of time needed to perform the service.

6. **Speak clearly.** Don't mumble or shout. Use correct English and avoid slang.

7. **Be tactful** and **courteous** when speaking. Refer to clients by their last name.

8. If you are busy enough to have appointments made in advance, it is a good practice to call your clients the night before the appointment to remind them and confirm the time. This will reduce your number of no-shows.

9. Always ask your clients at the end of their appointment if they wish to reschedule.

ADVERTISING YOURSELF

The first thing you might want to do when you begin a job in the salon is to make a list of every service you offer. Write a brief description of the service, length of time needed to perform it, and the cost of the service.

A copy of your service list should be kept near the appointment book so there will be no confusion among your clients about these facts. Give your coworkers a copy of your list of services and encourage them to offer your services to their clients.

COLLECTING PAYMENT FOR SERVICES

In some salons, the nail technician collects payments from clients. In others, the receptionist handles all payments. In either case, you will probably be required to prepare a ticket detailing the services you have performed for that client. The ticket should include the client's name, the date, the service provided, and the cost. The ticket will make it clear to clients what they are paying for and provide an accurate record of the transaction.

Do not offer reduced prices to special clients. This can lead to a difficult situation if your other clients are denied a price reduction.

Common Courtesy

No one likes to be kept waiting—and that includes your clients. When a customer comes through the door, make an effort to greet her right away. If you happen to be with another client when your next customer arrives, offer her a beverage and give her an estimate of when you will be with her. Furthermore, if you are running more than fifteen minutes late for the entire day, call each of your clients and alert them. This allows them to push back their appointments or rebook. Incorporating these simple, courteous gestures shows the client that her time is important and you value her business.

REVIEW QUESTIONS

1. What are the advantages and disadvantages of working in a full-service salon?

2. What are the advantages and disadvantages of working in a nails-only salon?

3. What are ten questions that will help you determine if a salon is right for you?

4. What are eight questions that will help you determine if a salon has safe working conditions?

5. Explain the difference between income and expenses and give two examples of each.

6. List four practical uses for business records that are required by local, state, and federal laws.

7. List five types of information that a salon can gather by keeping accurate business records.

8. Discuss the advantages of keeping proper service, inventory, and personal appointment records.

9. List nine guidelines that should be followed in booking appointments.

Chapter 18
SELLING NAIL PRODUCTS AND SERVICES

LEARNING OBJECTIVES

After you have studied this chapter, you should be able to:

1. List the basic steps in selling.
2. Describe the difference between product features and benefits.
3. Demonstrate your ability to turn product features into benefits.
4. List the questions you should try to answer as you determine your client's needs and wants.
5. Explain how you can sell while you work.
6. List and describe the steps in closing the sale.

INTRODUCTION

If you want to be a successful nail technician, you need to be a good salesperson too. You are responsible for selling both nail services and the products that will help your clients maintain those services. You will be successful if you reach one basic selling goal—to meet the needs of your clients.

The five basic steps in meeting your clients' needs and selling your products and services are described in this chapter. The basic steps to selling include:

1. Know your products and services.
2. Know what your client needs and wants.
3. Present your products and services.
4. Answer your client's questions and objections properly.
5. Close the sale.

KNOW YOUR PRODUCTS AND SERVICES

In the nail salon, products and services are very closely related. When you perform a nail service for your client, you select the products that are best for that person. Then you use them to perform a service that meets your client's needs and wants.

When you have finished with the nail service, you sell your client the products needed to maintain the service between visits to the salon.

There are two ways to know your products and services. One way is to know the features, and the other way is to know the benefits.

FEATURES

A *feature* is a specific fact about a product or service that describes it. Read labels, product bulletins, and industry literature to learn the features of your nail products. You look for information such as the ingredients your products contain, safety precautions you should follow when using them, how to apply them, and how to maintain them. Features of nail services include the procedures and how long they take to perform, the chemicals used, how much the services cost, what effect they have on the clients' nails, and how often they need maintenance.

The features of colored gel nails over tips include the fact that they are durable, lightweight, and come in a variety of colors. Light-cured gels take about 30 minutes to perform, use acrylic-based gel with a special light source, will not harm healthy nails, and need maintenance every two to three weeks. (Fig. 18.1)

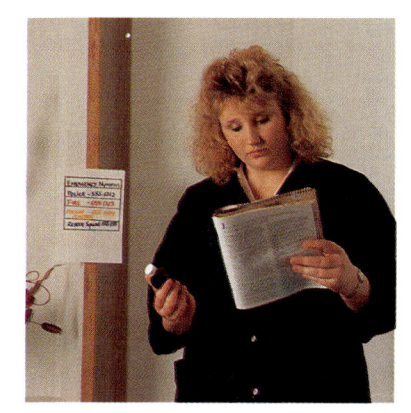

18.1 — Read about your retail products.

BENEFITS

The *benefits* of a product or service are what it will do for your client or how it will fulfill your client's needs and wants. The benefits of colored gel nails over tips are long, beautiful nails that save you both time and money. They give you nails that always look freshly polished, and lightweight and comfortable to wear, and require maintenance every two to three weeks instead of once a week.

You will be a good salesperson when you can turn the features of your products and services into benefits that meet the needs and desires of your clients.

KNOW WHAT YOUR CLIENT NEEDS AND WANTS

It is important to know your clients' nail needs if you want to sell them nail products and services that meet those needs. You can discover those needs during the client consultation (see Chapter 9).

As you observe your client and communicate with him or her, you will want to answer questions such as these:

1. **Does your client have special nail problems?** Clients with nail problems will need special nail services. Does your client have short bitten nails or nails that crack and tear easily? These clients may need services that strengthen or cover up their natural nails.

2. **What is your client's lifestyle?** The kind of life your client leads will determine what type of nail services they need. A business person may want nails that have a well-groomed look and are short and polished in a pale conservative color. A jewelry or cosmetics salesperson may want long, acrylic nails. A gardener or pianist might need short, natural-looking nails. A quilter might need short nails but want them polished in the latest fashion color. Be sure you give your clients the services and products that suit their activities and image. (Fig. 18.2)

   Nail "look" is one important consideration, but there are others. Wearability is another. A client whose hands are in water frequently may ask you for linen wraps. You would caution that client against linen wraps because they retain water and the dampness encourages the growth of mold and fungus on the wrap. You might suggest another service that would be more appropriate for this client, such as acrylic or gel nails.

3. **Is your client preparing for a special occasion?** A client who is going to a wedding might want nails that are the same color

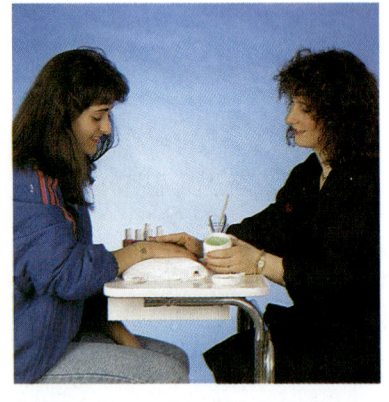

18.2 — Determine which services or products best suit your clients by discussing their lifestyles with them.

as the dress she is wearing. A client who is going on a job interview will probably want nails that look natural but well groomed. If your client is wearing a witch's costume to a Halloween party, she might want extra long acrylic nails painted black.

PRESENT YOUR PRODUCTS AND SERVICES

There are two powerful opportunities to sell your products and services to your clients. One way is while you are performing the service. The other way is to have the products and services displayed attractively near your work station.

SELL WHILE YOU WORK

When you are performing a service, tell your clients what you are doing, what products you are using, and why. If one of the procedures, such as nail filing and polish touch-up, can be done by your clients, suggest the type of abrasive and polish they should buy and tell them how to use the products.

While you are giving one service to a client, discuss other services and the features, benefits, and costs of each. If you are giving an acrylic nail service, compare it with linen wraps or gel nails. Your clients may want to try other services in the future.

DISPLAY A LIST OF YOUR SERVICES

Have your service list prominently displayed near your table. The card should be attractive and clear. It should list your services and the cost of each. You may put in other information you think would be helpful to your clients, such as length of time for each service, its features, and its benefits.

DISPLAY YOUR PRODUCTS

Display the nail products sold by your salon attractively and in view of your clients when they are having a service performed. (Fig. 18.3) Have written promotional materials about the products within easy reach of your clients so they can take information with them. Also, have free samples of nail products, when possible, and encourage your clients to take some and try them.

Don't pass up the opportunity to sell your clients polish, top coat, hand cream, polish remover, cuticle oil, and other products they will need to maintain their nail services between visits to the salon.

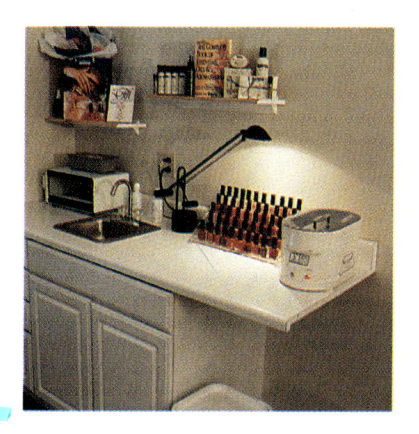

18.3 — Manicure station with retail display

232 ◆ PART V   THE BUSINESS OF NAIL TECHNOLOGY

ANSWER QUESTIONS AND OBJECTIONS

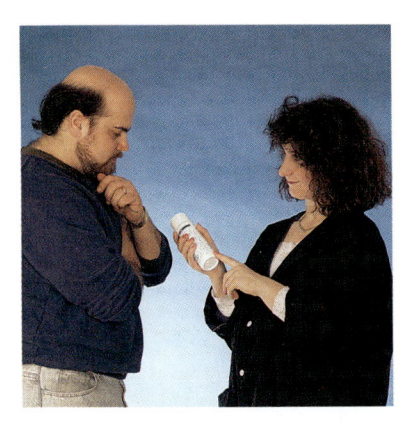

Be ready to answer any questions or objections your clients have about your products and service. (Fig. 18.4)

QUESTIONS

Clients may want to know what type of polish has the most unusual colors, how nail art is done and what materials are used, or how long a service takes. They may want to know the advantages and disadvantages of a service or what they should do when their nail breaks. Be as knowledgeable as you can about your products and services, but don't be afraid to say you don't know the answer and will find it for your client.

18.4 — Be ready to answer a client's questions about your products.

OBJECTIONS

Don't be afraid of client objections to a product or service. A client may object to the price, length of time a service takes, the results of a service, or the frequent maintenance of a particular service. Answer the objection honestly and pleasantly, describing the advantages of the product or service and weighing them against the disadvantages. When a client has valid objections to a product or service, suggest another option that will serve his or her needs better.

CLOSE THE SALE

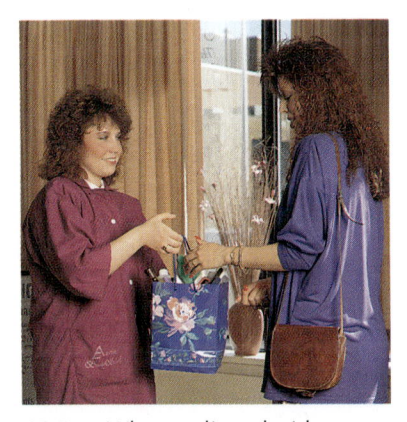

When a client decides to buy a product or service, you have closed the sale. There are three basic steps to closing a sale for nail products and services: suggestion selling, wrap-up, and scheduling another appointment. (Fig. 18.5)

SUGGESTION SELLING

Suggestion selling occurs when you suggest products or services for your client to buy. You will be successful at suggestion selling when you can match your products and services with your client's needs and wants. After performing a service, you should try to sell your clients the products needed to maintain their nails until their next appointment.

You might suggest that a client buy an additional service before leaving. As an example, for clients with rough hands, suggest they get a paraffin waxing treatment to soften them.

18.5 — When a client decides to buy a product or service, you have closed the sale.

WRAP-UP

After the client has decided what to buy, you can close the sale by saying, "Should I wrap this up for you?" or "Will this be cash or charge?"

SCHEDULING ANOTHER APPOINTMENT

Before a client leaves the salon, schedule another appointment for maintenance of the service you just performed or for another service. Confirm future appointments by giving each client your business card with the date and time of the next appointment. Advance scheduling is a good way to build a steady, happy clientele.

Easy Homecare Sales

Grouping products together into pre-made packages is a natural way to sell retail around the holiday time, but what about creating such kits for everyday home use? It's a great way to push products, plus clients love the convenience of having all the essentials at their fingertips. Don't know where to start? Gather together the components for your best-selling service—such as the ever-popular French manicure, the natural manicure or the pedicure—for home use. The trick is to anticipate what clients will need in order to care for their specific type of manicure or pedicure between visits, then assemble those items in different homecare kits—one for every type of nail service.

REVIEW QUESTIONS

1. What are the five basic steps in selling.
2. Describe the difference between product features and benefits.
3. Choose one of the nail services you have learned about in this book. Describe two features and two benefits of that service.
4. What are three questions you should try to answer as you determine your client's needs and wants?
5. Explain how you can sell while you work.
6. List and describe the three steps in closing the sale.

ANSWERS TO REVIEW QUESTIONS

CHAPTER 1

1. What is salon conduct?

   Salon conduct is the way you act when working with clients, your employer, and coworkers in the salon.

2. Give ten examples of professional salon conduct toward clients.

   Examples of professional salon conduct toward clients are: 1) being on time; 2) being prepared; 3) planning your day; 4) arranging appointments carefully; 5) keeping clients informed of schedule changes; 6) being courteous; 7) performing all tasks willingly and efficiently; 8) communicating with clients; 9) never complaining or arguing with a client; 10) using good judgment; 11) never chewing gum, smoking, or eating where you can be seen by clients. (Only 10 are needed.)

3. Explain why a salon might lose clients if nail technicians do not exhibit professional salon conduct.

   A salon might lose clients if nail technicians do not exhibit professional salon conduct because clients want to be treated well. if you are late, or you seem disorganized or uncaring, clients might feel uncomfortable. Clients shouldn't feel that their appointments inconvenience you. Chewing gum, smoking, or eating in front of clients can annoy them. Smoking can also be potentially dangerous around chemicals.

4. Give ten examples of professional salon conduct toward employers and coworkers.

   Examples of professional salon conduct toward employers and coworkers are: 1) being willing to learn; 2) communicating; 3) giving credit to others; 4) respecting the opinions of coworkers; 5) taking the initiative; 6) using good judgment; 7) leaving personal problems at home; 8) never borrowing money from employers or coworkers; 9) promoting the salon; 10) developing your ability to sell.

5. Define professional ethics.

   Professional ethics is your sense of right and wrong when you interact with your clients, employer, and coworkers. The essential values in professional ethics are honesty, fairness, courtesy, and respect for the feelings and rights of others.

6. Give seven examples of professional ethics toward clients.

   Examples of professional ethics toward clients are: 1) suggesting services that meet clients' needs; 2) keeping your word and fulfilling all obligations; 3) treating all clients fairly; 4) following state regulations for sanitation and safety; 5) being loyal; 6) not criticizing others; 7) not abandoning clients.

7. Give five examples of professional ethics toward employers and coworkers.

   Five examples of professional ethics toward employers and coworkers are: 1) being honest; 2) fulfilling obligations; 3) respecting the talents of your employer and coworkers; 4) not inviting criticism of coworkers; 5) never gossiping or starting rumors among coworkers.

8. Describe the type of appearance you should have as a professional nail technician.

   As a nail technician one should be clean and fresh, have fresh breath and healthy teeth, wear clean clothes that are appropriate for the salon, and pay attention to hair, skin, and nails.

9. Explain why a salon might lose clients if it employs nail technicians who have an unprofessional appearance.

   A salon might lose clients if it employs nail technicians who have an unprofessional appearance because, as a member of the beauty industry, a nail technician should be pleasant to be around. If you are not clean and pleasant smelling, clients may object to having you touch them while performing nail services.

CHAPTER 2

1. What are bacteria? What do bacteria look like?

   Bacteria are microscopic organisms that live almost everywhere. They can be round, grow in chains, or look like the spiral of a corkscrew.

2. Are all bacteria harmful? Give examples to explain your answer.

   No, at least 70% of all bacteria are nonpathogenic or non-disease-producing. Many bacteria aid in the digestion of food an make oxygen.

3. What are the three main groups of pathogenic bacteria? Describe them.

   The three main groups of pathogenic bacteria are cocci, bacilli, and spirilla. Cocci grow in clusters, chains, or pairs; bacilli are the most common and are rod-shaped; spirilla are spiral or corkscrew-shaped.

4. Why can bacteria reproduce so quickly?

   They grow to maturity and then divide into two bacterium. The newly formed cells begin to grow and divide almost immediately.

5. Give examples of common infections caused by viruses.

   Hepatitis, chicken pox, influenza, colds, measles, and mumps are the most common examples.

6. Is it likely that salon services can cause AIDS?

   The chance of transmitting HIV in the salon is near zero! It is virtually impossible.

7. Describe the appearance of bacterial infection on the nail plate?

   Bacterial infections often appear as greenish yellow spots on the nail plate beneath the enhancement.

8. Do molds and mildew grow on or under the nail plate?

   No, molds and mildew do not infect the fingernail.

9. What is immunity? Name three types of immunity.

   Immunity is the ability of the body to resist disease and destroy microorganisms when they have entered the body. Immunity can be natural, naturally acquired, or artificially acquired.

10. Name five common sources of infection in the salon.

    a. Contaminated manicuring tools and equipment.
    b. Clients' nails, hands, and feet.
    c. Your clients', coworkers', and your own mouth, nose, and eyes.
    d. Open wounds or sores on you or your client.
    e. Objects throughout the entire salon.

CHAPTER 3

1. What is the difference between disinfection and sanitation?

   Sanitation is the lowest form of decontamination. It is designed to significantly lower the number of pathogens on a surface. Disinfection is a much higher level of decontamination. Disinfection kills all pathogens, except bacterial spores.

2. Disinfection is almost identical to _____ except disinfection does not kill bacterial spores.

   Sterilization.

3. What is an antiseptic?

   Antiseptics reduce the number of pathogens in a cut and the immune system kills what is left.

4. What is the best type of disinfectant to use in a salon?

   EPA registered, hospital-level disinfectants are perfect for salons.

5. What are the two most commonly used types of disinfectants?

   Quats and phenolics.

6. Once implements are properly _____, they must be stored where they will remain free from _____.

   Disinfected, contamination

7. Can tuberculosis (TB) be transmitted by salon implements?

   It is impossible to transmit TB on a salon implement nor will tuberculocidal disinfectants prevent the spread of TB in salon.

8. Formaldehyde is a strong _____ _____.

   Allergic sensitizer.

9. What must you use to remove implements from disinfectant containers?

   Rubber gloves or tongs.

10. Describe Universal Sanitation in your own words.

    Universal Sanitation means you do everything that is required to sanitize and disinfect the salon and your implements. No short cuts!

CHAPTER 4

1. List five early warning signs of chemical overexposure.

   Rash and other skin irritation, lightheadedness, insomnia, runny nose, sore throat, watery eyes, tingling toes, fatigue, irritability, sluggishness, breathing problems.

2. What does MSDS stand for?

   Material Safety Data Sheet

3. Name four simple and inexpensive things you can do to reduce vapors in the salon.

   a. Keep all products tightly sealed when not in use.
   b. Use a covered dappen dish or pump to limit the vapors in the air.
   c. Avoid using pressurized sprays. They create finer mists and are difficult to control.
   d. Empty your waste container often. It is one of the best sources of vapors.

4. Define breathing zone.

   Your breathing zone is an invisible sphere about the size of a beach ball that sits directly in front of your mouth.

5. Describe how a local exhaust system works. Why is it best?

   Local exhaust uses a moveable exhaust vent, hose, or tube to capture vapors, dusts, and mists. Specially designed blowers pull contaminants from the breathing zone down the exhaust tube and expel them from the building. They are best because they work. They don't try to do the impossible...clean the air and return it to the salon. That isn't possible in the salon environment.

6. What is the best and least expensive way to prevent excessive inhalation of dusts?

   Use a dusk mask. It filters air as the air goes into your mouth.

7. Why should products be stored away from heat and pilot lights?

   Excessive heat will ruin them and some are more flammable than gasoline.

8. Why should smoke not be allowed in the salon?

    Many salon products are more flammable than gasoline.

9. What is CTD? Explain how this happens.

    Cumulative trauma disorder. It is caused by repetitive motions which can damage sensitive nerves, especially in the hands.

10. List seven symptoms of CTD.

    Pain, numbness, aching, stiffness, tingling, weakness, and swelling.

CHAPTER 5

1. Nail plates are mostly protein made from chemicals called _____ _____.

    Amino acids

2. Define molecules.

    A molecule is a chemical in its simplest form.

3. What are catalysts and why are they important to nail chemistry?

    Catalysts are chemicals that speed up chemical reactions. They make enhancements and overlays harden much more quickly.

4. A _____ is anything that dissolves another substance called a _____.

    Solvent, solute

5. True or False? Primers can eat the nail plate. Explain your answer.

    False, no enhancement product will dissolve or eat the nail plate. Heavy abrasives and overfiling strip the nail plate away and make it thin.

6. Define monomers.

    The individual molecules that join to make the polymer are called monomers.

7. What are the two main differences between irritations and allergic reactions?

   Allergic reactions become worse with each exposure, irritations do not. Also, irritations are temporary and allergic reactions last a lifetime.

8. What six things can you avoid or do to ensure that clients never suffer from product allergy?

   a. *Never* smooth the enhancement surface with more liquid monomer.

   b. *Never* use monomer to "clean up" the edges, under the nail or sidewalls.

   c. *Never* touch any monomer liquids, gels, or adhesives to the skin.

   d. *Never* touch the hairs of the brush with your fingers.

   e. *Never* mix your own special product blends

   f. *Always* follow instructions—exactly!

9. Only _____ and _____ skin contact can cause a client to become allergic to products.

   Prolonged, repeated

10. In your own words explain what Paracelus discovered about toxic substances. How can you use this knowledge to work safely?

    Paracelus said that everything can be poisonous if we overexpose ourselves. So, learning to prevent overexposure would make a nail technician's job safe.

CHAPTER 6

1. How can an understanding of anatomy and physiology help you become a better nail technician?

   An understanding of anatomy and physiology can help you become a better nail technician because it will give you a scientific background for many of the nail service you provide. It will help you decide which services are better for clients' nail or skin conditions and how to adjust and control the service for best results.

2. What is the purpose of cells within the human body?

   Cells are the basic functional units of all living things. Cells carry on all life processes and reproduce new cells, enabling the body to replace worn or injured tissues.

3. What is cell metabolism?

   Cell metabolism is a complex chemical process in which cells are nourished and supplied with the elements necessary to carry on their many activities.

4. Name the five types of body tissue and explain the function of each.

   Five types of body tissues are: 1) connective tissue, which supports, protects, and binds the body tissues together; 2) muscular tissue, which contracts and moves various parts of the body; 3) nerve tissue, which carries messages to and from the brain and coordinates all body functions; 4) epithelial tissue, which is a protective covering on body surfaces; 5) liquid tissue, which carries food, wastes, and hormones by means of blood and lymph.

5. What are the five most important organs of the body? Explain the function of each.

   The five most important organs of the body are: 1) the brain, which controls the body; 2) the lungs, which supply oxygen to the blood; 3) the liver, which removes toxic products of digestion; 4) the kidneys, which excrete water and other waste products; 5) the stomach and intestines, which digest food; 6) the heart, which circulates the blood. (Only five are needed.)

6. List the ten systems that make up the human body. What is the function of each system?

   Ten systems making up the human body are: 1) the integumentary system, which functions as a protective covering and contains sensory receptors; 2) the skeletal system, which serves as a means of support, movement, and protection; 3) the muscular system, which produces all movement of the body; 4) the nervous system, which controls and coordinates the functions of all other body systems; 5) the circulatory system, which supplies blood throughout the body; 6) the endocrine system, which secretes hormones into the bloodstream; 7) the excretory system, which eliminates waste from the body; 8) the respiratory system, which supplies oxygen to the body; 9) the digestive system, which changes food into substances that can be used by the body cells; 10) the reproductive system, which allows humans to reproduce.

7. What are four ways in which muscles are stimulated?

    Muscles are stimulated by: 1) massage; 2) electric current; 3) light rays; 4) heat rays; 5) moist heat; 6) nerve impulses; 7) chemicals. (Only four are needed.)

8. What are four types of muscles that are affected by massage?

    Four types of muscles that are affected by massage are: 1) shoulder and upper arm; 2) forearm; 3) hand; 4) lower leg and foot.

9. What are the three divisions of the nervous system? What is the function of each division?

    Three divisions of the nervous system and their functions are: 1) the central nervous system, which controls the voluntary actions of the five senses; 2) the peripheral nervous system, which carries messages to and from the central nervous system; 3) the autonomic nervous system, which regulates the activities of smooth muscles, glands, blood vessels, and the heart.

10. What are the chief functions of the blood?

    The chief functions of the blood are: to carry water, oxygen, food, and secretions to cells; to carry away carbon dioxide and waste products; to help equalize body temperature; to aid in protecting the body from harmful bacteria and infection; and to clot, preventing the loss of blood.

CHAPTER 7

1. What are the three parts that make up the nail?

    Three parts making up the nail are: 1) nail body (plate); 2) nail root; 3) free edge.

2. Define nail disorder.

    A nail disorder is a condition caused by injury to the nail, disease, or an imbalance in the body.

3. What is the golden rule for dealing with nail disorders?

   The golden rule states that if the nail or skin to be worked on is infected, inflamed, broken, or swollen, a nail technician should refer the client to a doctor.

4. List five nail disorders that can be serviced by a nail technician.

   Five nail disorders that can be serviced by a nail technician are: 1) hangnails; 2) discolored nails; 3) eggshell nails; 4) furrows; 5) leukonychia; 6) onychatrophia or atrophy; 7) onychauxis; 8) onychophagy; 9) onychorrhexis; 10) ptergium. (Only five are needed.)

5. List five nail disorders that cannot be serviced by a nail technician.

   Five nail disorders that cannot be serviced by a nail technician are: 1) mold; 2) onychia; 3) onychogryposis; 4) onycholysis; 5) onychoptosis; 6) paronychia; 7) pyrogenic granuloma. (Only five are needed.)

CHAPTER 8

1. What are the characteristics of healthy skin?

   Healthy skin is characterized by being slightly moist and acid, soft, and flexible. healthy skin also has elasticity, a smooth, fine-grained texture, and is free of blemishes and diseases.

2. What are five functions of the skin?

   Five functions of the skin are: 1) protection; 2) prevention of fluid loss; 3) response to external stimulus; 4) heat regulation; 5) secretion; 6) excretion; 7) absorption; 8) respiration. (Only five are needed.)

3. Describe the epidermis and dermis.

   The epidermis is the outermost protective covering of the skin. It contains no blood vessels, but does contain many small nerve layers. The dermis is the deep layer of the skin. It contains blood vessels, lymph vessels, nerves, sweat glands, and oil glands in an elastic network made up of collagen.

4. How is the skin nourished?

   The skin is nourished by blood and lymph.

5. What are the functions of sweat glands?

   The functions of sweat glands are to regulate body temperature and eliminate waste products through perspiration.

6. Name five type of lesions.

   Five types of lesions are: 1) bulla; 2) crust; 3) cyst; 4) excoriation; 5) fissure; 6) macule; 7) papule; 8) pustule; 9) scales; 10) scars; 11) stain; 12) tubercule; 13) tumor; 14) nodules; 15) ulcers; 16) vesicles; 17) wheals. (Only five are needed.)

7. What are the characteristics of eczema and psoriasis?

   Eczema is characterized by itching, burning, and the formation of scales and oozing blisters. Psoriasis is characterized by a chronic inflammation with round, dry patches covered with coarse silvery scales.

CHAPTER 9

1. What is the purpose of a client consultation?

   The purpose of a client consultation is to discuss the client's general health, the health of his or her nails and skin, and the client's lifestyle in order to select the most appropriate nail service.

2. What are the characteristics of healthy nails?

   Healthy nails are not inflamed, infected, swollen, or broken.

3. How would your services differ for a runner or a guitar player?

   A guitar player may need short nails on the left hand and longer nails on the right. He or she will also need calluses on the fingertips of the left hand. A runner may have calluses on the feet that protect feet while running.

4. Under what circumstances would you refer a client to a physician?

   If an infection, swelling, broken skin, or an inflammation is evident, one should refer a client to a physician.

5. What are the three types of information on the client health/record card?

The general information asks for the client's name, address, telephone number, and best appointment hours. The client profile asks for information about the type of work and leisure activities the client participates in. The medical record asks for information about the client's general health. This information will help you determine whether it is safe to perform hand and foot massage on the client.

CHAPTER 10

1. When you give a manicure, you need equipment, implements, materials, and nail cosmetics. Give three examples of each of these manicuring supplies.

    Three examples of equipment used in nail technology are: 1) manicure table with an adjustable lamp; 2) client's chair and nail technician's chair or stool; 3) fingerbowl; 4) disinfection container; 5) client's cushion; 6) sanitized cotton container; 7) supply tray; 8) electric nail dryer. (Only three are needed.)

    Implements used in nail technology are: 1) orangewood stick; 2) steel pusher; 3) metal nail file; 4) emery board; cuticle nipper. (Only three are needed.)

    Materials needed for a manicure include: 1) disposable towels or terry towels; 2) cotton or cotton balls; 3) plastic bags; 4) 70% ethyl alcohol; 5) powder alum or styptic powder. (Only three are needed.)

    Nail cosmetics include: 1) polish remover; 2) cuticle cream; 3) cuticle oil; 4) cuticle solvent; 5) nail bleach; 6) nail whitener; 7) dry nail polish; 8) colored polish; 9) liquid enamel or lacquer; 10) base coat; 11) nail strengthener; 12) top coat or sealer; 13) liquid nail dry; 14) hand cream or lotion. (Only three are needed.)

2. What are two reasons for having a manicuring table that is sanitary and properly equipped?

    Two reasons for having a manicuring table that is sanitary and properly equipped are: 1) anything needed during a service will be at your fingertips; 2) having an orderly table will give you and your client confidence during the manicure.

3. Describe the four basic nail shapes.

   Four basic nail shapes are: 1) rectangular or square; 2) round; 3) oval; 4) pointed.

4. List the six steps in the water manicure pre-service.

   The six steps in the water manicure pre-service are: 1) pre-service sanitation procedure; 2) set up standard manicuring table; 3) greet client; 4) have client wash hands with an antibacterial soap; 5) do client consultation; 6) begin working with the hand that is not the client's favored hand.

5. Briefly describe the water manicure procedure.

   The water manicure procedure is as follows: 1) remove polish; 2) shape nails; 3) soften cuticles; 4) clean nails; 5) dry hand; 6) apply cuticle remover; 7) loosen cuticles; 8) nip cuticles; 9) clean under free edge; 10) repeat steps 4-9 on other hand; 11) bleach nails (optional); 12) buff with chamois buffer (optional); 13) apply cuticle oil; 14) bevel nails; 15) apply hand lotion and massage hand and arm; 16) remove traces of oil; 17) choose color; 18) apply polish.

6. Name the five types of polish applications.

   Five types of polish applications are: 1) full coverage; 2) free edge; 3) hairline tip; 4) half moon or lunula; 5) slimline or free walls.

7. List the five steps in the water manicure post-service.

   The five steps in the water manicure post-service are: 1) make another appointment; 2) sell retail products; 3) clean up around your table; 4) discard used materials; 5) sanitize table and implements.

8. List the four steps in the French manicure procedure.

   Four steps in the French manicure are: 1) apply base coat; 2) apply white polish; 3) apply sheer pink, natural, or peach polish; 4) apply top coat.

9. What are the three benefits of the reconditioning hot oil manicure? How often should clients receive a reconditioning hot oil manicure?

   Three benefits of the reconditioning hot oil manicure are: 1) it is recommended for clients with ridges and brittle nails; 2) it is also recommended for clients with dry cuticles; 3) it improves the hands by leaving the skin soft and adding moisture to hands and nails. A reconditioning manicure is recommended once a week.

10. What type of polish application is included in a man's manicure?

    A man's manicure is the same as a woman's except that a colored polish is not used in a man's manicure.

11. Name five hand massage techniques and five arm massage techniques.

    Five hand massage techniques are: 1) relaxer movement; 2) joint movement on fingers; 3) circular movement in palm; 4) circular movement on wrist; 5) circular movement on back of hand and fingers. Five arm massage techniques are: 1) distribute cream or lotion; 2) effleurage on arms; 3) wringing movements on arm-friction massage movement; 4) kneading movement on arm; 5) rotation of elbow-friction massage movement.

12. What are two safety cautions for hand and arm massage?

    Two safety cautions for hand and arm massage are: 1) avoid vigorous joint massage if your client has arthritis; 2) do not massage if your client has high blood pressure, a heart condition, or has had a stroke.

CHAPTER 11

1. Name five pedicure supplies.

    Five pedicure supplies are: 1) pedicure station; 2) pedicure stool and footrest; 3) client's chair; 4) rinse and soap baths; 5) toe separators; 6) foot file; 7) toenail clippers; 8) antiseptic fungal foot spray; 9) antibacterial soap; 10) foot lotion; 11) foot powder; 12) pedicure slippers. (Only five are needed.)

2. List the seven steps in the pedicure pre-service.

    The steps in the pedicure pre-service include: 1) pre-service sanitation procedure; 2) setting up the pedicure station; 3) spread one terry cloth towel on the floor in front of the client's chair, spread another over the stool to dry feet; 4) set up standard manicuring table in pedicure station; 5) both basins should be filled with warm water and antibacterial soap in one and antiseptic in the other; 6) greet client; 7) complete client consultation.

3. Briefly describe the pedicure procedure.

   The pedicure procedure includes: 1) removing shoes and socks; 2) spraying feet; 3) soaking feet; 4) rinsing feet; 5) drying feet; 6) removing polish; 7) clipping nails; 8) inserting toe separators; 9) filing nails; 10) using foot file to remove dry skin and callus growths; 11) rinsing the foot; 12) repeating steps 7-11 on other foot; 13) brushing nails; 14) applying cuticle solvent; 15) pushing back the cuticle; 16) brushing the foot; 17) applying lotion; 18) massaging foot; 19) proceed with steps 13-19 on other foot; 20) remove traces of lotion; 21) apply polish; 22) powder feet.

4. Describe the proper technique to use in filing toenails.

   Toenails are filed straight across, rounded slightly at the corners to conform to the shape of the toes. Do not file into the corners of nails. Rough edges are to be smoothed with the fine side of the emery board.

5. List the six steps in the pedicure post-service.

   Post service pedicure steps include: 1) scheduling another appointment; 2) advising client about foot care; 3) selling retail products; 4) cleaning pedicure area; 5) discarding used materials; 6) sanitizing table and implements.

6. Name six foot massage techniques.

   Six foot massage techniques include: 1) relaxer movement to the joints of the foot; 2) effleurage on the top of the foot; 3) effleurage on heel; 4) effleurage movement on toes; 5) joint movement for toes; 6) thumb impression-friction movement; 7) metatarsal scissors; 8) fist twist compression; 9) effleurage on instep; 10) percussion or tapotement movement. (Only six are needed.)

7. What is a safety caution for pedicuring?

   A safety caution for a pedicure is to ask clients if they are being treated for high blood pressure, heart condition, or diabetes.

CHAPTER 12

1. List the four supplies, in addition to your basic manicuring table, that you need for nail tip application.

   Four supplies needed for nail tip application, in addition to the basic manicuring table, are: 1) abrasive; 2) a buffer block; 3) nail adhesive; 4) nail tips.

ANSWERS TO REVIEW QUESTIONS ◆ **249**

2. Name the two types of nail tips.

   Three types of nail tips are plastic, nylon, and acetate. (Only two are needed.)

3. What portion of the natural nail plate should be covered by a nail tip?

   Nail tips should cover no more than one-half the natural nail plate.

4. What type of tip application is considered a temporary service? Why?

   Applying a tip without an overlay, such as a fabric wrap or acrylic nail, is considered a temporary service because a tip without such a service is very weak.

5. Briefly describe the procedure for nail tip application.

   The procedure for nail tip application is as follows: 1) remove all polish; 2) push back cuticle; 3) buff nail to remove shine; 4) clean nails; 5) size tips; 6) apply nail antiseptic; 7) apply adhesive; 8) slide on tips; 9) apply adhesive bead to seam; 10) trim nail tip; 11) blend tip into natural nail; 12) buff tip for perfect blend; 13) shape nail; 14) proceed with desired service.

6. Describe the proper maintenance of nail tips.

   The proper maintenance for nail tips is to follow with weekly or biweekly manicures for regluing and rebuffing. Non-acetone polish remover should be used because acetone dissolves the tips.

7. Describe the procedure for the removal of tips.

   The procedure for removing tips is as follows: 1) complete nail tip application pre-service procedure; 2) soak nails; 3) slide off tip; 4) buff nail; 5) condition cuticle and surrounding skin; 6) proceed with desired service; 7) complete nail tip application post-service if no further service is performed.

CHAPTER 13

1. List four kinds of nail wraps.

   Four kinds of nail wraps are 1) silk; 2) linen; 3) fiberglass; 4) paper wraps.

2. Explain the benefits of using silk, linen, fiberglass, and paper wraps.

   The benefits for silk, linen, fiberglass, and paper wraps are as follows: 1) silk wraps are strong, lightweight, and smooth when applied to nails; 2) linen is thicker than silk or fiberglass; linen is strong and lasts a long time; 3) fiberglass has a loose weave, which makes for easy penetration of the adhesive; it's especially strong and durable; 4) paper wraps are temporary.

3. Describe the procedure for fabric wrap application.

   The procedure for fabric wrap application is as follows: 1) remove old polish; 2) clean nails; 3) push cuticle back; 4) buff nail to remove shine; 5) apply nail antiseptic; 6) apply glue; 7) cut fabric; 8) apply fabric adhesives; 9) apply fabric; 10) trim fabric; 11) apply fabric adhesive; 12) apply fabric adhesive dryer; 13) apply second coat of adhesive; 14) apply second coat of adhesive dryer; 15) shape and refine nails; 16) buff nails; 17) apply hand lotion; 18) remove traces of oil; 19) apply polish.

4. Explain how a fabric wrap is used as a crack repair.

   A fabric wrap is used as a crack repair by cutting a repair patch to completely cover the crack or break.

5. Describe how to remove fabric wraps and what to avoid.

   The fabric wrap removal procedure is as follows: 1) complete nail wrap pre-service; 2) soak nails; 3) slide off softened wraps; 4) buff nails; 5) condition cuticles. Avoid damaging the nail plate when removing fabric wraps.

6. Describe the purpose of paper wraps and explain why they are not recommended for very long nails.

   The purpose of paper wraps is to provide a temporary method of strengthening the nail. Paper wraps are not recommended for very long nails because they do not provide the strength that long nails require.

7. List the materials used for paper wraps.

   The materials used in paper wraps are mending tissues, mending liquid, and ridge fillers.

8. Outline the procedures used in paper wraps.

   The procedure used in paper wraps is as follows: 1) complete nail wrap pre-service; 2) remove old nail polish; 3) clean nails; 4) push back cuticles; 5) buff nails to remove shine; 6) apply nail antiseptic; 7) tear mending tissue; 8) apply mending liquid to tissue; 9) apply paper wrap; 10) smooth the wrap; 11) cut tissue; 12) apply mending liquid under free edge; 13) smooth wrap; 14) refine nail; 15) apply mending liquid; 16) apply ridge filler; 17) apply polish; 18) complete nail wrap post-service.

9. Define liquid nail wrap and describe its purpose.

   Liquid nail wrap is a polish made of tiny fibers designed to strengthen and preserve the natural nail as it grows. After it has been brushed on the nail in several directions and allowed to harden, it creates a network that protects the nail.

CHAPTER 14

1. List the supplies needed for acrylic nail application.

   The supplies needed for acrylic nail application are: acrylic liquid, acrylic powder, primer, abrasive, small containers for liquid and powder acrylic, nail forms, sable brush, safety glasses, plastic gloves, and safety mask (optional).

2. Briefly describe the chemistry of acrylic nails.

   The chemistry of acrylic nails is broken down into three basic ingredients. A monomer is made up of many small molecules that aren't attached to each other. Liquid acrylic is a monomer. A polymer is made up of molecules that are attached to each other in long chains, usually forming something hard. Finished acrylic nails are polymers. A catalyst speeds up the hardening process. Powdered acrylic is a combination of ground up polymer and a catalyst. Polymerization is the process of forming the nail.

3. Describe the procedure for the application of acrylic nails over forms.

   The procedure for applying acrylic nails over forms is as follows: 1) complete acrylic application pre-service; 2) remove polish; 3) clean nails; 4) push back cuticle; 5) buff nail to remove shine; 6) apply nail antiseptic; 7) position nail form;

8) apply primer; 9) prepare acrylic liquid and powder; 10) dip brush into liquid; 11) form acrylic ball; 12) place ball of acrylic on free edge; 13) shape free edge; 14) place second ball of acrylic; 15) shape second ball of acrylic; 16) apply acrylic beads; 17) apply acrylic to remaining nails; 18) remove forms; 19) shape nails; 20) buff nail; 21) apply cuticle oil; 22) apply hand cream and massage hand and arm; 23) clean nails; 24) apply polish.

4. Describe the safety precautions for applying primer.

    The safety precautions for applying primer are: never use primer without plastic gloves and safety glasses; offer a pair of safety glasses to the client. Check primer on a regular basis to make sure it isn't contaminated with bacteria.

5. Describe the procedure for applying acrylic nails over tips.

    The procedure for applying acrylic nails over tips is as follows: 1) complete acrylic application pre-service; 2) remove polish; 3) clean nails; 4) push back cuticle; 5) buff nail to remove shine; 6) apply nail antiseptic; 7) apply tips; 8) apply primer; 9) prepare acrylic liquid and powder; 10) dip brush into liquid; 11) form acrylic ball; 12) place ball of acrylic on free edge; 13) shape free edge; 14) place second ball of acrylic; 15) shape second ball of acrylic; 16) apply acrylic beads; 17) shape and refine nail; 18) buff nail; 19) apply cuticle oil; 20) apply hand cream and massage hand and arm; 21) clean nails; 22) apply polish; 23) do standard post-service procedure.

6. How does the procedure for acrylic nail application over bitten nails differ from other acrylic nail procedures?

    The procedure for acrylic nail application over bitten nails requires you to create a portion of the nail plate before applying the nail form.

7. Describe the two basic types of maintenance for acrylic nails.

    The two basic types of maintenance for acrylic nails are fill-in and crack repair. Fill-in allows nails to look natural and even while growing out. Crack repair is the addition of extra acrylic to fill the crack in an acrylic nail and reinforce the rest of the nail.

8. Describe the proper procedure for acrylic removal.

    The proper procedure for acrylic removal is as follows: 1) fill bowl with acetone; 2) soak fingertips; 3) remove acrylic with orangewood stick; 4) buff nails; 5) condition cuticle.

9. Explain how the application of odorless acrylics differs from the application of traditional acrylics.

   The application of odorless acrylics is different from the application of traditional acrylics because odorless acrylics do not smell as strongly, they're wetter than traditional acrylics, and they require less shaping. When nails are dry, the surface has a tacky, gummy residue that rolls off as you refine the nails.

CHAPTER 15

1. Describe the two basic types of gel.

   The two basic types of gel are: 1) light-cured gels, which harden when exposed to a special light source such as an ultraviolet light or halogen light; 2) no-light gels, which harden when a gel activator is sprayed or brushed on, or when they are soaked in water.

2. List the supplies needed for light-gel application.

   The supplies needed for light-gel application are: light-cured gel, curing light, brush, nail forms, primer (if recommended by gel manufacturer), block buffer, nail tips, adhesive, and nail art supplies.

3. Describe the proper procedure and precautions for light-cured gel application.

   The proper procedure for light-cured gel is as follows: 1) remove polish; 2) clean nails; 3) push back cuticles; 4) buff nails to remove shine; 5) apply nail antiseptic; 6) apply tips if desired; 7) apply primer if recommended; 8) apply gel; 9) cure gel; 10) repeat steps 8 and 9 on the other hand; 11) apply second coat of gel to the first hand; 12) cure gel; 13) repeat steps 11 and 12 on the other hand; 14) repeat steps 11-13; 15) clean nails; 16) apply cuticle oil; 17) apply hand cream and massage hand and arm; 18) clean nails; 19) apply polish. The safety caution for light-cured gel application is that inadequately shielded ultraviolet lamps can damage skin and eyes.

4. Describe the proper procedure and precautions for light-gel application over forms.

   The proper procedure for light-cured gel application over forms is: 1) complete gel application pre-service; 2) apply nail forms; 3) apply gel to natural nail; 4) cure gel; 5) create free edge; 6) cure gel; 7) apply gel to entire nail; 8) cure gel; 9) remove forms; 10) shape free edge; 11) apply gel to entire nail without form; 12) cure gel; 13) remove residue; 14) apply cuticle oil; 15) apply hand cream and massage hand and arm; 16) clean nails; 17) apply polish; 18) complete gel application post-service.

5. Describe no-light gel application.

    No-light gel application includes: 1) gel application pre-service; 2) remove polish; 3) clean nails; 4) push back cuticles; 5) buff nails to remove shine; 6) apply nail antiseptic; 7) apply tips if desired; 8) apply gel; 9) cure gel with activator or water; 10) repeat steps 8 and 9 on the other hand; 11) apply second coat of gel and cure if necessary; 12) shape and refine nails; 13) buff nails to remove shine; 14) apply cuticle oil; 15) apply hand cream and massage hand and arm; 16) clean nails; 17) apply polish; 18) do gel application post-service.

CHAPTER 16

1. Why should you develop nail art skills?

    You should develop nail art skills because nail art is a creative part of a nail technician's job. It turns nails into small canvasses on which you can paint pictures, designs, and collages with tiny gems, foils, or tapes.

2. What is the technique called for airbrushing two or more colors on the nail at the same time?

    This technique is called a color fade or color blend.

3. How does the finished airbrushed French manicure differ from the traditional application?

    The airbrushed French manicure has no bumps or unevenness at the white tip. The application is very smooth and the white tip has a perfect shape every time.

4. Describe the parts of the airbrush and how they work together to release the paint.

    Each airbrush has a small cone shaped fluid nozzle, also called a tip, that a tapered needle fits into. When the needle fits snugly in the fluid nozzle, no paint is released when the trigger is depressed. When the needle is drawn back, the airbrush begins to release paint. The further the needle is drawn back, the more paint is released.

5. Describe the best airbrush to use for nails.

   An Airbrush that is designed for small quantities of paint, is gravity-fed (gravity pulls the paint into the airbrush) and mixes the paint with the air inside the airbrush (internal mix). This type of airbrush usually has a well or small color cup for the paint to be placed in the airbrush.

6. What is the most common choice for an air source for airbrushing nails?

   The most common choice for airbrushing nails is a small compressor.

7. What is the most common air pressure used by nail technicians when airbrushing?

   Most nail technicians work at a pressure between 25 pounds per square inch to 35 pounds per square inch.

8. Describe the procedure for an airbrushed version of a French manicure.

   The procedure for an airbrushed French manicure is as follows: 1) Apply a clear base coat to the nails. 2) Choose your French manicure airbrush paint and mist the French manicure color over the nail lightly. 3) Optional: Add a shimmer to your French manicure paint by misting a gold highlight or shimmer evenly over the French beige. 4) French tip application with a stencil. 5) Using the stencil, roll the finger sideways and carefully line up the stencil with the white tip already sprayed. 6) Optional: Mist the lunula slightly lighter than nail tip color. 7) Apply your nail paint bonder and let it dry for three minutes. Apply the airbrush paint protective glaze for durability.

CHAPTER 17

1. What are the advantages and disadvantages of working in a full-service salon?

   The advantages of working in a full-service salon are that you automatically get all of the nail business, your services make it convenient for clients to have their nails done while they're there for hair-care or skin-care services. You can also attract clients by offering special rates for nail care while they are having other services performed. Disadvantages of working in a full-service salon include not having other nail technicians to share ideas and experiences with. You may also be limited in the variety of services that you're allowed to perform if you work in a traditional salon. There also won't be someone to fill in for you when you're sick or on vacation.

2. What are the advantages and disadvantages of working in a nails-only salon?

   Advantages of working in a nails-only salon include having the opportunity to share ideas and experiences with other nail technicians and serving their clients when they are sick or on vacation. Disadvantages include competition for clients in a salon with many nail technicians.

3. What are ten questions that will help you determine if a salon is right for you?

   Ten questions that will help you determine if the salon is right for you are: 1) Will the salon provide additional training? 2) Will the salon help you build clientele? 3) Will you be considered an employee, or an independent contractor who rents a booth? 4) If you are an employee, how will the salon pay you? 5) Will the salon provide nail care products or will you have to bring your own? 6) Does the salon offer benefits? 7) Are there fixed or flexible working hours? 8) What is the dress code? 9) Does the salon close for regular vacation periods or does each employee take a separate vacation? 10) What is the salon's reputation? 11) Does the salon have safe working conditions? (Only ten are needed.)

4. What are eight questions that will help you determine if a salon has safe working conditions?

   Eight questions that will help you determine if a salon has safe working conditions are: 1) Does it have proper ventilation? 2) Does it provide separate refrigerators for food and nail product storage? 3) Are MSDS sheets on display or within easy access to employees? 4) Are work stations well-equipped and clean? 5) Are nail technicians required to wear dust masks? 6) Are nail technicians required to wear safety glasses? 7) Are aerosol cans used or are safer application methods used? 8) Are salon workers ready for emergencies?

5. Explain the difference between income and expenses and give two examples of each.

   Income is the money you make. It includes salary, commission from services, commission from retail product sales, and tips.

(Only two are needed.) Expenses are what you spend. They include equipment, supplies, books explaining techniques, comfortable shoes, uniforms, and tuition for courses on nail techniques. (Only two are needed.)

6. List four practical uses for business records that are required by local, state, and federal laws.

   Four practical uses for business records required by local, state, and federal laws are: 1) determining income, profits, losses, or expenses; 2) providing the value of your clientele, or the salon's worth to prospective buyers; 3) getting a bank loan; 4) computing income tax, social security, unemployment, and disability insurance.

7. List five types of information that a salon can gather by keeping accurate business records.

   Five types of information that can be gathered by keeping accurate records are: 1) profit and loss comparisons with other weeks, months, or years; 2) changes in demands for services; 3) inventory; 4) net income; 5) material and supply levels.

8. Discuss the advantages of keeping proper service, inventory, and personal appointment records.

   The advantages of keeping proper service, inventory, and personal appointment records are that service records can help another nail technician fill in for a client's usual technician; service records can record client's personal information; inventory records should be kept for use and retail value; personal records will help you arrange your work time for the client's convenience.

9. List nine guidelines that should be followed in booking appointments.

   Nine guidelines that should be followed in booking appointments are: 1) keep a supply of appointment books, pencils, erasers, pens, a calendar, and message pad within reach; 2) be prompt; 3) identify yourself and the salon when answering the phone; 4) be pleasant; 5) take the client's home phone number, type of service to be performed, and date and time of appointment when scheduling appointments; 6) speak clearly; 7) be tactful and courteous when speaking; 8) if you have appointments made in advance, call the night before to remind clients; 9) at the end of the appointment, ask clients if they wish to reschedule.

CHAPTER 18

1. What are the five basic steps in selling.

   Five basic steps in selling are: 1) knowing your products and services; 2) knowing the needs and wants of your clients; 3) presenting your products and services; 4) answering your client's questions and objections properly; 5) close the sale.

2. Describe the difference between product features and benefits.

   A product's feature is a specific fact about it (or a service) that describes it. The benefits of a product or service are what it will do for your client or how it will fulfill your clients wants and needs.

3. Choose one of the nail services you have learned about in this book. Describe two features and two benefits of that service.

   Two features of colored gel nails over tips include the fact that they are lightweight and come in a variety of colors. Two benefits of colored gel nails over tips are long, beautiful nails that will save you both time and money. (Check with your instructor for other correct answers.)

4. What are three questions you should try to answer as you determine your client's needs and wants?

   Three questions that you should try to answer as you determine your client's needs and wants are: 1) Does your client have special nail problems? 2) What is your client's lifestyle? 3) Is your client preparing for a special occasion?

5. Explain how you can sell while you work.

   You can sell while you work by displaying a list of your services and displaying a list of your products. Tell clients what you are doing, what products you are using, and why.

6. List and describe the three steps in closing the sale.

   Three steps in closing a sale are: 1) suggestion selling, which occurs when you suggest services or products for your client to buy; 2) wrap up, which can be used to ask if you can wrap up a product and ask how the client will be paying for the product; 3) schedule another appointment for maintenance of the service you have performed.

GLOSSARY/INDEX

Note: Boldface entries are definitions.

A

Abductor, 75
   hallucis (ab-DUK-tohr ha-LU-sis, 75
Abductors (ab-DUK-tohrs) separate the fingers, 74
Acetone, 52
Acrylic nails
   maintenance/removal, 186-89
   odorless, 190
   over bitten nails, 184-86
   over tips or natural nails, 182-84
   post-service, 181-82
   pre-service, 177
   procedures, 177-81
   supplies for, 176-77
Adductors (a-DUK-tohrs) draw the fingers together, 74
Adhesion chemicals, 53-55
Adhesive is a chemical that causes two surfaces to stick together, 53
Adipose (AD-i-pohs) is the tissue that gives smoothness and shape to the body, contains a store of fat to be burned for energy, and acts as a protective cushion for the outer skin, 100
Advertising, self, 226
Afferent (AF-fer-ent nerves) carry impulses or messages from sense organs to the brain, 77
Airbrush, 207-9
   nail color/art and, 206-15
   set-up/practice, 209-11
      on clients, 211-13
   two-color fade, 214-15
Albinism (AL-bi-niz-em) is a congenital absence of melanin pigment in the body, including the skin, hair, and eyes, 105
Alcohol, as a disinfectant, 30-31
Allergic contact dermatitis is caused by an ingredient in a product, 58
Allergic reactions, from prolonged/repeated contact, 59-60
Alum, powdered, 121
Anabolism (ah-NAB-o-liz-em) is the process of building up larger molecules from smaller molecules, 66
Anterior tibial (TIB-ee-al) artery supplies blood to the foot, 82
Antibacterial soap, 121
Antibacterial soap contains a soap or detergent and an antibacterial agent to sanitize the client's hands, 121
Appearance, professional, 12
Appointments
   booking, 225-26
   records of, 223
Arm
   blood supply to, 81-82
   bones of, 69-70
   massage, 140-43
Arrector pili (a-REK-tohr PIGH-ligh) muscles are attached to the hair follicles. These muscles can cause goose bumps, 100
Arteries are thick-walled muscular and elastic tubes that carry oxygen-filled blood from the heart to the capillaries throughout the body, 80
Athlete's foot is a fungus infection of the foot, 105
Atrium (AY-tree-um) make up the upper chambers of the heart, 80
Autonomic (aw-toh-NAHM-ik) nervous system is the portion of the nervous system that functions without conscious effort and regulates the activities of the smooth muscles, glands, blood vessels, and heart, 76
Axon (AK-son) sends messages to other neurons, glands, or muscles, 77

B

Bacilli (bah-SIL-i) are the most common bacteria. They are rod-shaped and produce such diseases as tetanus, influenza, typhoid, tuberculosis, and diphtheria, 16
Bacteria (bak-TEER-ee-ah), are one celled microorganisms, 15
   growth/reproduction of, 17
   movement of, 17
   types of, 15-16
Bactericides kill harmful bacteria, 29
Ball-and-socket joint such as the hip or shoulder, one bone is rounded and fits into the socket of another bone, 69
Balls, cotton, 121
Base coat is colorless and is applied to the natural nail before the application of colored polish, 123
Bead, sterilizers, 33
Belly is the middle part of the muscle, 73
Biceps (BEYE-cseps) is the muscle on the front of upper arm that lifts the forearm, flexes the elbow and turns the palm up, 73
Birthmark is a malformation of the skin due to abnormal pigmentation or dilated capillaries, 106
Bleach
   as a disinfectant, 30-31
   nail, 122
Blood
   is a nutritive fluid that moves throughout the circulatory system, 80
      circulation of, 80
      composition of, 81
      functions of, 81
   platelets (PLAY-tel-lets) play an important roll in the clotting of blood, 81
   spills, sanitation and, 34-35
   vessels transport blood to and from the heart and to various tissues of the body, 80
Bone is white on the outside and deep red on the inside, 69
   structure of, 69
Booking appointments, 225-26
Brain, 76-77
   controls the body, 67
Bruised nails is a condition in which a clot of blood forms under the nail plate, 89
Bulla (BYOO-lah) is a blister containing watery fluid, 103
Business records, 224-25

259

C

Calcaneous (kal-KAY-nee-us) of the foot are long and slender like the metacarpal bones of the hand, 70
Callus is an acquired superficial, round and thickened patch of epidermis due to pressure or friction on the hands and feet, 106
Capillaries are tiny, thin-walled blood vessels that connect the smaller arteries to the veins, 80
Cardiac (CAR-dee-ak) muscle is the heart muscle, 72
Carpal tunnel syndrome is the most common cumulative trauma disorder, 46
Carpus (KAHR-pus) or wrist, is a flexible joints composed of eight small, irregular bones held together by ligaments, 70
Cartilage (CAR-tih-ledg) is a tough elastic substance similar to bone but it has no mineral content, 69
Catabolism (kah-TAB-o-liz-em) is the breaking down of larger substances or molecules into smaller ones, 67
Catalyst is a chemical that can make a chemical reaction go faster, 52
CDT (Cumulative trauma disorders is also known as repetitive motor disorder), 46-47
Cells are the basic units of all living things, 65
   growth of, 66
   metabolism of, 66-67
Central nervous system consists of the brain and spinal cord, 76
Centrosome (SEN-tro-sohm) encloses the cytoplasm. It controls the transportation of substances and out of the cells, 65
Cerebro-spinal (ser-EE-broh SPEYE-nahl) system consists of the brain and spinal cord, 76
Chamois (SHAM-ee) buffer, 119-20
Chemicals
   adhesion/adhesives and, 53-55
   catalysts and, 52
   commonly used, 38-39
   fingernail coatings, 55-58
   learning about, 39-40
   odors from, 43
   reactions of, 52
   understanding, 51-63
Chloasma (kloh-AZ-mah) are brown spots on the skin, 106
Circulatory (SUR-kyoo-lah-tohr-ee) vascular (VAS-kyoo-lahr) system controls the steady circulation of the blood through the body by means of the heart and the blood vessels, 68, 79
Clavicle (KLAV-i-kul) is known as the collar bone, 69
Clients
   conduct toward, 7-9
   cushion for, 117
   ethics toward, 10-11
   health/record card, 110-13
   needs,
      determining, 109, 230
      meeting, 109-10
   records, keeping, 225
Coatings
   evaporation, 57-58
   fingernail, 55-58
Cocci (KOK-si), are round, pus-producing bacteria, 16
Common peroneal (per-oh-NEE-al) nerve is located behind the knee and supplies impulses to the skin of the foot and toes, 78
Connective tissue serves to support, protect, and bind together tissues of the body, 67
Contact dermatitis is caused by touching certain substances to the skin, 58
Contaminant is a substance that causes contamination, 26
Contamination, control of, 26
Cosmetics, nail, 121-23
Cotton, 121
Coworkers
   conduct toward, 9-10
   ethics toward, 11
Crack repair, acrylic nails, 188-89
Cross-linker monomer, is a monomer that joins different polymer chains together, 57
Crust is an accumulation of serum and pus mixed with epidermal flakes, 103
Cumulative trauma disorders (CTD) is also known as repetitive motor disorder, 46-47
Cuticle is the outermost protective covering of the skin, 99
   cream/oil, 122
   solvent/remover, 122
Cyst (SIST) is a semisolid or fluid lump above or below the skin surface, 103
Cytoplasm (SEYE-toh-plaz-em) is found outside of the nucleus and contains food materials necessary for the growth, reproduction, and self-repair of the cell, 65

D

Decontamination is the elimination of contaminants, including pathogens, from implements or other surfaces, 26
Deep peroneal nerve passes down the back of the leg and provides impulses to the skin of the leg and foot, 78
Deltoid (DEL-toid) is a large, thick triangular muscle that covers the shoulder and lifts and turns the arm, 73
Dendrites (DEN-dreyets) receive messages from other neurons, 77
Dermatitis, means skin inflammation, 58
Dermis is the deep layer of the skin and is also called "true skin", 100
Diaphragm is a muscular partition that controls breathing and separates the chest from the abdominal region, 84
Digestion is the process of converting food into a form that can be used of the body, 84
Digestive enzymes are chemicals that change certain kinds of food into a form capable of being used by the body, 84
Digestive system changes food into soluble form, suitable for use by the cells of the body, 68, 84
Digital (DIF-it-al) nerve and its branches supply all fingers of the hand, 78
Digits consist of three phalanges in each finger and two in the thumb, 70
Diplococci (deye-ploh-KOK-si) grow in pairs and cause pneumonia, 16
Discolored nails is a condition in which the nails turn a variety of colors, 89
Disinfectants are substances that destroy pathogens on implements and other nonliving surface, 29
   containers for, 29-30
   safety with, 35

types of, 30-31
use of, 29-30
Disinfection, 28-31
  container, 117
Disposable towels, 121
Dorsal (DOOR-sal) nerve supplies impulses to the top of the foot, 78
Dorsalis pedis artery supplies blood to the foot, 82
Dry nail polish is used with the chamois buffer to add shine to the nail, 122
Dust, overexposure to, preventing, 43

E

Eczema (EK-se-mah) is a chronic, long-lasting disorder of unknown cause, 104
Efferent (EF-fer-ent nerves) carry impulses from the brain to muscles, 77
Eggshell nails are thin, white, and curved over the free edge, 89
Electric manicure, 139-40
Emery board, 119
Enamel, liquid, 122
Endocrine (EN-doh-krin) system is made up of ductless glands that secrete substances into the bloodstream, 68, 83
Endocrine glands secrete hormones, 83
Energy has no substance, but can affect matter in many ways, 51
  chemistry and, 57
Environment, working, 221-26
Enzymes are responsible for the chemical changes in food, 84
Epidermis (ep-i-DUR-mis) is the outermost protective covering of the skin, 99
Epithelial (ep-i-THE-le-al) is a protective covering on body surfaces, such as the skin, mucous membranes, linings of the ear, digestive and respiratory organs, and glands, 67
Equipment, 117-18
Erythrocytes carry oxygen to the cells, 81
Esophagus (i-SOF-a-gus), or food pipe through which food passes to the stomach, 84
Ethics
  toward clients, 10-11
  toward coworkers, 11
Evaporation coatings, 57-58
Excoriation (ed-skohr-i-AY-shun) is a sore or abrasion caused by scratching or scraping, 103
Excretory (EK-skr-tohr-ee) system purifies the body by eliminating waste matter, 83
Exhale carbon dioxide is expelled, 84
Exhaust, local, 42
Expense records, 223
Extensor digitorum brevis (ek-STEN-sur dij-it-TOHR-um BREV-us), 75
Extensor digitorum longus (eck-STEN-sur dij-it-TOHR-um LONG-us) bends the foot up and extends the toes, 75
Extensors (eck-STEN-sur) straightens the wrist, hand, and fingers to form a straight line, 73
Eyes, protecting, 43-45

F

Fabric wraps
  are made from silk, linen, or fiberglass, 165
  maintenance, 169-71
  post-service, 168
  pre-service, 165-66
  procedure, 166-68
  removal, 171-72
  repairs, 171
  supplies, 165
Femur (FEE-mur) is a heavy, long bone that forms the leg above the knee, 70
Fiberglass, is a very thin synthetic mesh with a loose weave, 165
Fibula (FIB-ya-lah) is the smaller of the two bones that form the leg below the knee, 70
Fingerbowl, 117
Fingernails. See Nails
Fingers consist of three phalanges in each finger and two in the thumb, 70
Fissure (FISH-ur) is a crack in the skin that penetrates the dermis, 103
Flexors (FLEKS-ors) bend to the wrist, draw the hand upward, and close the fingers toward the forearm, 73
Foil, nail art and, 203
Foot
  blood supply to, 82
  bones of, 70-71
  massage, 151-53
  muscles of, 74
  nerves of, 78
Forearm, muscles of, 73
Formaldehyde
  avoid using, 34
  strengthening nails with, 123
Formalin, avoid using, 34
Free edge is the end of the nail that extends beyond the fingertip, 87
Free edge polish application, 131
Free walls polish application, 131
Freehand nail painting, 206
French manicure, 133, 216-17
Full coverage polish application, 131
Full-station salon, 221
Fundus (FUN-dus) glands are tubelike and end at the skin surface to form a sweat pore, 101
Fungicides destroy fungus, 29
Furrows on nails, also known as corrugations, are long thin ridges that run either lengthwise or across the nail, 89-90

G

Gastrocnemius (gas-truc-NEEM-e-us) is attached to the lower rear surface of the heel and pulls the foot down, 75
Gel
  application,
    no-light, 198-99
    post-service, 196
    pre-service, 193-94
    procedure, 194-96
  maintenance/removal, 199
  over forms, 196-97
  supplies, 193
Gems, nail art and, 202-3
General is the blood circulation from the heart throughout the body and back to the heart again, 80
Gland is a specialized organ that secretes substances, 83

Gold leaf application, 205

H

Hairline tip polish application, 131
Half moon polish application, 132
Hand
  blood supply to, 81-82
  bones of, 69-70
  cream/lotion, 123
  massage, 140-43
  muscles of, 74
  washing, sanitation and, 27
Hangnails, 90
Health/record card, client, 110-13
Heart is a muscular, cone shaped organ which pumps blood throughout the circulatory system, 67, 79-80
Heat, nail chemistry and, 57
Herpes simplex is a skin infection common in dental staff and others involved with the care of the mouth, 105
Hinge joints which are found in the elbow and knee, two or more bones connect like a door, 69
Histamines enlarge the vessels around an injury, 60
Homeostasis (ho-me-oh-STAY-sus) is the breaking down, energy-releasing reactions are balanced with the building-up, energy-consuming reactions, 67
Hormones are chemicals that affect metabolism and other body processes, 83
Horny layer consists of tightly packed, scalelike cells that are continually shed and replaced, 99
Hot oil manicure, 133-35
Humerus (HYOO-mo-rus) is the uppermost and largest bone in the arm, 69

I

Implements, 118-20
  sanitation and, 31
  sanitation of, 120
Income records, 223
Infection (in-FEK-shun) will have evidence of pus, 89
Inflammation (in-flam-MAY-shun) is red and sore, 89
Ingrown nails is when the nail grows into the sides of tissue around the nail, 91
Inhale, oxygen is absorbed into the blood, 84
Insertion is the part of the muscle which moves, 72-73
Integumentary (in-TEG-yoo-men-ta-ree) system is made up of the skin and its various accessory organs, 68
Intestines digest food, 67
Inventory records, 225
Irritant contact dermatitis is caused by a substance causing irritation to the skin, 58, 60-61

J

Joints are junctions where bones meet, 69

K

Keratin (KER-a-tin) is the protein which makes up nails, skin and hair, 87
Keratoma is an acquired superficial, round and thickened patch of epidermis due to pressure or friction on the hands and feet, 106
Kidneys excrete water and other waste products, 67, 83

L

Lacquer (LAK-er) contains a solution of nitrocellulose in a volatile solvent, 122
Large intestines evacuates decomposed and undigested food, 83
Left atrium (AY-tree-um) is the upper left chamber of the heart, 80
Left ventricle (VEN-tri-kel) is the lower left chamber of the heart, 80
Leg
  blood supply to, 82
  bones of, 70-71
  muscles of, 74
  nerves of, 78
Lentigines (len-ti-JEE-neex) are small brown or yellow spots, 106
Lesion (LEE-zhun) is a structural change in tissue caused by injury or disease, 103
Leucocytes (LOO-ko-seyets) perform the function of destroying disease-carrying germs, 81
Leucoderma (loo-ko-DER-ma) is a general term for the abnormal lack of pigmentation, 105
Leukoncyhia (loo-ko-NIK-ee-ah) is a condition in which white spots appear on the nail, 90
Ligaments (LIG-e-mentz) are bands of fibrous tissue that support the bones at the joints, 69
Light-cured gel. See Gel
Liquid enamel, 122
Liquid nail dry is used to prevent smudging of the polish, 123
Liquid nail wrap is a polish made up of tiny fibers designed to strengthen and preserve the natural nail as it grows, 173
Liquid tissue carries food, waste products, and hormones by means of the blood and lymph, 67
Liver removes toxic products of digestion, 67, 83
Local exhaust, 42
Lungs are spongy tissues composed of microscopic cells that take in air, 67, 84
  exhale carbon dioxide, 83
Lunula polish application, 132
Lymph (LIMF) vascular system consists of lymph glands and vessels through which lymph circulates, 79, 82-83

M

Macule (MAK-ul) is a small, discolored spot or patch on the surface of the skin, 103
Manicure
  electric, 139-40
  French, 133, 216-17
  hot oil reconditioning, 133-35
  man's, 135-38
  table, 117
  water, 126-32
    post-service, 132
    pre-service, 126-27
    procedure, 127-32
Massage
  foot, 151-53
  hand/arm, 140-43
  muscles affected by, 73-75
Material Safety Data Sheets (MSDS), 39-40
Materials, 120-21

GLOSSARY/INDEX ◆ 263

Matrix (MAY-triks) contains nerves together with lymph and blood vessels that produce nail cells and control the rate of growth of the nail, 88
Matter takes up space or occupies an area, 51
  forms of, 51-52
Median (MEE-di-an) with its branches supplies the arm and hand, 78
Melanin (MIL-a-nin) determines skin color and protects cells below from the destructive effects of excessive ultraviolet rays, 99
Melanotic sarcoma is a fatal skin cancer that begins with the growth of a mole, 106
Men, manicure for, 135-38
Metacarpals (met-a-KAHR-puls) are the bones of the palm of the hand, are long and slender, 70
Microorganisms (meye-kroh-OR-gah-niz-ems), are organisms, such as bacteria, which are so small they can only be seen through a microscope, 15
Mixed nerves have both sensory and motor fibers and have the ability to both send and receive messages, 77
Mold is a fungus infection of the nail, 93
Mole is a small, brown spot on the skin, 106
Monomers (MON-uh-murs) are individual molecules that join to make the polymer, 56
Motor nerves carry impulses from the brain to muscles, 77, 100
MSDS (Material Safety Data Sheets), 39-40
Muscles
  affected by massage, 73-75
  parts of, 72-73
  stimulation of, 73
Muscular (MUS-kyoo-lahr) system covers, shapes, and supports the skeleton, 71-75
Muscular tissue contracts and moves various parts of the body, 67
Myology (meye-OL-oh-jee) is the study of the structure, functions, and diseases of the muscles, 71

N

Nail
  acrylic,
    odorless, 190
    over bitten nails, 184-86
    over tips or natural nails, 182-84
    post service, 181-82
    pre-service, 177
    procedure, 177-81
    supplies for, 176-77
  art,
    airbrush, 206-15
    foil, 203
    freehand painting, 206
    gems, 202-3
    gold leaf application, 205
    striping tape, 203
      application, 203-4
  bed is the portion of skin beneath the nail body that the nail plate rests upon, 87
  bleach, 122
  body or plate is the main part or plate of the nail, 87
  brush, 119
  cosmetics, 121-23
  determining condition of, 108
  disorder is a condition caused by injury to the nail or disease or imbalance in the body, 88
  disorders,
    not treated by nail technicians, 93-95
    serviceable by nail technicians, 88-93
  dryer, 118
  file, 118
  lacquer, 122
  liquid enamel, 122
  maintenance/removal, 184-87
  parts of, 87-88
  polish,
    colored, 122
    dry, 122
    types of, 131-32
  root is where the nail growth begins, 87
  shape, choosing, 125-26
  strengthener/hardener, 123
  structures beneath, 87-88
  tips,
    application, 158-61
    maintenance of, 162
    post-service, 161
    removal of, 162
    supplies for, 157-58
  whitener, 122
  wraps are nail-size pieces of cloth or paper that are bonded to the front of the nail plate with nail adhesive, 165-68
Nails-only salon, 221-22
Neevus (NEE-vus) is a brown or black stain on the nail caused by a pigmented mole that occurs in the nail, 90
Nerve cell is the primary structural unit of the nervous system, 77
Nerve is made of cordlike fibers and sends messages from the body organs to the central nervous system, 100
Nerve tissue carries to and from the brain, and controls and coordinates all body functions, 67
Nerves
  arm/hand, 77-78
  types of, 77
Nervous system controls and coordinates the functions of all the other systems of the body, 68, 76-78
Neurology is the branch of medicine that deals with the nervous system and its disorders, 76
Neuron (NOOR-on) is the primary structural unit of the nervous system, 77
Nevus (NEE-vus) is a malformation of the skin due to abnormal pigmentation or dilated capillaries, 106
Nodules are small tumors, 104
No-light gel application, 198-99
Nonpathogenic (non-path-o-JEN-ik), non-disease causing bacteria, 15
Non-striated muscles are involuntary muscles, 72
Nucleus (NOO-klee-us) is made of dense protoplasm and is found in the center of the cell within the nuclear membrane, 65
Nylon fiber nail hardener, 123

O

Objective symptoms are those that are visible, 103
Oil glands secrete an oily substance called sebum, 101
Onychatrophia (on-i-kah-TROH-fee-ah), also known as atro-

phy, describes the wasting away of the nail, 90
Onychauxis (on-i-KIK-sis) or hypertrophy (hy-PER-troh-fee) is the overgrowth of nails, 90-91
Onychia (on-NIK-ee-ah) is an inflammation somewhere in the nail, 93
Onychocryptosis (on-i-koh-krip-TOH-sis) is when the nail grows into the sides of tissue around the nail, 91
Onychogryposis (on-i-koh-greye-POH-sis) is a condition in which the nail curvature is increased and enlarged, 93
Onycholysis (on-i-KOL-i-sis) is a condition in which the nail loosens from the nail bed, but does not come off, 94
Onychomycosis (oni-koh-meye-KOH-sis) tinea unguium (TIN-ee-ah UN-gwee-um) is an infectious disease caused by a fungus, 93-94
Onychophagy (on-i-KOH-fa-jee) is the medical term for nails that have been bitten enough to become deformed, 91
Onychophosis (on-ih-KOH-foh-sis) refers to a growth of horny epithelium in the nail bed, 92
Onychophyma (on-ih-koh-FEE-mah) denotes the swelling of the nail, 92
Onychoptosis (on-i-kop-TOH-sis) is a condition in which part or all of the nail sheds periodically and falls off the finger, 94
Onychorrhexis (on-i-kohr-REK-sis) refers to split or brittle nails that also have a series of lengthwise ridges, 92
Onychosis (on-ih-KOH-sis) is a technical term applied to nail disease, 92
Onyx (ON-iks) is the technical terms for nails, 87
Opponent muscles are located in the palm of the hand and act to bring the thumb toward the fingers, allowing the grasping action of the hand, 74
Orangewood stick, manicures and, 118
Organs are structures designed to accomplish a specific function, 67
Origin is the part of the muscle which does not move, 72
Oval nail, 126
Overexposure, 59
  avoiding, 41-44
  principle, 62
  signs of chemical, 38-39

P

Paper wraps, are made of very thin paper and dissolve in both acetone and non-acetone remover, 165, 172-73
Papillae (pa-PIL-e) are little cone-like projections which extend upward into the epidermis, 100
Papillary (PA-pil-ah-ry) layer lies directly under the epidermis and contains the papillae (pa-PIL-e), little cone-like projections that extend upward into the epidermis, 100
Papule (PAP-yool) is a small pimple that does not contain fluid, but can develop pus, 103
Paraffin wax, use of, 140
Parasympathetic nervous system, 76
Paronychia (par-oh-NIK-ee-ah) is a bacterial inflammation of the tissue around the nail, 94-95
Patella (pah-TEL-lah), also called the accessory bone forms the knee cap, 70
Pathogenic (path-o-JEN-ik), disease causing bacteria, 16
  classifications of, 16
Pedicure, 146-51
  post-service, 150-51
  pre-service, 146-47
  procedure, 147-50
  supplies for, 145-46
Pericardium (per-i-KAHR-dee-um) is the membrane which encloses the heart, 79
Periosteum (pe-ree-OS-tee-um) is a pink fibrous membrane that covers and protects the bone, 69
Peripheral (pe-RIF-er-al) system is made up of the sensory and motor never fibers that extend from the brain and spinal cord and are distributed to all parts of the body, 76
Peroneus longus (per-oh-NEE-us LONG-us) covers the outer side of the calf and inverts the foot and turns it outward, 75
Personal records, keeping, 223
Pharnyx (FAR-ingks), 84
Phenolics, 30
Phalanges are bones of the toes, 71
Pivot (PIH-vut) joints like the neck, one bone turns on another bone, 69
Plasma is the fluid part of the blood in which the red and white blood cells and blood platelets flow, 81
Plastic
  bags, 121
  spatula, 121
Pointed nail, 126
Polish
  colored, 122
  dry nail, 122
  remover, 122
  types of, 131-32
Polymer chains, simple versus cross-linking, 56-57
Polymerizations (puh-lim-uh-ruh-ZAY-shuns) are chemical reactions that make polymers, 56
  understanding, 56
Polymers (POL-uh-murs) are long chains of molecules which can be liquid, but are usually solids, 55-56
Popliteal (pop-lih-TEE-ul) artery supplies blood to the foot, 82
Primers are substances that improve adhesion, 53-54
Products
  features of, 229
  presenting, 231
Professional appearance, 12
Pronator (PRO-nay-tor) turns the hands inward, so the palm faces downward, 73
Protein hardener, 123
Protoplasm (PROH-toh-plaz-em) is a colorless, jellylike substance that contains food elements such as protein, fat, carbohydrates, andmineral salts, 65
Psoriasis (so-REYE-a-sis) is a chronic inflammation with round, dry patches covered with coarse silvery scales, 104
Pterygium (te-RIJ-ee-um) describes the condition of the forward growth of the cuticle on the nail, 92
Public relations, 232
Pulmonary (PUL-mo-ner-ee) circulation is the blood circulation that goes from the heart to the lungs to be purified, 80
Pumace (PUM-is) powder is used with the chamois buffer to add shine to the nail, 122
Pustule (PUS-chool) is a lump on the skin with an inflamed base and a head containing pus, 103
Pyogenic granuloma is a severe inflammation of the nail in which a lump of red tissue grows up from the nail bed to the nail plate, 95

Q

Quaternary ammonium compounds (Quats), 30
Quats (Quaternary ammonium compounds), 30

R

Radial (RAY-dee-al) nerve and its branches supply the thumb side of the arm and the back of the hand, 77
Radial (RAY-dee-ul) artery supplies blood to the arm and hand, 81
Radius (RAY-dee-us) is the small bone in the forearm on the same side as the thumb, 69
Rebalancing acrylic nails, 186-88
Receptors are sensory nerve endings, 77
Reconditioning hot oil manicure, 133-35
Record/health care, client, 110-13
Records
  business, 224-25
  clients, 225
  inventory, 225
  personal, keeping, 223
Rectangular nail, 126
Red blood cells carry oxygen to the cells, 81
Red corpuscles (KOR-pus-els) carry oxygen to the cells, 81
Reflex is an automatic response to a stimulus, 77
Repetitive motor disorder is also known as cumulative trauma disorder, 46-47
Reproductive system enables human beings to reproduce, 68
Respiratory (RES-pi-rah-toh-ree) system supplies oxygen to the body, 68
Respiratory system is situated within the chest cavity, 84
Reticular (re-TIK-u-lar) layer contains fat cells, blood and lymph vessels, sweat and oil glands, hair follicles, and the arrector pili, 100
Right atrium (AY-tree-um) the right upper chamber of the heart, 80
Right ventricle (VEN-tri-kel) is the lower right chamber of the heart, 80
Ringworm of the hand is a highly contagious disease caused by a fungus, 105
Round nail, 126

S

Safety guidelines, 44-45
Sales, closing, 232-33
Salon
  clients, conduct toward, 7-9
  coworkers, conduct toward, 9-10
  full-station, 221
  nails-only, 221-22
Sanitation, 27-28
  blood spills and, 34-35
  disinfection and, 28-31
  of implements, 120
  pre-service, 32-33
  universal, 35-36
Sanitizers
  bead, 33
  ultraviolet ray, 33
Saphenous (sa-feen-us) nerve supplies impulses to the skin of the inner side of the leg and foot, 78
Scales are produced during the shedding of the epidermis, 103

Scapula (SKAP-yoo-lah) forms part of the shoulder, 69
Scar is a light-colored, slightly raised mark on the skin formed after an injury or lesion of the skin has healed, 104
Scarf skin is the outermost protective covering of the skin, 99
Sebaceous (si-BAY-shus) glands secrete an oily substance called sebum, 101
Secretory (se-KREE-e-ree) nerves are the nerves of the sweat and oil glands, 101
Sensitization is a greatly increased or exaggerated sensitivity to products, 59
Sensory nerves carry impulses or messages from sense organs to the brain, 77, 100-101
Services
  benefits, 230
  collecting payment for, 226
  features of, 229
  presenting, 231
Silk, is a thin natural material with a tight weave that becomes transparent when adhesive is applied, 165
Simple polymer chains are long chains of monomers attached head to tail, 56
Sinews (SIN-yooz) join muscles together, 73
Skeletal system is the physical foundation or framework for the body, 68-71
Skin
  determining condition of, 108
  disorders, 102-5
  elasticity of, 102
  eliminates perspiration, 83
  function of, 97-98
  glands of, 101-2
  infections of, 105
  inflammation of, 104
  lesions of, 103-4
  nerves of, 100-101
  pigmentation of, 105-6
  structure of, 98-101
Skin problems, 58-62
  dermatitis, 58
  precautions concerning, 61-62
Slimline polish application, 131
Soleus (SO-lee-us) originates at the upper portion of the fibula and bends the foot down, 75
Solvent is anything which dissolves another substance, 52
Spatula, manicures and, 121
Spills, blood, sanitation and, 34-35
Spinal cord, 76-77
Spirilla (spi-RIL-a) are spiral or corkscrew-shaped bacteria, 16-17
Square nail, 126
Stain is an abnormal discoloration that remains after moles, freckles, or liver spots disappear, or after certain diseases, 104
Staphylococci (staf-lo-KOK-si), grow in clusters and are present in local infections, such as abscesses, pustules, and boils, 16
Statum corneum (STRAT-um KOHR-nee-um) consists of tightly packed, scalelike cells that are continually shed and replaced, 99
Steel pusher, 118
Sterilization, 27

Stomach digests food, 67
Stratum germinativum (STRAT-um jur-mi-hah-TIV-um) is composed of several layers of differently shaped cells. The deepest layer is responsible for supplying new cells to make up for the ones that are continually worn away, 99
Stratum granulosum (STRAT-um gran-yoo-LOH-dum) consist of cells that look like granules. These cells change into keratin near the surface of the skin, 99
Stratum lucidum, (STRAT-um LOO-si-dum) is a small layer of clear cells that light can pass through, 99
Streptococci (strep-to-KOK-si) grow in chains and cause strep throat and infections or diseases that spread throughout the body such as blood poisoning or rheumatic fever, 16
Striated (STRY-ate-id) muscles are voluntary muscles that you can move whenever you want, 71
Striping tape, nail art and, 203-4
Stypic (STIP-tik) powder is used to contact the skin to stop minor bleeding that may occur during a manicure, 121
Subcutaneous (sub-kyoo-TAY-nee-us) tissue is made up of fatty tissue known as adipose (AD-i-pohs), 100
Subjective symptoms are those that can be felt, 103
Sudoriferous (su-dohr-IF-er-us) glands or sweat glands, regulate body temperature and eliminates waste products through perspiration, 101
Superficial peroneal nerve passes downward in front of the fibula and supplies impulses to the leg and foot, 78
Supinator (SUE-pi-nay-tor) turns the hand outward so the palm faces upward, 73
Supplies, 117-23
  equipment, 117-18
  implements, 118-20
  materials, 120-21
  pedicuring, 145-46
Supply tray, 118
Sural nerve supplies impulses to the outer side and back of the foot and leg, 78
Sympathetic nervous system, 76
Synovial (sy-NOV-ee-al) fluid is the lubrication that prevents friction at the joints where bones meet, 69
Systemic circulation is the blood circulation from the heart throughout the body and back to the heart again, 80
Systems are groups of organs that cooperate for a common purpose, namely the welfare of the entire body, 68

T

Table, basic set-up of, 124-25
Tactile corpuscles (TAK-til KOR-puh-sils) are nerve endings, 100
Tan is the darkening of the skin caused by exposure to the ultraviolet rays of the sun, 106
Tarsal (TAR-sul) bones make up the ankle, 70
Tendons (TEN-dunz) join muscles together, 73
Terry cloth towels, 121
Thrombocytes (throm-BOH-syts) play an important roll in the clotting of blood, 81
Tibia (TIB-ee-ah) is the larger of the two bones that form the leg below the knee, 70
Tibial (TIB-ee-al) nerve supplies impulses to the knee, the muscles of the calf, the skin of the leg, and the sole, heel, and underside of the toes, 78
Tibialis anterior (tib-ee-AHL-is an-TEHR-ee-ohr) muscle covers the front of the skin. It bends the foot upward and inward, 75
Tinea of the hand is a highly contagious disease caused by a fungus
Tinea pedis (TIN-ee-ah PEH-dus) is a fungus infection of the foot, 105
Tissues are composed of groups of cells of the same kinds, 67
Top coat or sealer is a colorless polish applied over colored polish to prevent chipping and add a shine to the finished nail, 123
Towels
  disposable, 121
  terry cloth, 121
Treponema pallida (trep-o-NE-mah PAL-i-dah) is the bacteria which causes syphilis, 16
Triceps (TREYE-seps) are muscles that cover the entire back of the upper arm and extend the forearm forward, 73
Tubercle (TOO-ber-kyool) is a solid lump larger than a papule, 104
Tumor is an abnormal cell mass that varies in size, shape, and color, 104
Tweezers, 119
Two-color fade, 214-15

U

Ulcer (UL-ser) is an open lesion on the skin or mucous membrane of the body, 104
Ulna (UL-nah) is the large bone on the small-finger side of the forearm, 69
Ulnar (UL-ner) arteries supply blood to the arm and hand, 81
Ulnar (UL-ner) nerve and its branches supply the small finger side of the arm and palm of the hand, 77
Ultraviolet ray sanitizers, 33
Universal sanitation, 35-36

V

Vagus (VAYgus) nerve regulates the heartbeat, 79
Valves allow the blood to flow in one direction, 80
Veins carry blood that lacks oxygen from the capillaries back to the heart, 80
Ventilation control, 41-42
Ventricles (VEN-tri-kels) are the lower chambers of the heart, 80
Vesicle (VES-i-kell) is a blister containing clear fluid, 104
Viricides kill pathogenic viruses, 29

W

Water manicure, 126-32
  post-service, 132
  pre-service, 126-27
  procedure, 127-32
Wax, paraffin, use of, 140
Wheals (HWEELS) or hives are swollen, itchy bumps on the skin that last for several hours, 104
White corpuscles (KOR-pus-els) perform the function of destroying disease-causing germs, 81
Whitener, nail, 122
Wipe container, 117
Working, environment, 221-26
Working guidelines, 44-45